Prosthodontics and Restorative Dentistry

This helpful resource explains many digital technologies in prosthetics, restorative dentistry, and oral tissue engineering. It covers the latest advances in digital workflow for making complete denture prosthodontics, removable partial denture prosthodontics, fixed prosthodontics (crowns and bridges, veneers, inlays, and onlays), implant prosthodontics, and maxillofacial prosthodontics. This text will be useful for dental students and practitioners seeking a guide for integrating digital technologies in clinical dentistry applications.

Prosthodontics and Restorative Dentistry
Latest Advances in Digital Technologies

Edited by
Zohaib Khurshid BDS, MRes, FDTFEd, FHEA, MFDS RCPS (Glasgow), Dental Education PGCert (Dundee)
Department of Prosthodontics and Dental Implantology, College of Dentistry, King Faisal University, Al Ahsa, Saudi Arabia
Center for Artificial Intelligence and Innovation (CAII), Faculty of Dentistry, Chulalongkorn University, Bangkok, Thailand

Co-Editors
Muhammad Sohail Zafar PhD, MSc, BDS, PGDip (Med Edu), FDTFEd, FHEA, MFDSRCPSG
College of Dentistry, Ajman University, United Arab Emirates
Dinesh Rokaya BDS, MSc, PhD
College of Dentistry, Ajman University, United Arab Emirates

CRC Press
Taylor & Francis Group
Boca Raton London New York

CRC Press is an imprint of the
Taylor & Francis Group, an **informa** business

Designed cover image: Editors

First edition published 2026
by CRC Press
2385 NW Executive Center Drive, Suite 320, Boca Raton FL 33431

and by CRC Press
4 Park Square, Milton Park, Abingdon, Oxon, OX14 4RN

CRC Press is an imprint of Taylor & Francis Group, LLC

ISBN: 978-1-032-55014-5 (hbk)
ISBN: 978-1-032-55015-2 (pbk)
ISBN: 978-1-003-42854-1 (ebk)

DOI: 10.1201/9781003428541

Typeset in Palatino
by KnowledgeWorks Global Ltd.

Table of Contents

Contributors

Muhammad Adeel Ahmed
Department of Restorative Dental Sciences
College of Dentistry, King Faisal University
Al-Ahsa, Saudi Arabia

Mario Alberto Alarcón-Sánchez
Molecular Biology in Medicine Program
and
Department of Integral Dental Clinics
Institute of Research in Dentistry, University Center of Health Sciences, University of Guadalajara (CUCS-UdeG)
Guadalajara, Mexico

Mohammed Ahmed Alghauli
Department of Prosthodontics, Faculty of Dentistry
Ibb University
Ibb, Yemen

Mahdieh Alipour
Department of Oral and Craniofacial Sciences
School of Dental Medicine, University of Pittsburgh
Pittsburgh, Pennsylvania, USA

Gustavo Moreira de Almeida
Head of the Endodontics Postgraduate Program
Faculdade FAIPE
Ilhéus, Brazil

Ahmed Yaseen Alqutaibi
Substitutive Dental Sciences Department
College of Dentistry, Taibah University
Al-Madinah, Saudi Arabia
and
Department of Prosthodontics, Faculty of Dentistry
Ibb University
Ibb, Yemen

Marina Amaral
Department of Dentistry
University of Taubate
Taubate, Brazil

Pokpong Amornvit
Department of Restorative Dentistry
College of Dentistry, Taibah University
Al Madina Al Munawwarrah, Saudi Arabia

Heba Ashi
Faculty of Dentistry
King Abdulaziz University
Jeddah, Saudi Arabia

Kusai Baroudi
RAK College of Dental Sciences, RAK Medical & Health Sciences University
Ras Al Khaimah, United Arab Emirates

Leonardo dos Santos Barroso
University of Volta Redonda (UNIFOA)
Rio de Janeiro, Brazil

Sompop Bencharit
Workman School of Dental Medicine
High Point University
High Point, North Carolina, USA

Aybike Cengiz Dagtekin
Department of Prosthodontics, Faculty of Dentistry
Firat University
Elazig, Turkey

Bekir Eser
Department of Prosthodontics, Faculty of Dentistry
Firat University
Elazig, Turkey

Taha Fayad
Faculty of Dentistry
Sinai university
Al-Arish, Egypt

Deepa Gurunathan
Department of Paediatric Dentistry
Saveetha Dental College
Chennai, India

Mohamad Syahrizal Halim
Conservative Dentistry Unit
School of Dental Sciences, Health Campus, Universiti Sains Malaysia
Kota Bharu, Kelantan, Malaysia

Artak Heboyan
Department of Prosthodontics, Faculty of Stomatology
Yerevan State Medical University after Mkhitar Heratsi
Yerevan, Armenia

Amir I. O. Ibrahim
Department of Restorative Dental Sciences
College of Dentistry, King Faisal University
Al-Ahsa, Saudi Arabia

Rizwan Jouhar
Department of Restorative Dental Sciences
College of Dentistry, King Faisal University
Al-Ahsa, Saudi Arabia

Suchada Kongkiatkamon
Bangkok Hospital Dental Center
Bangkok Hospital
Bangkok, Thailand

Walter Y. H. Lam
Faculty of Dentistry
The University of Hong Kong
Hong Kong Special Administrative Region, China

Stephan Lampl
Department of Paediatric Dentistry
Saveetha Dental College
Chennai, India

Katherine C. M. Leung
Faculty of Dentistry
The University of Hong Kong
Hong Kong Special Administrative Region, China

Raveena Makker
Dept of Prosthodontics and Crown & Bridge
Index Institute of Dental Sciences
Indore, India

Ana Maria Estivalete Marchionatti
Odontologia, CNEC Faculty of Santo Ângelo
Rio Grande do Sul, Brazil

Desigar Moodely
Smile and Education Centre
Scinmed, Cape Town, South Africa

Adriana Marques Nunes
University of Volta Redonda (UNIFOA)
Rio de Janeiro, Brazil

Yu Pan
Department of Dentistry
Shenzhen People's Hospital (The Second Clinical Medical College, Jinan University; The First Affiliated Hospital, Southern University of Science and Technology)
Shenzhen, Guangdong, China

Edmond H. N. Pow
Faculty of Dentistry
The University of Hong Kong
Hong Kong Special Administrative Region, China

Prashanthi Reddy
Department of Oral Medicine
Government Dental College
Indore, India

Mayson Salih
Department of Prosthodontics, Faculty of Dentistry
University of Science and Technology
Umburman, Sudan

Laís Regiane Silva-Concílio
Department of Dentistry
University of Taubate
Taubate, Brazil

Juan Manual Taboas
Department of Oral and Craniofacial Sciences
School of Dental Medicine, University of Pittsburgh
Pittsburgh, Pennsylvania, USA

Samet Tekin
Department of Prosthodontics, Faculty of Dentistry
Firat University
Elazig, Turkey

João Paulo Mendes Tribst
Department of Reconstructive Oral Care
Academic Centre for Dentistry Amsterdam (ACTA), University of Amsterdam and Vrije Universiteit
Amsterdam, The Netherlands

Marco Tudts
Cosmident Oral Design Centre
Lier, Belgium

Vinícius Felipe Wandscher
Odontologia, CNEC Faculty of Santo Angelo
Rio Grande do Sul, Brazil

1 Introduction to Digital Dentistry

Dinesh Rokaya, Suchada Kongkiatkamon, Zohaib Khurshid, Pokpong Amornvit, and Muhammad Sohail Zafar

1.1 INTRODUCTION

Digital dentistry utilizes any dental technology that involves the use of computer-based technologies consisting of hardware devices and software for examination, diagnosis, treatment planning, and treatment. Recently, there has been significant progress in digital dentistry. Various digital technologies and devices include intraoral scanners (IOSs), computerized occlusal analysis devices, digital jaw trackers, virtual reality (VR), computerized dental simulators (CDSs), etc. Utilizing these technologies has increased clinical success [1]. IOSs enable dentists to take impressions, perform diagnostics, or plan treatment without the use of mechanical tools. Various IOSs are available in the market varying in terms of their accuracy [2, 3].

The advantages of digital technologies in dentistry include predictable planning, time savings, reliability, less cost due to reduced treatment sequences and laboratory work, good patient satisfaction, and high patient comfort [4]. Furthermore, the utilization of digital tomography of the bony structures, planning software, and computer-aided design (CAD)/computer-aided manufacturing (CAM)–generated temporaries and prototypes makes the treatment process simpler [4, 5]. The clear and precise digital workflow has simplified the manufacturing and fabrication process with less human input, reducing the risk of infection, and the technique avoids errors, including cast deformation, errors in articulator settings, and acrylic resin deformation. Finally, digital dentistry has increased the quality of life of patients [6].

1.2 CAD/CAM AND DIGITAL WORKFLOW

Dentists and lab technicians use dental software to design restorations or prostheses such as crowns, bridges, veneers, inlays, onlays, dentures, etc. Although the general digital dental workflow is similar for all cases, it may slightly vary depending on the case, type of treatment needed, complexity, and complicating factors. The standard digital dental workflow consists of the following three steps (**Figure 1.1**):

1. *Taking or Scanning the Digital Impression*: The first step is making the digital impression using an IOS, which can take approximately 2–4 minutes. However, the digital workflow can start with a conventional impression that is digitized in the lab by scanning dental impressions or casts with a desktop scanner. The patient can see the 3D image of their teeth displayed on the screen.
2. *Planning and Designing*: The dentists use CAD/CAM software to design restorations and other treatments. Based on need, the design or treatment plan can be revised or refined.
3. *Manufacturing*: The approved digital designs can be sent to 3D printers or milling machines for the fabrication of crowns, veneers, bridges, dentures, splints, or appliances such as aligners and retainers.

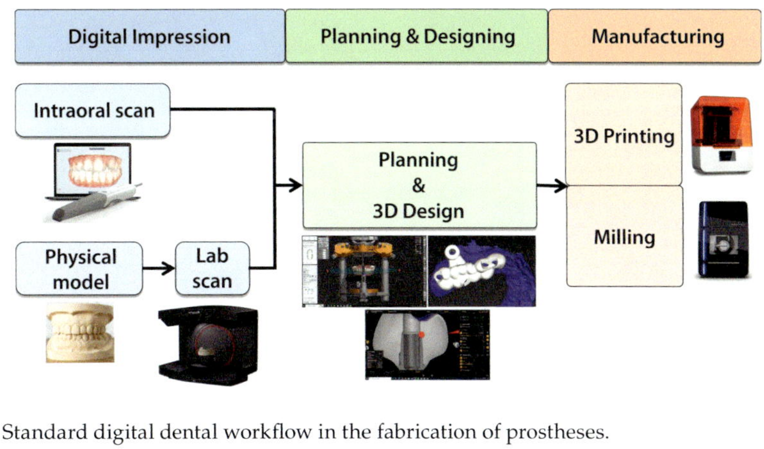

Figure 1.1 Standard digital dental workflow in the fabrication of prostheses.

DOI: 10.1201/9781003428541-1

1.3 DIGITAL TECHNOLOGIES IN PROSTHETIC AND RESTORATIVE DENTISTRY

Various applications of digital dentistry are shown in **Figures 1.2–1.9**. **Figure 1.2** shows the CAD design in computer software for a full-mouth restoration case. **Figure 1.3** shows the CAD for implant restoration. The material thickness and dental implant part can be determined from the software. **Figure 1.4** shows the design of an implant placement guide using CAD software.

Similarly, **Figure 1.5** shows the design of the endodontic surgical guide using CAD software in a case that is complex due to access difficulty and root proximity. **Figure 1.6** shows the printable esthetic crown lengthening surgical guide fabricated by using 3D printing. **Figure 1.7** shows

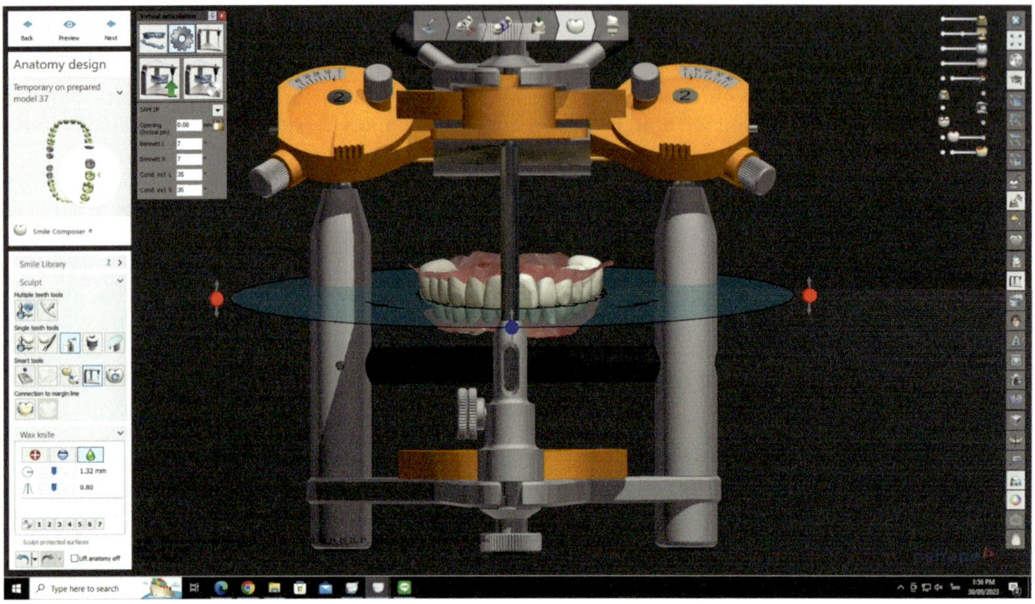

Figure 1.2 CAD software for full-mouth restoration.

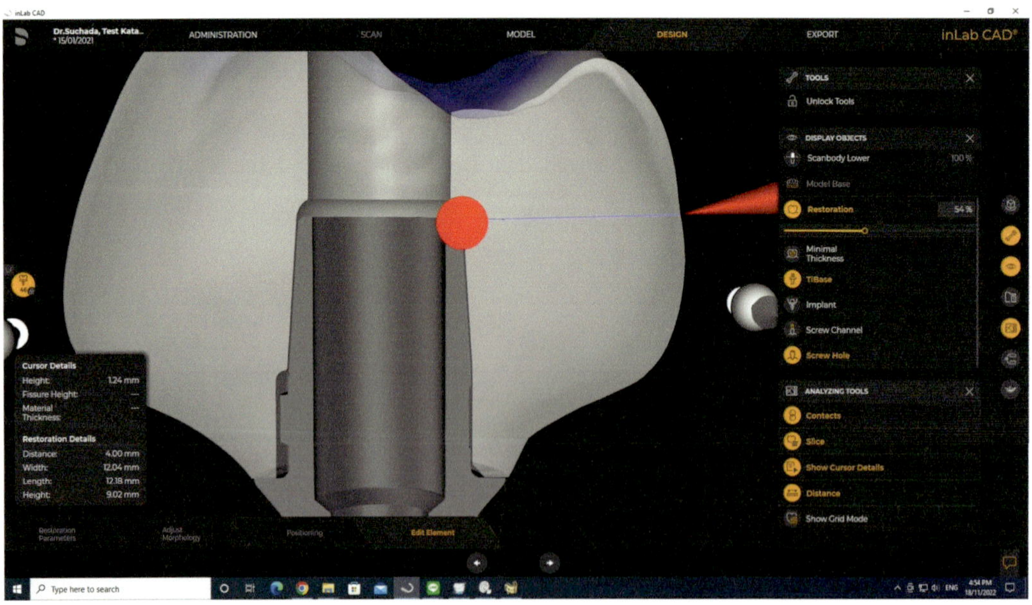

Figure 1.3 CAD for implant restoration showing the determination of the material thickness and dental implant part.

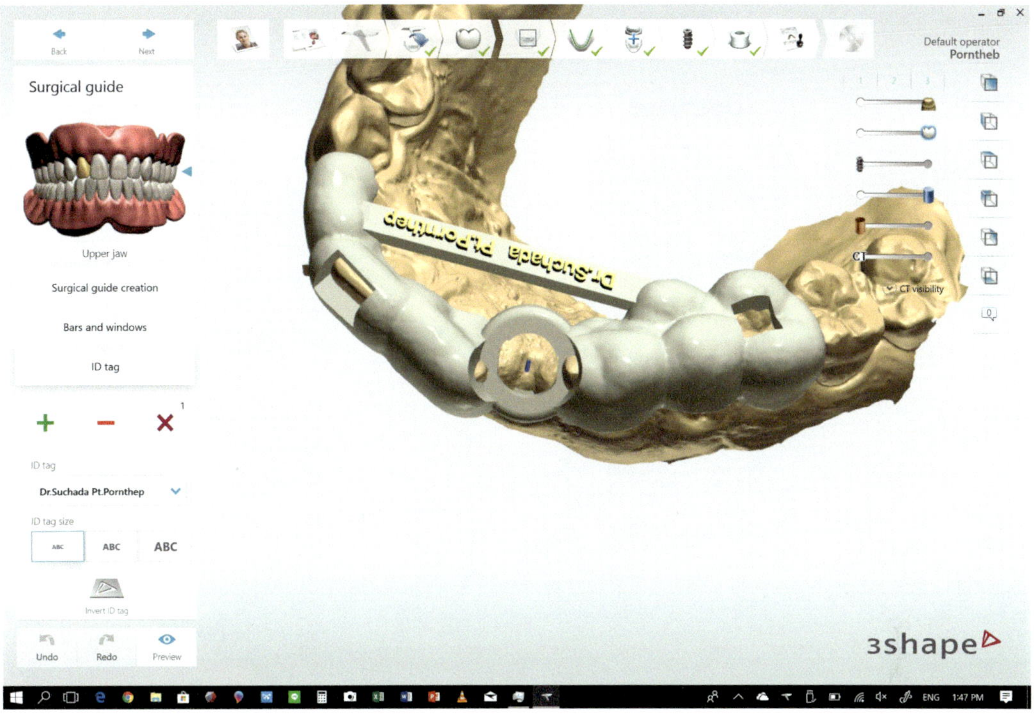

Figure 1.4 Digital design of an implant placement guide using CAD software.

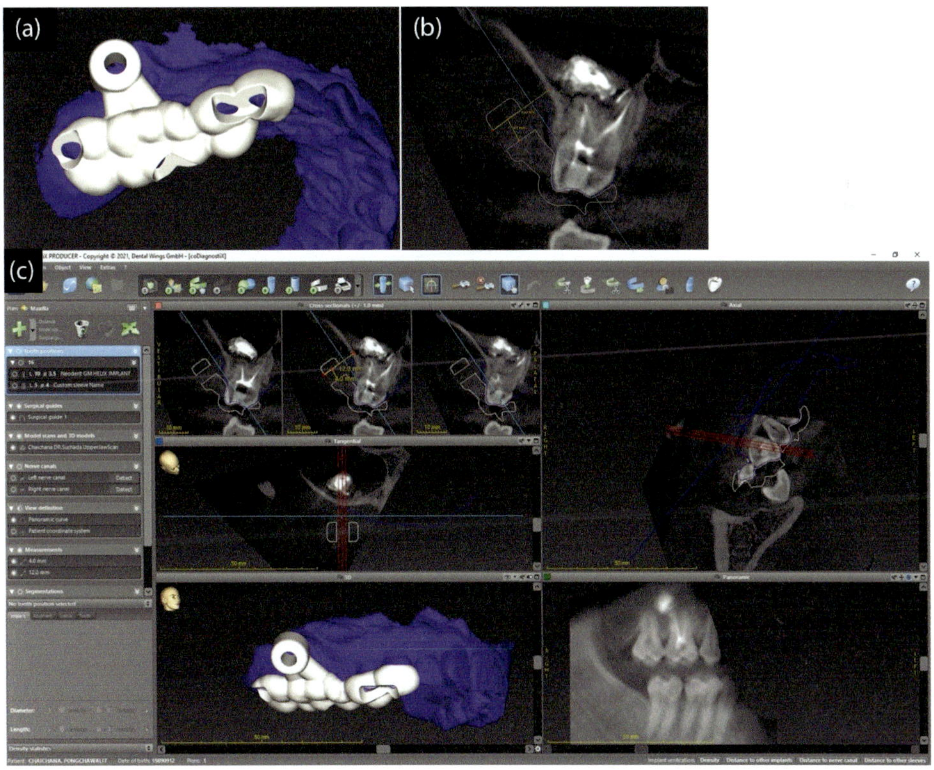

Figure 1.5 CAD of an endodontic surgical guide (a) using CAD in a complex case due to access difficulty and root proximity (b and c).

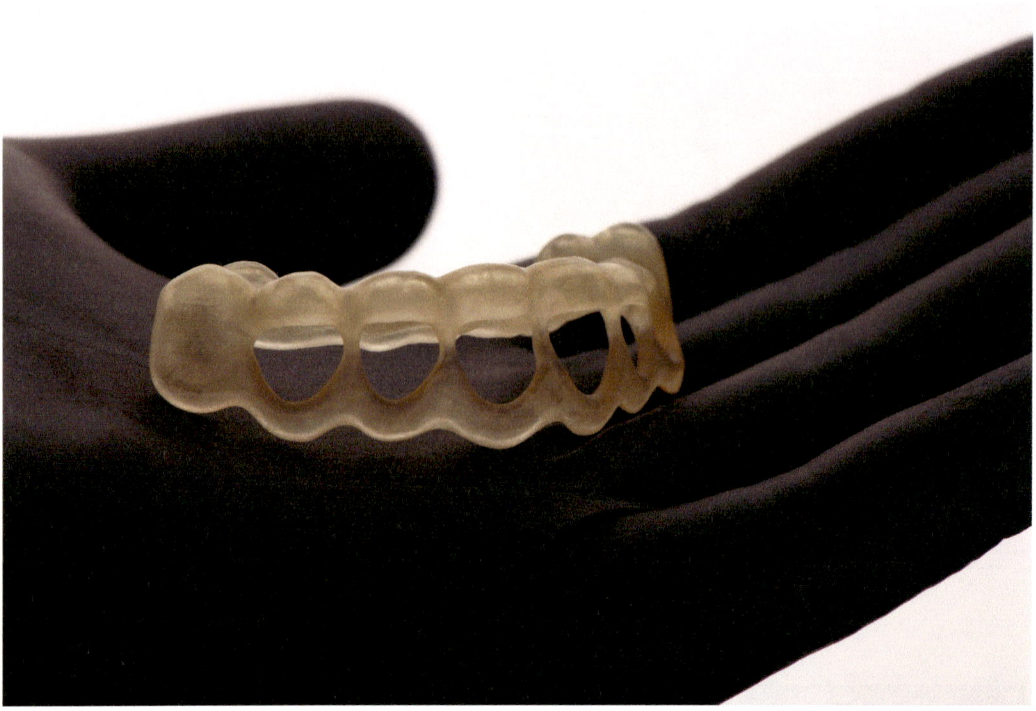

Figure 1.6 Printable esthetic crown lengthening surgical guide fabricated by using a 3D printing machine.

the printing temporary and mock-up for a veneer case using resin tooth color material. **Figure 1.8** shows the milled CAD/CAM zirconia crowns from zirconia discs, and **Figure 1.9** shows the milled CAD/CAM dental ceramic for veneer restoration from zirconia blocks.

At present, it is possible to fabricate the restoration on a single visit that employs CAD software (CAD-on method) for the ceramic restoration [7]. Recently, millable lithium-disilicate glass–ceramic

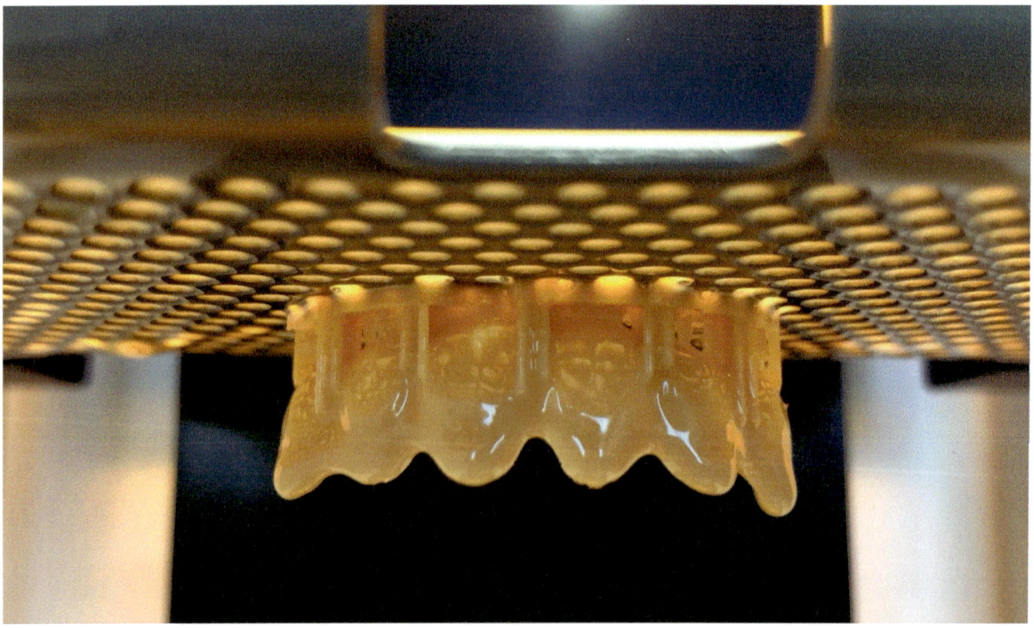

Figure 1.7 Printing temporary and mock-up for veneer case by using resin tooth color material.

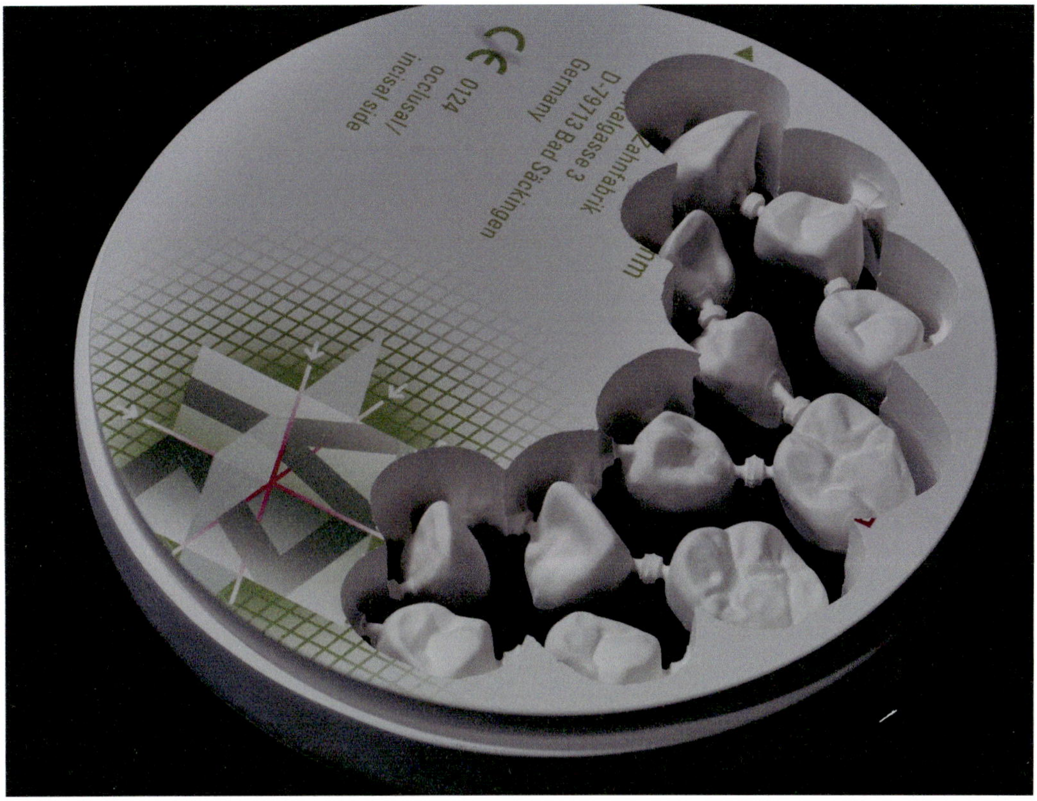

Figure 1.8 Milled CAD/CAM zirconia crowns from zirconia discs.

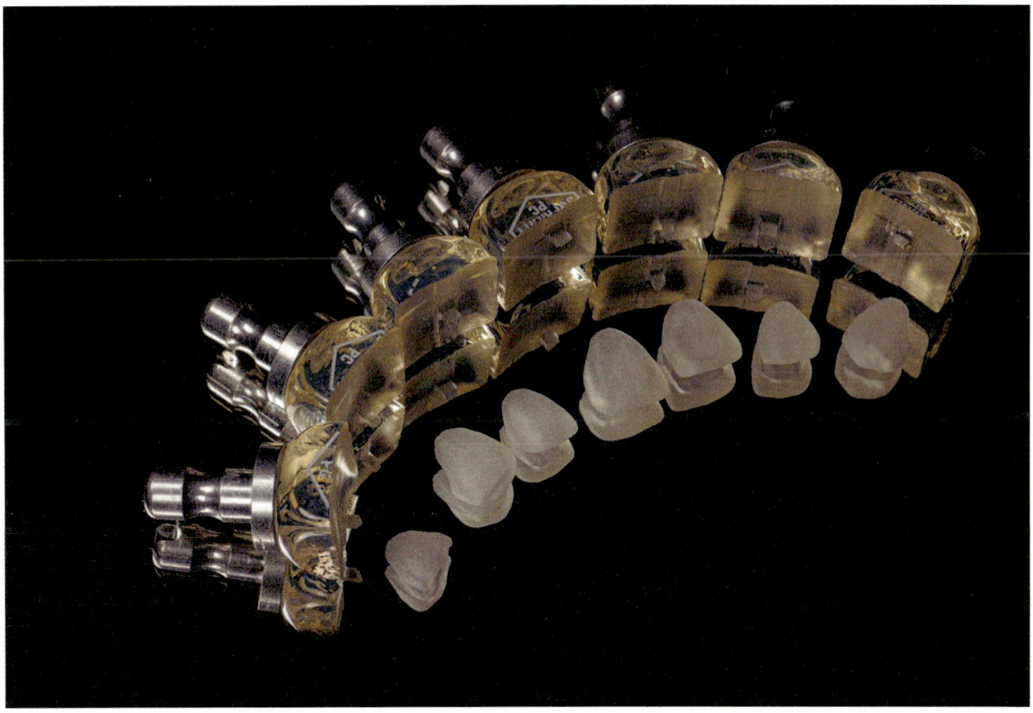

Figure 1.9 Milled CAD/CAM dental ceramic for veneer restoration from zirconia blocks.

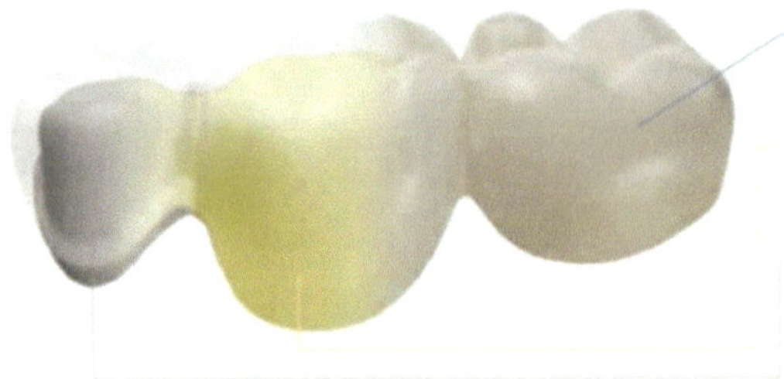

Figure 1.10 CAD-on bridge design components. (Adapted with permission from Ref [7].)

blocks have been used to fabricate high-strength, multilayer zirconia crowns [8]. Graiff et al. [7] described a process of joining multilayer CAD/CAM zirconia components (**Figures 1.10–1.13**). In this technique, the zirconia framework and the veneering ceramic structure are designed using CAD software and milled using CAD/CAM technology (**Figure 1.11**), and the zirconia framework is sintered [7]. Finally, these components are then assembled and joined with the fusion of a glass–ceramic. The final product has high flexural strength (approximately 900 MPa) and is resistant to fracture under occlusal loads. This process produces a precise restoration that requires only minor retouching and accurately fits in the patient's mouth. The CAD-on method is suitable for fabricating single crowns and three to four bridge units on either natural teeth or implants.

Generally, the milling process of the zirconia always results in the framework being approximately 20–25% bigger than actually needed [8]. Then, the high-temperature sintering of the zirconia

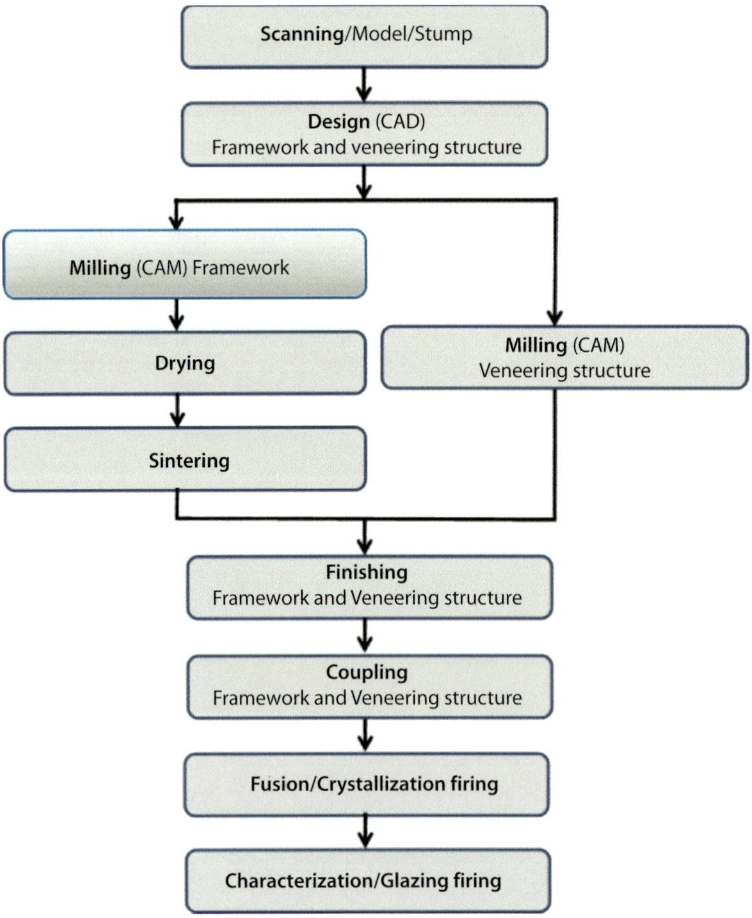

Figure 1.11 Fabrication of a CAD-on prosthesis. (Adapted with permission from Ref [7].)

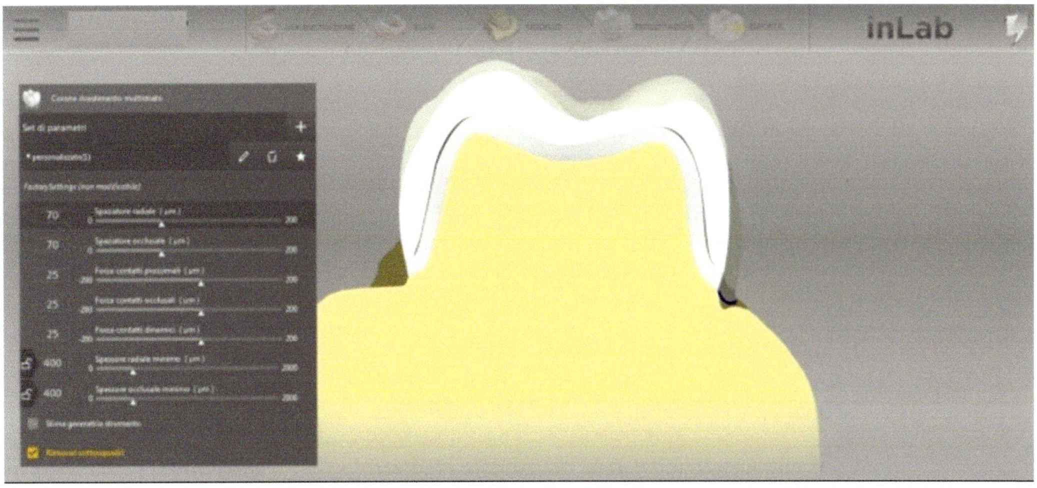

Figure 1.12 CAM design showing the gap setting of 70 μm in computer software for the manufacture of prostheses. (Adapted with permission from Ref [7].)

framework in a ceramic furnace at around 1500°C results in the contraction of the bigger framework that was previously milled. The glass–ceramic fusion between the two milled prosthetic components is attained with a fusion glass–ceramic material and occurs due to the crystallization of the lithium disilicate at 840–850°C. During this firing process, approximately 0.2% linear contraction of the lithium disilicate occurs.

Marginal adaptability is important for the long-term success of such zirconia restoration, and inadequate marginal adaptation results in plaque retention, gingival inflammation, risk of microleakage, and secondary caries. In addition, the internal gap can compromise the fracture resistance of restorations.

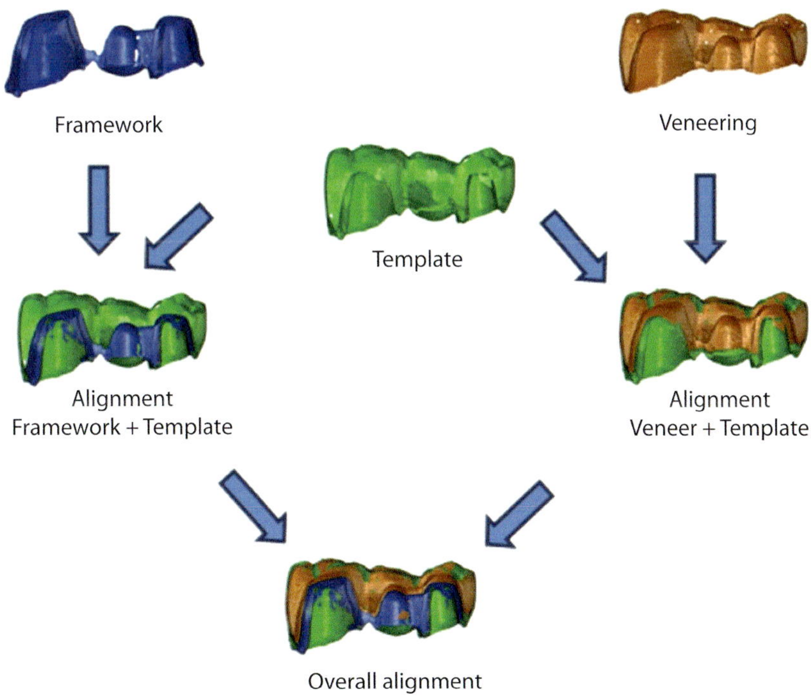

Figure 1.13 Assembling the CAD-on prosthetic components. (Adapted with permission from Ref [7].)

1.4 DIGITAL TECHNOLOGIES IN DENTAL OCCLUSION

In dental occlusion, a virtual articulator and jaw motion analyzer can be used to transfer jaw relations for an accurate record of the occlusal relationships and a balanced occlusion [9–12]. It has been shown that the use of digital technologies allows more precise examination, visualization, fabrication of the occlusal splints, and records of occlusal relationships [11, 13, 14]. Correct diagnosis is important in the management of occlusal problems. At present, various digital technologies are used in clinical dentistry for oral rehabilitation and occlusal adjustments [1, 15, 16]. **Figure 1.14** shows the management of a bruxism patient with a splint fabricated using 3D technologies [17]. Digital technologies (intraoral scan and software) were used to fabricate a splint and 3D model with clear resin. An occlusal splint of 2.7 mm thickness was fabricated, and the T-Scan Novus system was used for the examination of the occlusion digitally (**Figure 1.14g**).

1.5 DIGITAL TECHNOLOGIES IN ORTHODONTICS

Cone-beam computed tomography (CBCT), face scanner, intraoral scanner, CAD software, and 3D printing have a great impact on orthodontics and maxillofacial surgery [18]. These technological advancements help in diagnosis and treatment. Digital technologies have allowed the customization of orthodontic appliances. Teeth can be scanned to create digital models (**Figure 1.15**). Then, all

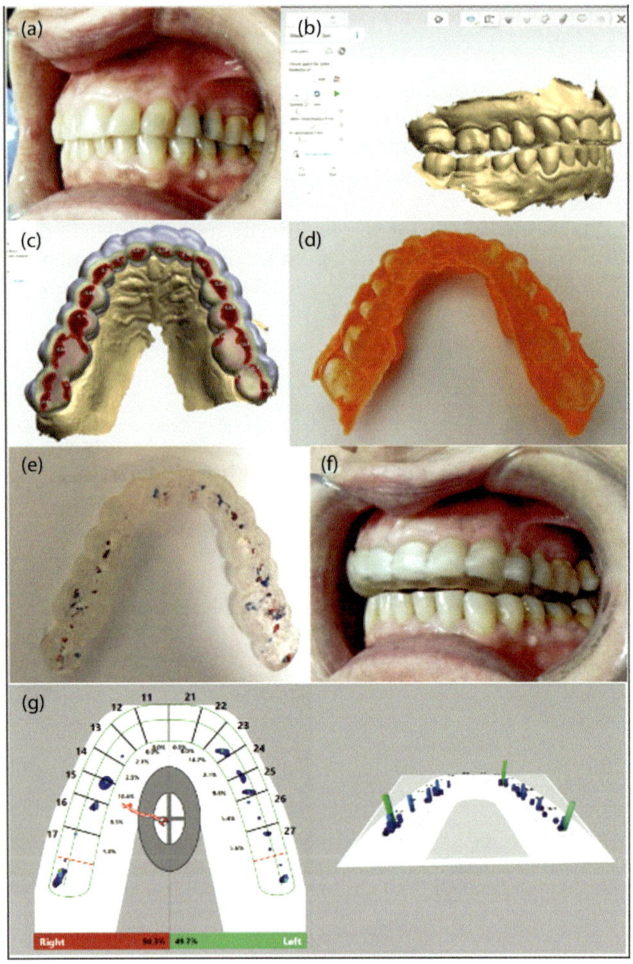

Figure 1.14 Picture of a patient showing an occlusal problem and its treatment using digital technologies. (a) Intraoral picture of the patient with occlusal problems. (b) Intermaxillary relation in the software for fabrication of the splint. (c) Balanced occlusion from the software. (d) Silicone bite. (e) Fabricated splint and its occlusal registration. (f) Splint in the patient's mouth. (g) Occlusal registration in T-Scan software. (Adapted with permission from Ref [17].)

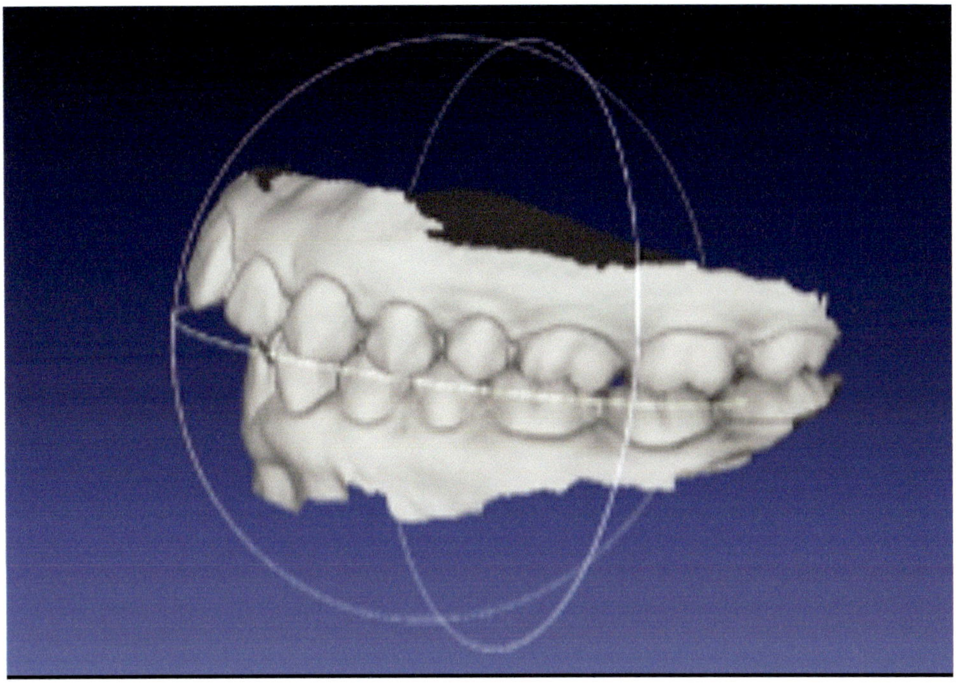

Figure 1.15 A 3D digital model. (Adapted with permission from Ref [19].)

appliances are designed and manufactured digitally. In addition, intraoral and facial scans create a "virtual patient" and help in treatment planning. Advanced imaging and orthodontic analysis software gathers digital data obtained from the various digital units and the clinical examination. CAD software is used in designing customized appliances, which are manufactured using 3D printing. The orthodontic aligners can be designed and manufactured in the orthodontic office, whether it is printing aligners or thermoformed aligners. With the digital technology, the simulation process has become more practical and faster. This allows greater predictability irrespective of the orthodontic appliance [19, 20].

CAD software has helped to design customized fixed orthodontic brackets and print them in the clinic. The virtual assembly of the appliance can be done in the Ortho Analyzer™ software (3Shape, Copenhagen, Denmark) [21]. The brackets can be selected in from the software's library **(Figure 1.16)** [19].

In orthodontics, the digital workflow of the fixed appliances has resulted in greater precision in the placement of the brackets and reduced the time for bonding [22, 23]. This can be done using an indirect bonding guide (**Figure 1.17**), and this technique allows correct bracket placement, minimizes isolation, helps to see the difficulties of the procedure, and results in faster bonding appointments and more comfort for patients [24–26]. The indirect bonding tray can be fabricated by two techniques: A pressure-forming technique and a direct 3D-printed model (**Figure 1.18**). The indirect bonding guide can be made on the printed resin model with brackets by the pressure-forming method [26]. However, virtual movements in digital software are unpredictable and unrealistic [27].

In maxillofacial surgery and orthodontics, digital technologies have gradually changed the means of diagnosis, treatment plans, and assessment of the results. Airway 3D measurements can be done from CBCT. This is useful for patients with obstructive sleep apnea syndrome, as the airway constriction can be evaluated, and the treatment outcome can be compared before and after treatment (**Figure 1.19**).

1.6 DIGITAL TECHNOLOGIES IN ESTHETIC DENTISTRY AND BIOMATERIALS

Esthetics is the primary consideration for prosthetic patients [29, 30]. Digital dentistry has also aided esthetic dentistry. For facial and dental esthetics, various facial landmarks (nose, eyes, chin, zygoma, etc.) and maxillary anterior teeth play an important role. Furthermore, the golden proportion of teeth should be considered for the digital smile design to improve the esthetics [31].

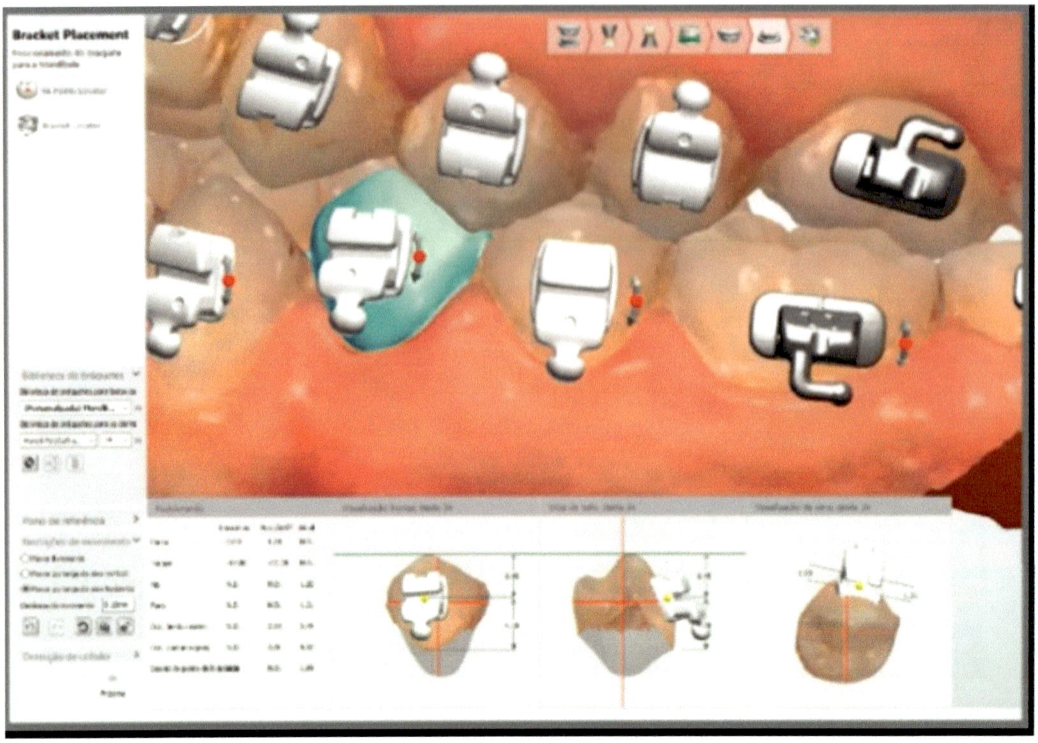

Figure 1.16 Virtual bracket placement in Ortho Analyzer™ software. (Adapted with permission from Ref [19].)

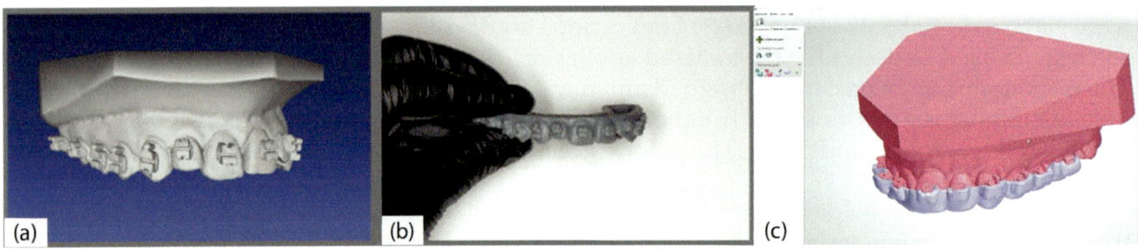

Figure 1.17 (a) 3D model with brackets placed virtually. (b) 3D printed model used to create a transfer tray. (c) Transfer tray designed with the Appliance Designer™ software. (Adapted with permission from Ref [19].)

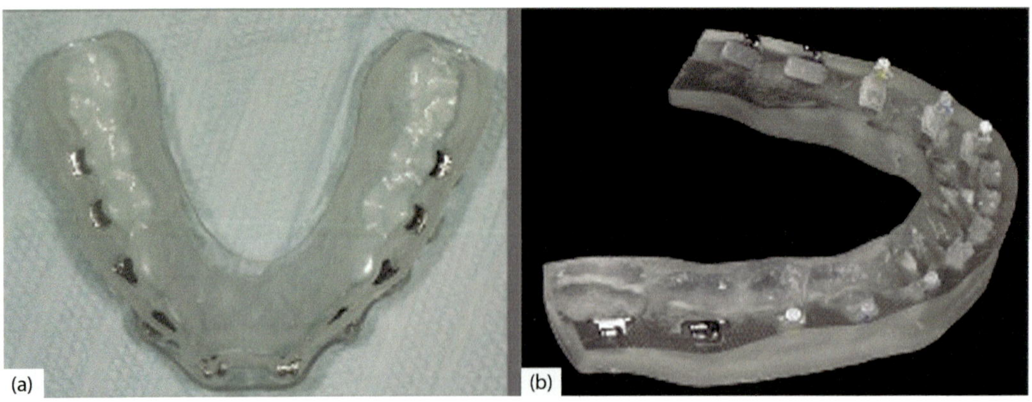

Figure 1.18 (a) Pressure-formed indirect bonding double tray and placed brackets. (b) 3D-printed bonding tray and placed brackets. (Adapted with permission from Ref [19].)

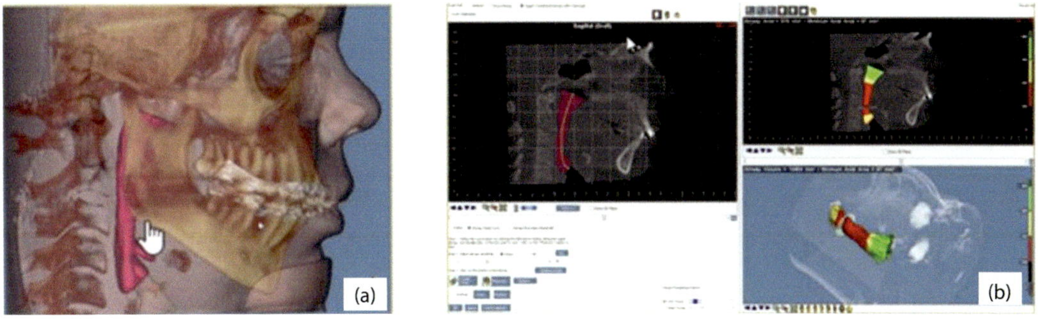

Figure 1.19 View of airway tract in CBCT. The upper pharyngeal airway (pink; a). Segmentation of the upper airways: Oropharynx (red), nasopharynx (green), and hypopharynx (lower yellow; b). (Adapted with permission from Ref [28].)

Currently, the trends have shifted from conventional removable prostheses toward implants and implant-supported prostheses for the replacement of missing teeth [32].

There is increasing use of metal-free materials these days, such as ceramic-based and poly-ether-ether-ketone (PEEK) [32, 33]. Various types of ceramic and zirconia are available on the market, and dentists can choose based on their requirements [34]. The prostheses can be fabricated chairside via CAD/CAM systems for restorations ranging from single to full-mouth reconstruction.

1.7 DIGITAL TECHNOLOGIES IN DENTAL EDUCATION

VR and CDSs are also gaining popularity in dental education [5]. One popular VR, DentSim (DenX Ltd., Australia), has evaluated students' preparations by using computer tracking and showed that VR simulator–enhanced training can improve the development of technical skills of future dentists [35]. VR technology has proven an effective training method in dental implant education for both dental students and dentists [36]. Furthermore, utilizing a CDS has also improved student performance in preclinical operative dentistry [37]. VR technology also has been used in surgery education. VR technology can build realistic human body models and can create tools to view, touch, feel, hear, and manipulate the models [38]. Using such technologies, students can learn in less time as they develop their skills quickly [5].

1.8 LIMITATIONS OF THE DIGITAL TECHNOLOGIES

The major limitation of utilizing various digital technologies includes the cost of implementing them. Hence, there can be a financial burden for some dental clinics to incorporate these technologies into practice. In addition, to be able to use the technologies of digital dentistry, dentists, technicians, and dental staff should have the requisite knowledge. These may require additional training to learn and use such technologies. Other concerns are regarding privacy and data security of the patient in digital systems [39].

Furthermore, every dental procedure cannot be fully replaced by digital technologies, and in many cases, we still need traditional approaches [39]. In addition, there is no guarantee that using digital procedures and techniques will result in 100% success of a treatment [4]. The accuracy of these advancing digital technologies needs further analysis [40–42].

Some failures have been associated with 3D-printed prostheses. The 3D-printed dentures have lower bond strength and higher failure rates [33]. The combination of milled and conventional techniques seems to be a safer and better choice. These limitations should be addressed before utilizing digital technologies and devices such as IOSs, computerized occlusal analysis devices, digital jaw trackers, etc.

1.9 CONCLUSION

Digital technologies are useful diagnostic and design tools for various areas of dentistry including prosthodontics, orthodontics, and restorative care. VR and CDSs are also gaining popularity in dental education. Digital technologies have allowed the customization of orthodontic appliances. Teeth can be scanned to create digital models, and appliances are designed and manufactured digitally. Various limitations of digital technologies in dentistry should be addressed before utilizing such techniques.

REFERENCES

1. Humagain, M, Rokaya, D. Integrating digital technologies in dentistry to enhance the clinical success. Kathmandu Univ Med J (KUMJ). 2019;17(68):256–257.
2. Mangano, F et al. Intraoral scanners in dentistry: a review of the current literature. BMC Oral Health. 2017;17(1):149.
3. Amornvit, P et al. Comparison of accuracy of current ten intraoral scanners. Biomed Res Int. 2021;2021:2673040.
4. Gollner, MG. Digital transformation: analog expertise and digital optimization. Int J Comput Dent. 2022;25(4):407–419.
5. Prithviraj, DR et al. Revolutionizing restorative dentistry: an overview. J Indian Prosthodont Soc. 2014;14(4):333–343.
6. Schierz, O et al. Digital dentistry and its impact on oral health-related quality of life. J Evidence-Based Dent Pract. 2024;24(1, Supplement):101946.
7. Graiff, L et al. Coupling of multilayer CAD-CAM prosthetic components: computing the user interaction influence on the adhesion interface geometry. Int J Interactive Design Manufacturing (IJIDeM). 2023;17(6):3321–3331.
8. D'Addazio, G et al. Fracture resistance of zirconia-reinforced lithium silicate ceramic crowns cemented with conventional or adhesive systems: an in vitro study. Materials (Basel, Switzerland). 2020;13(9):2012.
9. Wang, J et al. Fully digital workflow for replicating treatment dentures: a technique for jaw relation transfer and dynamic occlusal adjustment. J Prosth Dent. 2023;130(3):288–294.
10. Kim, JE et al. Complete assessment of occlusal dynamics and establishment of a digital workflow by using target tracking with a three-dimensional facial scanner. J Prosthodont Res. 2019;63(1):120–124.
11. Solaberrieta, E et al. Comparison of a conventional and virtual occlusal record. J Prosthet Dent. 2015;114(1):92–97.
12. Kongkiatkamon, S, Rokaya, D. Full digital workflow in the esthetic dental restoration. Case Rep Dent. 2022;2022:8836068.
13. Stavness, IK et al. Simulation of dental collisions and occlusal dynamics in the virtual environment. J Oral Rehabil. 2016;43(4):269–278.
14. Krahenbuhl, JT et al. Accuracy and precision of occlusal contacts of stereolithographic casts mounted by digital interocclusal registrations. J Prosthet Dent. 2016;116(2):231–236.
15. Peng, T et al. Comparative evaluation of the volume of occlusal adjustment of repositioning occlusal devices designed by using an average value digital articulator and the jaw movement analyzer. J Prosthet Dent. 2025;133(5):1268–1274.
16. McBeath, KCC et al. Digital technologies to support better outcome and experience of care in patients with heart failure. Curr Heart Fail Rep. 2022;19(3):75–108.
17. Shopova, D et al. Case report: digital analysis of occlusion with T-scan novus in occlusal splint treatment for a patient with bruxism. F1000Res. 2021;10:915.
18. Panayi, NC et al. Digital orthodontics: present and future. AJO-DO Clinical Companion. 2024;4(1):14–25.
19. Cunha, T et al. Orthodontic digital workflow: devices and clinical applications. Dental Press J Orthodont. 2021; 26(6):e21spe26.
20. Barreto, FAM, Santos, J. Virtual orthodontic setup in orthodontic camouflage planning for skeletal class III malocclusion. Dental Press J Orthodont. 2018;23(2):75–86.
21. Spitz, A et al. CAD/CAM technology for digital indirect bonding. J Clin Orthodont. 2018;52(11):621–628.
22. Oliveira, NS et al. Comparison of the accuracy of virtual and direct bonding of orthodontic accessories. Dental Press J Orthodont. 2019;24(4):46–53.
23. Duarte, MEA et al. Reproducibility of digital indirect bonding technique using three-dimensional (3D) models and 3D-printed transfer trays. The Angle Orthodont. 2020;90(1):92–99.
24. Deahl, ST et al. Practice-based comparison of direct and indirect bonding. Am J Orthodont Dentofac Orthoped. 2007;132(6):738–742.
25. Nawrocka, A, Lukomska-Szymanska, M. The indirect bonding technique in orthodontics-a narrative literature review. Materials (Basel, Switzerland). 2020;13(4):986.
26. Nojima, LI et al. Indirect orthodontic bonding–a modified technique for improved efficiency and precision. Dental Press J Orthodont. 2015;20(3):109–117.
27. Camardella, LT et al. Virtual setup: application in orthodontic practice. J Orofac Orthoped. 2016;77(6):409–419.
28. Francisco, I et al. Application of three-dimensional digital technology in orthodontics: the state of the art. Biomimetics (Basel, Switzerland). 2022;7(1):23.
29. Mack, MR. Perspective of facial esthetics in dental treatment planning. J Prosthet Dent. 1996;75(2):169–176.
30. Humagain, M et al. Gender based comparison of gingival zenith esthetics. Kathmandu Univ Med J (KUMJ). 2016; 14(54):148–152.
31. Levin, EI. Dental esthetics and the golden proportion. J Prosthet Dent. 1978;40(3):244–252.
32. Saeed, F et al. Prosthodontics dental materials: from conventional to unconventional. Mater Sci Eng C Mater Biol Appl. 2020;106:110167.
33. Tzanakakis, EG et al. Adhesion of conventional, 3D-printed and milled artificial teeth to resin substrates for complete dentures: a narrative review. Polymers (Basel). 2023;15(11).
34. Kongkiatkamon, S et al. Current classification of zirconia in dentistry: an updated review. PeerJ. 2023;11:e15669.
35. LeBlanc, VR et al. A preliminary study in using virtual reality to train dental students. J Dent Educ. 2004;68(3):378–383.
36. Huang, Y et al. Student perceptions toward virtual reality training in dental implant education. PeerJ. 2023;11:e14857.
37. Urbankova, A. Impact of computerized dental simulation training on preclinical operative dentistry examination scores. J Dent Educ. 2010;74(4):402–409.
38. Lange, T et al. Virtual reality in surgical training. Surg Oncol Clin N Am. 2000;9(1):61–79, vii.
39. Khurshid, Z. Digital dentistry: transformation of Oral health and dental education with technology. Eur J Dent. 2023;17(4):943–944.
40. Revilla-León, M et al. An overview of the digital occlusion technologies: intraoral scanners, jaw tracking systems, and computerized occlusal analysis devices. J Esthet Restor Dent. 2023;35(5):735–744.
41. Revilla-León, M et al. Accuracy of the maxillomandibular relationship at centric relation position recorded by using 3 different intraoral scanners with or without an optical jaw tracking system: an in vivo pilot study. J Dent. 2023;132:104478.
42. Revilla-León, M et al. Differences in maxillomandibular relationship recorded at centric relation when using a conventional method, four intraoral scanners, and a jaw tracking system: a clinical study. J Prosthet Dent. 2024;132(5):964–972.

2 Materials for Digital Dentistry

Aybike Cengiz Dagtekin, Samet Tekin, Bekir Eser, Zohaib Khurshid, and Heba Ashi

2.1 INTRODUCTION

In recent years, the development of new technologies has paralleled the rapid evolution of restorative materials in digital dentistry (DD), thereby opening new horizons for digital dental materials (DDMs). The use of state-of-the-art technologies, such as computerized design/computerized manufacturing (CAD/CAM), laser sintering, and three-dimensional (3D) printing in everyday practice has contributed significantly to the development of a new technology of dental substances. Materials such as high-strength ceramics, hybrid composites, reinforced polymers, high-strength alloys, and metal-free ceramics offer advantages such as acceptable optical properties, reliable mechanical properties, and accuracy. Excellent compatibility, lower costs, and fast production are the main factors that have made digitization popular [1].

The digital era brought changes in the manufacturing of dental restorations, including crowns and bridges and the usage of dental CAD/CAM systems. These new technologies are rapidly becoming more widespread in the market. Subtractive manufacturing techniques are used more in prosthesis manufacturing; however, additive manufacturing methods such as fused deposition modeling, stereolithography, selective laser sintering, and 3D printing are also increasingly being used [2]. Dental ceramics and their processing strategies have advanced notably over the past decade, with much of the development associated with CAD/CAM methods. Clinicians have used all-ceramic restorations for several years. Monolithic restorations began to develop more rapidly as multilayered restorations, which were intended to be more aesthetic, became more prone to deformation. During these developments, CAD/CAM resin composites have become more attractive than ceramics and polymers because they can be easily milled and polished [3].

DDMs are mainly used in additive and subtractive manufacturing technologies.

The advantages of the growing use of additive production in dental area consist of the following:

- More accurate production in a shorter time.
- Available cost.
- Ease in determining tooth size and shape.
- Production of custom implant abutments.
- Reduced production time.
- The production of physical models with the information stored in the digital environment is not necessary.
- Patient comfort and motivation.
- More accurate decision making in the selection of implant sizes [4, 5].

Many different materials have been used in additive manufacturing. Examples of such materials include polymers, composites, ceramics, and metal alloys [4, 5]. Additive manufacturing produces dental models with a high accuracy [6].

In general, additive manufacturing produces much less substance waste. It is more energy-efficient than subtractive manufacturing. Such characteristics make them suitable for use in restorations made from hard-to-machine hard substances, like chromium-cobalt. The restriction of this system contains the difficulty caused by the layering of the materials on top of each other. Three-dimensional additive manufacturing can be considered an alternative to the milling method known as subtractive manufacturing. These systems, known as rapid prototyping, are different methods for producing restorations. Additive manufacturing has more benefits than subtractive manufacturing. The variety of additive procedures allows the usage of different basic materials for the fabrication of structures. These substances may be grouped into binder/powder material combinations, which include polymers (resins and thermoplastics), ceramics, and metals [7].

Studies have shown that the accuracy of dental restorations produced by the use of additive production strategies is better than that of subtractive production. Therefore, additive manufacturing methods are good alternatives to subtractive methods [8].

DOI: 10.1201/9781003428541-2

The aim of additive manufacturing is to enable the production of dental restorations and implant abutments using 3D data. This application can be used to fabricate detailed dental crowns, bridges, and orthodontic braces. In addition, different models, tools, and instruments can be produced in less time and cost. This system, which has developed rapidly with technology, produces patient data in the most accurate way using a dental 3D scanner. This technique has recently been investigated for purposes such as surgical guidance for implant prostheses, precise production of jaw model templates, and preoperative jaw positioning [6].

Materials, which include plastics, metals, and ceramics, may be produced using diverse techniques. Three-dimensional printing has been used for approximately three decades. Currently, this technology is developing faster than many other technologies. In the transition to clinical application in dentistry, the development of DDMs is recognized not only with precision manufacturing and accuracy but also with the development of physical and biological properties [9].

2.2 MATERIALS USED IN ADDITIVE MANUFACTURING IN DENTISTRY

2.2.1 Polymers

This group includes traditional temporary materials, monomethacrylates, acrylic resins, dimethacrylates, and bis-acryl/composite resins like bisphenol A-glycidyl dimethacrylate and light polymerizable urethane dimethacrylate [10].

Polymer temporary restorations are made to solve a patient's dental problems for a period of time. These substances ought to have good enough mechanical properties in shape accuracy, color stability, and enough hardness to satisfy their roles [11–13].

It is difficult to make recommendations regarding the minimum dimensions required for the connector areas of a temporary fixed prosthesis made of printable polymers or the possible number of pontics. The life of these materials in the clinic compared to those of permanent restorations is also lacking [14].

2.2.2 Ceramics

Ceramics are materials prone to cracking and fracturing at high temperatures, complicating additive manufacturing, which must be produced at high melting points. Fractures and cracks are common during postprocess cooling. In addition, temperature changes increase the porosity of the ceramics. Crack propagation and pores weaken the ceramic and degrade its mechanical properties [15].

In most studies on 3D-printed zirconia restorations, zirconia is usually produced by polymerization techniques such as digital light processing (DLP) and stereolithography (SLA) [16, 17]. In both of these techniques, the restorations are produced with high accuracy and resolution, smooth surface finish, and fine details [18–20].

Because zirconia offers a high refractive index, significant scattering by light (UV or laser) can occur during the DLP and SLA. The penetration depth of the incident light can be reduced during polymerization of the resin containing it. Therefore, additive manufacturing is required to produce materials with sufficient density after sintering. The values of hardness and fracture toughness in these products are in the range of 1038–1556 HV and 3.43–6.42 MPa, respectively. These values are normally lower than those of conventionally produced zirconia. For the theoretical density of the materials, values between 98 and 99.8% were obtained, which were similar to those of the conventional ones [21–24].

SLA printing techniques have additionally been used to supply zirconia implant abutments. The dimensional accuracy of the produced abutment grew high, and the acquired mechanical residences confirmed a bending strength (943 Mpa) close to that of conventionally produced ceramics (milled zirconia 800–1000 MPa) [25].

In addition, the challenges that exist in 3D printing system should not be underestimated. Characteristics such as surface quality, dimensional accuracy, and mechanical properties must be improved to enable the production of high-quality products [26].

2.2.3 Metals

Selective laser sintering is the main method used to fabricate metal-based restorations from titanium, chromium-cobalt (Cr-Co), and other alloys. Early trials of this generation created restorations that were porous, had negative surface coverage, and were not resistant to occlusal forces. The main goal of this technology is to create metallic structures with the most accurate mechanical properties and minimal surface irregularities that increase osteointegration in implant cases [27, 28].

Laser sintering has been used to overcome challenges such as the shrinkage of metals such as Cr-Co during casting and its high hardness during grinding. Active forces cannot be applied during the production of structures. In addition, substance waste is lower than that with other methods, making this technology particularly popular for precious alloys [29, 30].

2.2.4 Resins

UV resins consist of a polymer monomer, a prepolymer, an active diluent, a photoinitiator, and a photosensitizer. Under UV light with a wavelength of 250–300 nm, the polymerization reaction begins immediately, and the dispersed polymers combine into cross-linked polymers, transforming from a liquid to a solid 3D structure. UV resin applications include crowns, bridges, surgical guides, and prostheses [31–33].

The DLP is used for production. For DLP printers to process the material layer by layer, the viscosity of the resin must be appropriate. Bisphenol A-glycidyl methacrylate (Bis-GMA)-containing UV resins have high viscosity, which limits 3D printing. Alternatively, a more fluid triethylene glycol dimethacrylate (TEGDMA) monomer is used as a diluent [34–37].

Permanent resins were first introduced in February 2020 [38]. These resins are much cheaper than ceramic restorations, which can be obtained using the subtractive method. 3D-printed resins consist of silica particles of different sizes and shapes, and various methacrylate-containing resins [39]. It can be used with monomers, such as Bis-GMA and urethane dimethacrylate (UDMA), which are used in traditional light-cured composites. Bisphenol A-dimethacrylate (Bis-EMA) and TEGDMA can be used to adjust the viscosity of liquid resins [40]. Although the monomer content can be improved mechanically, ceramic fillers are also added [41, 42]. Increasing the percentage and size of the filler material limits the amount of light absorption; therefore, the filler material is added in limited quantities [43].

The resin 3D crowns used in fixed prosthesis applications were first used as provisional crowns. In these studies, the bending strength of 3D provisional materials was lower than that of milled provisional crowns [44].

Permanent crowns, inlays, and onlays can be produced by using these materials. In one study, it was reported that the crowns produced (Varseo Smile Crown Plus; BEGO, Bremen, Germany) had very good restoration compatibility and an aesthetically excellent appearance. In addition, composite-containing materials adapt more easily to the color structure of the tooth, resulting in a very natural appearance. For an even more natural appearance, occlusal colorants (Optiglaze Color, GC Germany, Bad Homburg) can be used for restorations [45].

With the rapid development of 3D-printed resins, studies are underway to use them not only in single-member restorations but also in long, fixed prostheses [45].

These changes are inevitable with the rapid development of technology and materials at the same time. The number of missing areas requiring attention is also increasing. Additive manufacturing is a promising alternative production method for dental restorations and appliances. Additive manufacturing techniques allow the production of uniformly structured restorations without the need for excessive force and with less non-recyclable waste than subtractive manufacturing techniques. Materials produced using subtractive systems have longer clinical lives than additive materials. However, clinical studies on recently introduced materials are insufficient. Studies and methods should be evaluated on a cost-benefit basis [14].

2.3 MATERIALS USED IN SUBTRACTIVE MANUFACTURING IN DENTISTRY

Using additive strategies for production is more beneficial due to fewer problems related to subtractive production. The fundamental gain of this kind of production is that it lets in for easier gaps and complicated inner geometries to be obtained [2].

In addition, the tools used in subtractive manufacturing show signs of wear after repeated use, which can cause cracks in the objects produced and consume excessive amount of material [9, 46].

2.3.1 Wax

Wax materials for various restorative procedures, mainly composed of acrylate polymers, can now be digitally designed and milled. This makes them both time- and cost-effective. Traditional wax modeling is both skilled and time-consuming. The most recent wax materials are created with metallic casting or pressed with a ceramic. Many producers offer millable wax blocks (VITA CAD-Waxx Blocks, VITA North America, Yorba Linda, California, USA). The marginal accuracy of restorations produced with traditional and CAD/CAM wax-up strategies was changed compared to traditional wax-up strategies and wax fashions produced with additive technology. As a result, the wax models produced by additive manufacturing were found to be more accurate [14].

2.3.2 Polymethyl Methacrylate

Polymethyl methacrylate (PMMA) is an artificial polymer produced via polymerization of methyl methacrylate. PMMA blocks had been used for constant prostheses and crowns. In a previous study, it was reported that PMMA and glass ceramics have similar properties when compared in terms of margin fit and aesthetics [47].

Increasing interest in PMMA restorations led to improvement of PMMA blocks with optical and bodily properties (e.g., Telio CAD, Ivoclar Vivadent, Shaan, Liechtenstein, VITA CAD-Temp MultiColor Blocks, VITA Zahnfabrik, Bad Sackingen, Germany). Restorations made with PMMA can be comfortly polished after finishing. Recently, CAD/CAM has come to be the most frequently used system for milling PMMA blocks [14, 48, 49].

2.3.3 CAD/CAM Composite Resins

There are two types of CAD/CAM ceramic blocks: Blocks containing a polymer matrix with ceramic filler particles (e.g., Lava Ultimate, 3M ESPE, Katana Avencia Block, Kuraray Noritake, Tokyo, Japan, and Cerasmart, GC International AG, Lucerne, Switzerland) and blocks with a ceramic matrix infiltrated with a polymer (e.g., VITA Enamic). The main features of these blocks are their resistance to increased loads, high fatigue resistance, high modulus of elasticity, favorable milling properties with smooth margins, no need for processes such as crystallization or sintering, and no need for polishing after etching [50, 51].

The methods and materials used for cementation are different for each block. The ceramic structure of polymer-infiltrated ceramics requires roughening with 5% hydrofluoric acid for 60 seconds, followed by silane application. However, the highly polymerized resin matrix of polymer blocks with ceramic content, like Lava Ultimate, requires pretreatment of these ceramics with $\leq$ 50 µm aluminum oxide particle abrasion, followed by silane application [52].

When comparing the wear resistance, polymer-infiltrated ceramics are better than ceramic-infiltrated polymers. In addition, both materials have lower wear resistance than conventional ceramic restorations [53].

Ceramic-infiltrated blocks are recommended for bridges, inlays, and onlays, while polymer-infiltrated ceramic blocks may be used for single crowns. Studies evaluating these ceramics as good options for indirect restorations are still lacking [53–55].

2.3.4 High-Performance Polymers

High-performance polymers are used clinically because of their good mechanical, physical, and biocompatible features. Polyetheretherketone (PEEK) and polyetherketonketone (PEKK) have been used in crowns, fixed dental prostheses, custom abutments, telescopic crowns, removable partial dentures, and implants. The machining of these materials is mechanically possible and easier to handle because they can be milled more easily than metals. Because PEEK is radiolucent, it does not cause artifacts in magnetic resonance imaging procedures. Another advantage is that it does not cause abrasion of the opposing teeth [56]. The low specific gravity of the material allows for lighter prostheses that are easy to clean [57]. Studies have also shown that PEEK does not have any cytotoxic effects on cells and does not cause mutagenicity [58].

PEEK has a higher fracture resistance than zirconia and many other ceramics, and PEEK can be easily modified by the addition of other materials [59]. PEEK, which is also used as an obturator to close oro-nasal defects, is lighter, biocompatible, has good adhesion, and is easy to polish [60]. Since PEEK is grayish brown in color, it is not suitable for use in aesthetic restorations of anterior teeth [61, 62].

Additive manufacturing offers less time and cost for PEEK production [63]. Patient data can be easily scanned and recorded using a 3D scanner and printed in a short time [64, 65]. To optimize the 3D printing of PEEK, certain parameters must be satisfied. The optimal printing conditions for PEEK are 420–440°C nozzle temperature, 0° scan angle, and 0.3 mm layer thickness [66].

The success of PEEK in dentistry has aroused interest in PEKK, which belongs to the same family as PEEK. PEKK was first introduced in 1962 and has since been used in the military. In recent years, it has been applied in medicine and dentistry [60, 67]. PEKK belongs to a newly developed family of reinforced polymers. PEKK is an elastic material that reveals suitable pressure absorption and fracture resistance [68]. Because the PEKK material can be both amorphous and crystalline, it is suitable for the production of different materials. It melts at 305°C. Compared to PEEK, PEKK exhibits better mechanical and physical properties and better resistance to pressure, owing to its extra ketone group [69].

The combination of PEKK implant abutments and titanium implants can result in long-term implant-supported restorations [70]. It has been reported that the level of abrasion on the opposing teeth is low in crowns produced with PEKK. Although the PEKK material itself deforms, it does not damage the opposing tooth. For this reason, PEKK crowns exhibit more wear than zirconia crowns [71, 72].

In addition, since metal clasps are not very aesthetic in removable partial dentures, PEKK has been used as a clasp in digitally designed removable partial prostheses [73].

Post-core production has also been considered by exploiting its stress-absorbing properties [74, 75]. It exhibits superior biomechanical properties compared with metal and fiber posts. It has a lower elastic modulus, resulting in fewer root fractures than the others [74].

The best-known 3D printing technique used for processing PEEK/PEKK is fused deposition modeling (FDM). FDM is a type of additive manufacturing (AM) method that involves the creation of objects by adding layers of material through fusion or deposition. Its advantages include lower cost, ease of use, and lower probability of degradation. Optimal printing conditions for PEKK were a nozzle temperature of 380°C, a scan angle of 45°, and a layer thickness of 0.2 mm [76].

2.3.5 Metals

Precious grindable metals such as chromium-cobalt, titanium, and gold have become materials that can be used in CAD/CAM, because they eliminate the possibility of miscasting the final restoration. Chromium-cobalt provides a substructure for crowns and fixed partial dentures. It is a cheap, corrosion-resistant metal. Chromium-cobalt alloys can be produced in different forms. Solid chromium-cobalt disks can be ground in solid grinding machines, and softer chromium-cobalt materials can be ground like wax or sintered in an argon gas environment to produce solid chromium-cobalt metal. Titanium blocks can be milled to produce abutments that can adapt to the desired colors for more demanding aesthetic applications. Precious alloys are made into millables, eliminating the problems associated with burning and casting [14].

An additive manufacturing technique is more commonly used for the production of metallic structures made of titanium, chromium-cobalt, and nickel alloys. In addition, the first additive manufacturing machines did not use vacuum during the construction process, and the laser diameter and power were insufficient to produce the desired restoration. This makes the production of metallic structures inefficient with early machines [77–79].

Although nickel-containing alloys are no longer used in dental prostheses because of the risk of nickel allergy, research on titanium constructs produced using joining techniques has shown that, despite some surface roughness, they have suitable force strength, ultimate tensile strength, and flexibility [80]. Although there have been a number of well-designed studies on the properties of titanium alloys (specifically Ti6Al4V) fabricated using SLS, few studies has been carried out on different substances that may be produced using identical technology [80].

Additive production strategies, including DMLS, were used to conquer the problems encountered in conventional casting and milling strategies for tough substances, including Cr-Co. Although chromium-cobalt alloys have challenges, such as high hardness and shrinkage during milling, this problem is overcome by technology because no active force is used during manufacturing [81].

The low quantity of irreversible waste generated during the use of fabrication techniques will additionally increase using valuable metals for digital fabrication [82]. Additive manufacturing is promising method to produce restorations from chromium–cobalt metal [83]. However, DMLS, a variation of the technique, has shown promise because it produces a large amount of the final material. Studies comparing the accuracy of porcelain crowns connected to metallic produced through DMLS have shown that their quality has a marginal fit to be used in dental prostheses [84].

2.3.6 CAD/CAM Ceramics

One of the most significant changes with the development of computerized systems is the introduction of monolithic restorations fabricated from high-strength ceramics, like zirconia. This concept is not new, as ceramic substances were used with the manufacturing of monolithic restorations for a exceptionally lengthy time; however, dentists and technicians have begun to achieve more success with the introduction of zirconia to produce full-contour crowns [85].

2.3.6.1 Resin Composite Materials

Resin composites consist of inorganic or organic fillers embedded in an organic resin matrix that contains initiators, stabilizers, and pigments. Composite resins can be modeled, polymerized, and directly applied intraorally. Prepolymerized composite resins composed of grindable blocks exhibit less polymerization shrinkage and residual monomer release. They are designed, milled, and polymerized outside the mouth to overcome some of the shortcomings of directly applied composites owing to their enhanced mechanical properties. Millable composite resins can be used to manufacture restorations, like crowns, bridges, inlays, and onlays. After processing, they require polishing, polymerization, and addition of dyes. Their strengths and other features are compared to those of ceramic blocks without consensus on which material is superior [86, 87].

2.3.6.2 *Hybrid Ceramics*

Hybrid ceramics are a brand new substance of CAD/CAM chairside materials designed to take the benefit of the unique aesthetic features of ceramic materials, combined with the reduced brittleness and increased fracture resistance inherent in composite resins. These are divided into two categories.

- Nanoceramic resin blocks with composite resins (commonly available Bis-GMA, UDMA, UTMA, and Bis-EMA), produced under high-temperature and high-pressure conditions.
- Polymer-infiltrated ceramic network (PICN) blocks containing ceramics (86 wt%) and composite resin (14 wt %) [88].

Hybrid ceramics are easier to grind and exhibit high mechanical strength and sufficient hardness even at reduced thicknesses [89]. The first on the market with nanoceramic materials is Lava Ultimate, which contains up to 80% silica (20 nm) and zirconia (4–11 nm) particles by weight. (3M Ultimate; 3M Oral Care, USA). According to the producer, the advantage of nanoceramic material over CAD/CAM composite blocks is that it has more gloss after polishing. The material exhibits a bending force of approximately 200 MPa [90].

Nanoceramic blocks are recommended as occlusal veneers or inlays and onlays in the posterior region [91]. Nanoceramic blocks are intermediate between the mechanical strengths of adhesive ceramics and high-filler composites. It had a modulus of elasticity of approximately 30 GPa [91]. The polishing of this material is faster than that of other materials. Adhesives should be used for cementation of restorations made of such materials [91].

2.3.6.3 *Silicate Ceramics*

2.3.6.3.1 Feldspathic and Leucite-Reinforced Ceramics

Traditional feldspathic porcelain is considered the optimal material in terms of its optical properties. It is also considered to be the weakest among glass-based ceramics. This type of porcelain requires roughening with 9.6% hydrofluoric acid for 1 minute, followed by ultrasonic bathing of the restoration to remove salt residues and then application of silane. Cemented with adhesives leucite was added to the matrix to increase the strength of feldspathic ceramics. Leucite-reinforced feldspathic ceramics (IPS Empress CAD, Ivoclar Vivadent) have excellent optic properties, which make them perfect for restorations in the aesthetic area. In addition, they provide a minimal increase in strength compared to conventional feldspathic porcelains. For this reason, they are not preferred in cases where load bearing is required, as more durable materials are available. These materials are available in two different forms, monochromatic blocks or polychromatic blocks (Vitablocs Triluxe forte and Vitablocs RealLife, Vita ZahnFabrik), and they are available in translucent options that offer enamel-like properties [92].

The average survival charge for inlay and onlay leucite restorations within the posterior area was 96.7% after nine years [93]. An estimated survival rate of 92–95% at five years for feldspathic ceramic restorations (onlay, overlay) and 91% at ten years for 2154 restorations has been reported [94].

2.3.6.3.2 Lithium Disilicates (LS2) and Zirconia Reinforced Lithium Silicate

Lithium disilicates (LS2) and zirconia-reinforced lithium silicate is classified as a glass ceramic in the lithium-disilicate-particle-containing glass class. It was introduced in the 1990s under the name "IPS Empress 2" (Ivoclar Vivadent, Schaan, Liechtenstein). It consists of 65% lithium disilicate by volume and small, needle-shaped crystals (3–6 μm × 0.8 μm) embedded in a glass matrix with 1% porosity and good mechanical properties. The bending strength was 350 MPa [95–97].

Subsequently, LS2 ceramics containing 72% lithium and silicate oxide were introduced to the market. Owing to this development, the mechanical features of glass-based ceramics have improved. Simultaneously, optimal optical properties were maintained. LS2-containing glass ceramics were roughened using 4.9% hydrofluoric acid (HF) for 20 seconds. Silane was applied, cemented to the tooth surface with an adhesive, and then cleaned using ultrasonic instruments [14].

IPS e.max Press, an LS2 formula with smaller grains and homogeneous properties, was developed. This material has a flexural strength of 370–460 MPa and a fracture toughness of 2.8–3.5 MPa, which are much better those of older ceramics. The high mechanical performance of this material is attributed to the layered and tightly interconnected structure of the elongated di-silicate crystals. This feature prevents crack propagation between the planes [96].

The flexural strengths of IPS e.max Press and IPS e.max CAD have been reported to be similar. In addition, the producing process did not affect the mechanical features of the LS2 ceramics [98].

IPS e.max CAD showed optimal fracture resistance in posterior crown and monolithic restoration applications. It was more resistant to cyclic milling movements than zirconia, which is more prone to chipping [98, 99].

Monolithic restorations for implant-supported prostheses and posterior crowns are more resistant to fractures than double-layered restorations [100–102]. In terms of wear and abrasion, the LS2 restoration was very close to the enamel when polished using the correct method [103].

Another advantage of LS2 is its compatibility with soft tissues. This material is preferred because it provides very little plaque retention. It also shows high biocompatibility in terms of easy proliferation of fibroblasts and epithelial cells, owing to its glossy, smooth surface [104, 105]. No increase in gingival groove fluid or inflammation was detected in the teeth with LS2 restoration. Similar results were observed for zirconia restorations [106]. It exhibits excellent biocompatibility and translucency, 30% higher than that of conventional zirconia, and good aesthetic properties [107].

Acid etching was found to be the best roughening method for glass-ceramic materials. The best-known procedure was hydrofluoric acid. For LS2, etching with 5% hydrofluoric acid for 20 seconds is recommended. This time (20 seconds) was shorter than that for leucite-based and feldspathic ceramics. Etching time is usually recommended at 9–10% HF for 60 seconds. Longer etching times are aggressive and degrade the smoothness and internal microstructure of the restoration, thereby reducing its mechanical performance. Extra etching significantly reduces the flexural strength. It reduces the adhesion potential and negatively affects its long-term success, especially in restorations with insufficient thickness [108, 109].

Sandblasting with aluminum oxide particles was used for surface roughening. However, sandblasting, which is preferred for adhesion, can reduce the flexural strength [110, 111].

The increasing clinical use of LS2 can be explained by its excellent aesthetics and good mechanical properties. The advantage of this material is that it is metal-free with appropriate bonding to dental tissues owing to its silica content. LS2 ceramics can be used in anterior aesthetic crowns, posterior inlays, onlays, posterior crowns, and implant-supported restorations [98].

Very high survival rates have been demonstrated in implant-supported, single-member monolithic restorations with LS2 made entirely with digital system flow [112]. LS2 is considered a viable option when ceramic restorations are indicated under mechanically unfavorable conditions. In fact, more rigid ceramic materials have been reported to strengthen the tooth structure and framework material and act as shields in the restorative aspect [113].

LS2-based restorations can be used even in cases in which thickness reduction (1–1.5 mm) is required. This material has a low wear potential and allows adhesive bond strength. This material is indicated particularly for use in cases of severe wear, especially in the posterior teeth, or when a major occlusal correction is required [114–116].

There was no significant difference in the marginal fit of the restorations between the digital and conventional methods used for the fabrication of monolithic LS2 crowns [117–119].

2.3.6.4 *Oxide Ceramics*

2.3.6.4.1 Zirconia

In ceramic classification, zirconia (ZrO2) is a heterogeneous, highly durable, and highly resistant polycrystalline ceramic with suitable mechanical features (Toughness of 5–10 MPa, flexural strength of 500–1200 MPa, and Young's modulus of 210 GPa). It exhibited excellent optical properties [120–122]. As with glass ceramics, zirconia is not sensitive to etching [123]. It has been reported to exhibit great biocompatibility, lower plaque retention than titanium, and good radiopacity in both in vitro and in vivo studies. It is insoluble in water and is highly resistant to intraoral corrosion [120–122].

It exists in nature in three different crystal configurations at different temperatures:

- Cubic form (melting point 2680°C to 2370°C).
- Tetragonal (2370°C to 1170°C).
- Monoclinic (1170°C to room temperature).

These different allotropic patterns allow for many different prosthetic uses [122, 124].

During industrial production, zirconia in cubic form is stabilized by the addition of metal oxides like yttrium, magnesium, cerium, and lanthanum during industrial production to take advantage of its positive intraoral properties. The percentage of such oxides varies with reference to the producing technique and clinical use. These stabilizing oxides contribute to maintaining zirconia in a thermodynamically semi-stable phase, both in the crystalline tetragonal phase and at room temperature. However, such oxides may be lost after surface abrasion, modifications, sandblasting, polishing, etc. [121, 124, 125]. Monolithic tetragonal zirconia restorations may be subjected to aging after short observation periods, but this does not cause a major deterioration in the mechanical properties of tetragonal zirconia [125]. Owing to the high strength of zirconia, it is resistant to occlusal loads in molar areas even at 0.5 mm occlusal thickness [126, 127]. In addition, yttrium oxide is added to zirconia to improve its optical properties, which increases its resistance to refraction, but may reduce its mechanical properties after roughening [128].

The most commonly used method for zirconia production is milling using CAM-CAM. The presintered or fully sintered blocks were created on a computer-controlled machine to produce parts of a specific size and shape. However, this can also lead to some disadvantages: High material wastage, limitations in accurately producing restorations with complex structures, long processing times, and high manufacturing costs [22].

Conventional water-based bonding agents (glass ionomer cement and zinc phosphate cement) and hybrid cements (resin-modified glass ionomer cements) can be considered as good choices for cementation. In contrast, resin cement is preferred in the presence of partial coverage restorations, preparations that cannot be retentive (e.g., abutment teeth with reduced occlusocervical dimensions), and high masticatory loads [129–131].

Regarding the production of zirconia using additive manufacturing technology, the bond strength value of porcelain to zirconia was higher than that produced using subtractive manufacturing technology. In addition, scanning electron microscopy (SEM) revealed that the additively produced zirconia sample had a higher number of pits (implying a strong bond between porcelain and zirconia). Therefore, the potential for the use of dental prostheses produced using additive technology is high [132].

REFERENCES

1. Zarone, F et al. "Digitally oriented materials": focus on lithium disilicate ceramics. Int J Dent. 2016:9840594.
2. Van Noort, R. The future of dental devices is digital. Dent Mater. 2012;28:3–12.
3. da Silva, LH et al. Dental ceramics: a review of new materials and processing methods. Brazilian Oral Res. 2017;31:133–146.
4. Lu, Z et al. Microstructure and phase analysis of 3D-printed components using bronze metal filament. J Mater Eng Perform. 2020;29(3):1650–1656.
5. Ngo, TD et al. Additive manufacturing (3D printing): a review of materials, methods, applications and challenges. Compos B: Eng. 2018;143:172–196.
6. Javaid, M, Haleem, A. Current status and applications of additive manufacturing in dentistry: a literature-based review. J Oral Biol Craniofac Res. 2019;9(3):179–185.
7. Barazanchi, A et al. Additive technology: update on current materials and applications in dentistry. J Prosthodontics. 2017;26(2):156–163.
8. Bae, EJ et al. A comparative study of additive and subtractive manufacturing for dental restorations. J Prosthet Dent. 2017;118(2):187–193.
9. Kessler, A et al. 3D printing in dentistry – state of the art. Oper Dent. 2020;45(1):30–40.
10. Burns, DR et al. A review of selected dental literature on contemporary provisional fixed prosthodontic treatment: report of the committee on research in fixed prosthodontics of the academy of fixed prosthodontics. J Prosthet Dent. 2003;90(5):474–497.
11. Digholkar, S et al. Evaluation of the flexural strength and microhardness of provisional crown and bridge materials fabricated by different methods. J Indian Prosthodontist Soc. 2016;16(4):328–334.
12. Balkenhol, M et al. Provisional crown and fixed partial denture materials: mechanical properties and degree of conversion. Dent Mater. 2007;23(12):1574–1583.
13. Balkenhol, M et al. Mechanical properties of provisional crown and bridge materials: chemical-curing versus dual-curing systems. J Dent. 2008;36(1):15–20.
14. Sulaiman, TA. Materials in digital dentistry—a review. J Esthet Restor Dent. 2020;32(2):171–181.
15. Xing, H et al. Study on surface quality, precision and mechanical properties of 3D printed ZrO_2 ceramic components by laser scanning stereolithography. Ceram Int. 2017;43(18):16340–16347.
16. Turkyilmaz, I, Wilkins, GN. 3D printing in dentistry – exploring the new horizons. J Dent Sci. 2021;16:1037–1038.
17. Tsolakis, IA et al. Comparison in terms of accuracy between DLP and LCD printing technology for dental model printing. Dent J (Basel). 2022;10(10):181.
18. Shaukat, U et al. A review of multi-material 3D printing of functional materials via vat photopolymerization. Polymers. 2022;14(12):2449. MDPI.
19. Bahati, D et al. Vat photopolymerization additive manufacturing technology for bone tissue engineering applications. Adv Eng Mater. 2023;25. Wiley.
20. Emir, F, Ayyildiz, S. Accuracy evaluation of complete-arch models manufactured by three different 3D printing technologies: a three-dimensional analysis. J Prosthodont Res. 2021;65(3):365–370.

21. Kontonasaki, E et al. Strength and aging resistance of monolithic zirconia: an update to current knowledge. Japanese Dent Sci Rev. 2020;56:1–23.
22. Branco, AC et al. Recent advances on 3D-printed zirconia-based dental materials: a review. Materials. 2023;16(5):1860.
23. Hsu, HJ et al. A comparison of the marginal fit and mechanical properties of a zirconia dental crown using CAM and 3DSP. Rapid Prototyp J. 2019;25(7):1187–1197.
24. Tangsatchatham, S, Juntavee, N. Flexural strength of various types of computerized machinable ceramic veneered to yttria stabilized tetragonal zirconia polycrystalline ceramic upon different hybridized techniques. Clin Cosmet Investig Dent. 2019;11:61–71.
25. Galante, R et al. Additive manufacturing of ceramics for dental applications: a review. Dent Mater. 2019;35(6):825–846.
26. Figliuzzi, M et al. A novel root analogue dental implant using CT scan and CAD/CAM: selective laser melting technology. Int J Oral Maxillofac Surg. 2012;41(7):858–862.
27. Vichi, A et al. Translucency of ceramic materials for CEREC CAD/CAM system. J Esthet Restor Dent. 2014;26(4):224–231.
28. Mangano, FG et al. Immediate, non-submerged, root-analogue direct laser metal sintering (DLMS) implants: a 1-year prospective study on 15 patients. Lasers Med Sci. 2014;29(4):1321–1328.
29. Münker, TJAG et al. Effects of sterilization on the mechanical properties of poly(methyl methacrylate) based personalized medical devices. J Mech Behav Biomed Mater. 2018;81:168–172.
30. Revilla-León, M et al. A review on chemical composition, mechanical properties, and manufacturing work flow of additively manufactured current polymers for interim dental restorations. J Esthet Restor Dent. 2019;31:51–57.
31. Kim, GT et al. Cytotoxicity, colour stability and dimensional accuracy of 3D printing resin with three different photoinitiators. Polymers. 2022;14(5):979.
32. Vyas, A et al. Photopolymerizable resin-based 3D printed biomedical composites: factors affecting resin viscosity. Mater Today Proc. 2022;62:1435–1439.
33. Cai, HX et al. Dental materials applied to 3D and 4D printing technologies: a review. Polymers. 2023;15(10):2405. MDPI.
34. Goodacre, CJ et al. Tooth preparations for complete crowns: an art form based on scientific principles. J Prosthet Dent. 2001;85(4):363–376.
35. Gajewski, VES et al. Monomers used in resin composites: degree of conversion, mechanical properties and water sorption/solubility. Braz Dent J. 2012;23:508–514.
36. Gonçalves, F et al. Influence of BisGMA, TEGDMA, and BisEMA contents on viscosity, conversion, and flexural strength of experimental resins and composites. Eur J Oral Sci. 2009;117(4):442–446.
37. Lemon, MT et al. Hydrogen bonding interactions in methacrylate monomers and polymers. J Biomed Mater Res. 2007;83(3):734–746.
38. Graf, T et al. Influence of pre-treatment and artificial aging on the retention of 3D-printed permanent composite crowns. Biomedicines. 2022;10(9):2186.
39. Bora, PV et al. Characterization of materials used for 3D printing dental crowns and hybrid prostheses. J Esthetic Restorative Dent. 2024;36(1):220–230.
40. Mohammed, AH et al. Effect of crosslinking concentration on properties of 3-(trimethoxysilyl) propyl methacrylate/N-vinyl pyrrolidone gels. Chem Cent J. 2018;12(1):15.
41. Leyva del Rio, D, Johnston, WM. Effect of monomer composition and filler fraction on surface microhardness and depth of cure of experimental resin composites. Eur J Oral Sci. 2023;131(3):e12933.
42. Gad, MM, Fouda, SM. Factors affecting flexural strength of 3D-printed resins: a systematic review. J Prosthodontics. 2023;32(S1):96–110.
43. Fidalgo-Pereira, R et al. The influence of inorganic fillers on the light transmission through resin-matrix composites during the light-curing procedure: an integrative review. Clin Oral Investig. 2022;26:5575–5594.
44. Alzahrani, SJ et al. Mechanical properties of three-dimensional printed provisional resin materials for crown and fixed dental prosthesis: a systematic review. Bioengineering. 2023;10(6):663.
45. Schweiger, J et al. 3D printing in digital prosthetic dentistry: an overview of recent developments in additive manufacturing. J Clin Med. 2021;10(9):2010.
46. Davidowitz, G, Kotick, PG. The use of CAD/CAM in dentistry. Dent Clin North Am. 2011;55(3):559–570.
47. Ender, A et al. Marginal adaptation, fracture load and macroscopic failure mode of adhesively luted PMMA-based CAD/CAM inlays. Dent Mater. 2016;32(2):e22–e29.
48. Al-Dwairi, ZN et al. A comparison of the surface properties of CAD/CAM and conventional polymethylmethacrylate (PMMA). J Prosthodontics. 2019;28(4):452–457.
49. Al-Dwairi, ZN et al. A comparison of the flexural and impact strengths and flexural modulus of CAD/CAM and conventional heat-cured polymethyl methacrylate (PMMA). J Prosthodontics. 2020;29(4):341–349.
50. Shembish, FA et al. Fatigue resistance of CAD/CAM resin composite molar crowns. Dent Mater. 2016;32(4):499–509.
51. Spitznagel, FA et al. Resin bond to indirect composite and new ceramic/polymer materials: a review of the literature. J Esthetic Restorative Dent. 2014;26:382–393.
52. Matzinger, M et al. Polishing effects and wear performance of chairside CAD/CAM materials. Clin Oral Investig. 2019;23(2):725–737.
53. Blatz, MB et al. Resin-ceramic bonding: a review of the literature. J Prosthet Dent. 2003;89(3):268–274.
54. Hampe, R et al. Fracture toughness analysis of ceramic and resin composite CAD/CAM material. Oper Dent. 2019; 44(4):E190–E201.
55. Negm, EE et al. Virtual evaluation of the accuracy of fit and trueness in maxillary poly(etheretherketone) removable partial denture frameworks fabricated by direct and indirect CAD/CAM techniques. J Prosthodontics. 2019;28(7): 804–810.
56. Bathala, L et al. The role of polyether ether ketone (Peek) in dentistry – a review. J Med Life. 2019;12:5–9.
57. Neugebauer, J et al. The use of plastics in fixed prosthetic implant restoration. Zwr-German Dent J. 2013;122:242–245.
58. Katzer, A et al. Polyetheretherketone—cytotoxicity and mutagenicity in vitro. Biomaterials. 2002;23(8):1749–1759.
59. Beuer, F et al. Load-bearing capacity of all-ceramic three-unit fixed partial dentures with different computer-aided design (CAD)/computer-aided manufacturing (CAM) fabricated framework materials. Eur J Oral Sci. 2008;116(4):381–386.
60. Stawarczyk, B et al. Three-unit reinforced polyetheretherketone composite FDPs: influence of fabrication method on load-bearing capacity and failure types. Dent Mater J. 2015;34(1):7–12.

61. Uhrenbacher, J et al. The effect of surface modification on the retention strength of polyetheretherketone crowns adhesively bonded to dentin abutments. J Prosthet Dent. 2014;112(6):1489–1497.
62. Schmidlin, PR et al. Effect of different surface pre-treatments and luting materials on shear bond strength to PEEK. Dent Mater. 2010;26(6):553–559.
63. Haleem, A, Javaid, M. Polyether ether ketone (PEEK) and its manufacturing of customised 3D printed dentistry parts using additive manufacturing. Clin Epidemiol Glob Health. 2019;7(4):654–660.
64. Rahmitasari, F et al. PEEK with reinforced materials and modifications for dental implant applications. Dent J. 2017;5(4):35.
65. Haleem, A, Javaid, M. 3D scanning applications in medical field: a literature-based review. Clin Epidemiol Glob Health. 2019;7(2):199–210.
66. Zanjanijam, AR et al. Fused filament fabrication of peek: a review of process-structure-property relationships. Polymers. 2020;12(8):1665.
67. Sorte, N et al. Poly-ether-ether-ketone (PEEK): a review. Int J Recent Sci Res. 2017;8:19208–19211.
68. Alqurashi, H et al. Polyetherketoneketone (PEKK): an emerging biomaterial for oral implants and dental prostheses. J Adv Res. 2021;28:87–95.
69. Guo, R, McGrath, JE. Aromatic polyethers, polyetherketones, polysulfides, and polysulfone. In: Krzysztof Matyjaszewski K, Möller M. eds, Polymer Science: A Comprehensive Reference. Elsevier; 2012:377–430.
70. Passia, N et al. Long-term retention behaviour of resin matrix attachment systems for overdentures. J Mech Behav Biomed Mater. 2016;57:88–94.
71. Kotthaus, M et al. Investigation of the retention forces of secondary telescopic crowns made from Pekkton® ivory in combination with primary crowns made from four different dental alloys: an in vitro study. Biomed Tech (Berl). 2019;64(5):555–562.
72. Choi, JW et al. In vitro investigation of wear of CAD/CAM polymeric materials against primary teeth. Materials. 2017;10(12):1410.
73. Sun, F et al. A speech bulb prosthesis for a soft palate defect with a polyetherketoneketone (PEKK) framework fabricated by multiple digital techniques: a clinical report. J Prosthet Dent. 2020;124(4):495–499.
74. Lee, KS et al. Biomechanical evaluation of a tooth restored with high performance polymer PEKK post-core system: a 3D finite element analysis. Biomed Res Int. 2017;2017:1373127.
75. Güven, M et al. Custom and prefabricated PolyEtherKetoneKetone (PEKK) post-core systems bond strength: scanning electron microscopy evaluation. Microsc Res Tech. 2020;83(7):804–810.
76. El Magri, A et al. Effect of printing parameters on tensile, thermal and structural properties of 3D-printed poly (ether ketone ketone) PEKK material using fused deposition modeling. J Appl Polym Sci. 2023;140(29):e54078.
77. Khaing, MW et al. Direct metal laser sintering for rapid tooling: processing and characterisation of EOS parts. J Mater Process Technol. 2001;113(1):269–272.
78. Kathuria, YP. Microstructuring by selective laser sintering of metallic powder. Surf Coat Technol. 1999;116–119:643–647.
79. Osakada, K, Shiomi, M. Flexible manufacturing of metallic products by selective laser melting of powder. Int J Mach Tools Manuf. 2006;46(11):1188–1193.
80. Frazier, WE. Metal additive manufacturing: a review. J Mater Eng Perform. 2014;23:1917–1928.
81. Abduo, J et al. Trends in computer-aided manufacturing in prosthodontics: a review of the available streams. Int J Dent. 2014;2014 (1):783948.
82. Berman, B. 3-D printing: the new industrial revolution. Bus Horiz. 2012;55(2):155–162.
83. Liu, Q et al. Rapid prototyping in dentistry: technology and application. Int J Adv Manuf Technol. 2006;29(3–4):317–335.
84. Ucar, Y et al. Internal fit evaluation of crowns prepared using a new dental crown fabrication technique: laser-sintered Co-Cr crowns. J Prosthet Dent. 2009;102(4):253–259.
85. da Silva, LH et al. Dental ceramics: a review of new materials and processing methods. Brazilian Oral Res. 2017;31: 133–146.
86. Magne, P et al. In vitro fatigue resistance of CAD/CAM composite resin and ceramic posterior occlusal veneers. J Prosthet Dent. 2010;104(3):149–157.
87. Mörmann, WH et al. Wear characteristics of current aesthetic dental restorative CAD/CAM materials: two-body wear, gloss retention, roughness and martens hardness. J Mech Behav Biomed Mater. 2013;20:113–125.
88. Crăciunescu, EL et al, Indirect restorative polymeric dental materials. In: Ardealan LC, Rusu LC, eds, Advances in Dentures – Prosthetic Solutions, Materials and Technologies [Internet]. InTechOpen; 2023. www.intechopen.com/online-first/88239
89. Coldea, A et al. Mechanical properties of polymer-infiltrated-ceramic-network materials. Dent Mater. 2013;29(4):419–426.
90. Fasbinder, DJ. Chairside CAD/CAM: an overview of restorative material options. Compend Contin Educ Dent. 2012;33(1):50, 52–58.
91. Albero, A et al. Comparative characterization of a novel cad-cam polymer-infiltrated-ceramic-network. J Clin Exp Dent. 2015;7(4):e495–e500.
92. Lambert, H et al. Dental biomaterials for chairside CAD/CAM: state of the art. J Adv Prosthodontics. 2017;9(6):486–495.
93. Schulte, AG et al. Longevity of ceramic inlays and onlays luted with a solely light-curing composite resin. J Dent. 2005;33(5):433–442.
94. Morimoto, S et al. Survival rate of resin and ceramic inlays, onlays, and overlays: a systematic review and meta-analysis. J Dent Res. 2016;95:985–994.
95. Zarone, F et al. Digitally oriented materials; Focus on lithium disilicate ceramics. Int J Dent. 2016,2016:9840594.
96. Denry, I, Holloway, JA. Ceramics for dental applications: a review. Materials. 2010;3(1):351–368.
97. Albakry, M et al. Influence of hot pressing on the microstructure and fracture toughness of two pressable dental glass-ceramics. J Biomed Mater Res B Appl Biomater. 2004;71(1):99–107.
98. Fabian Fonzar, R et al. Flexural resistance of heat-pressed and CAD-CAM lithium disilicate with different translucencies. Dent Mater. 2017;33(1):63–70.
99. Willard, A et al. The science and application of IPS e.Max dental ceramic. Kaohsiung J Med Sci. 2018;34(4):238–242.
100. Dogan, DO et al. Fracture resistance of molar crowns fabricated with monolithic all-ceramic CAD/CAM materials cemented on titanium abutments: an in vitro study. J Prosthodontics. 2017;26(4):309–314.

101. Hamza, TA, Sherif, RM. Fracture resistance of monolithic glass-ceramics versus bilayered zirconia-based restorations. J Prosthodontics. 2019;28(1):e259–e264.
102. Choi, JW et al. In vitro study of the fracture resistance of monolithic lithium disilicate, monolithic zirconia, and lithium disilicate pressed on zirconia for three-unit fixed dental prostheses. J Adv Prosthodontics. 2017;9(4):244–251.
103. Lee, A et al. Wear behavior of human enamel against lithium disilicate glass ceramic and type III gold. J Prosthet Dent. 2014;112(6):1399–1405.
104. Tetè, S et al. Proliferation and adhesion capability of human gingival fibroblasts onto zirconia, lithium disilicate and feldspathic veneering ceramic in vitro. Dent Mater J. 2014;33(1):7–15.
105. Forster, A et al. Human epithelial tissue culture study on restorative materials. J Dent. 2014;42(1):7–14.
106. Ariaans, K et al. Use of molecular indicators of inflammation to assess the biocompatibility of all-ceramic restorations. J Clin Periodontol. 2016;43(2):173–179.
107. Baldissara, P et al. Translucency of zirconia copings made with different CAD/CAM systems. J Prosthet Dent. 2010; 104(1):6–12.
108. Murillo-Gómez, F et al. Effect of acid etching on tridimensional microstructure of etchable CAD/CAM materials. Dent Mater. 2018;34(6):944–955.
109. Prochnow, C et al. Hydrofluoric acid concentrations: effect on the cyclic load-to-failure of machined lithium disilicate restorations. Dent Mater. 2018;34(9):e255–e263.
110. Ataol, AS, Ergun, G. Repair bond strength of resin composite to bilayer dental ceramics. J Adv Prosthodont.2018;10(2):101–112.
111. Bajraktarova-Valjakova, E et al. Acid etching as surface treatment method for luting of glass-ceramic restorations, part 1: acids, application protocol and etching effectiveness. Open Access Maced J Med Sci. 2018;6(3):568–573.
112. Joda, T et al. Monolithic implant-supported lithium disilicate (LS2) crowns in a complete digital workflow: a prospective clinical trial with a 2-year follow-up. Clin Implant Dent Relat Res. 2017;19(3):505–511.
113. Sorrentino, R et al. Nonlinear visco-elastic finite element analysis of different porcelain veneers configuration. J Biomed Mater Res B Appl Biomater. 2009;91(2):727–736.
114. Schultheis, S et al. Monolithic and bi-layer CAD/CAM lithium-disilicate versus metal-ceramic fixed dental prostheses: comparison of fracture loads and failure modes after fatigue. Clin Oral Investig. 2013;17(5):1407–1413.
115. Dhima, M et al. Evaluation of fracture resistance in aqueous environment under dynamic loading of lithium disilicate restorative systems for posterior applications. Part 2. J Prosthodontics. 2014;23(5):353–357.
116. Vianna, ALSV et al. Effect of cavity preparation design and ceramic type on the stress distribution, strain and fracture resistance of CAD/CAM onlays in molars. J Appl Oral Sci. 2018;26:e20180004.
117. Haddadi, Y et al. Accuracy of crowns based on digital intraoral scanning compared to conventional impression-a split-mouth randomised clinical study. Clin Oral Investig. 2019;23(11):4043–4050.
118. Abdel-Azim, T et al. Comparison of the marginal fit of lithium disilicate crowns fabricated with CAD/CAM technology by using conventional impressions and two intraoral digital scanners. J Prosthet Dent. 2015;114(4):554–559.
119. Zeltner, M et al. Randomized controlled within-subject evaluation of digital and conventional workflows for the fabrication of lithium disilicate single crowns. Part III: marginal and internal fit. J Prosthet Dent. 2017;117(3):354–362.
120. Denry, I, Kelly, JR. State of the art of zirconia for dental applications. Dent Mater. 2008;24(3):299–307.
121. Zarone, F et al. From porcelain-fused-to-metal to zirconia: clinical and experimental considerations. Dent Mater. 2011;27(1):83–96.
122. Miyazaki, T et al. Current status of zirconia restoration. J Prosthodontic Res. 2013;57:236–261.
123. Zarone, F et al. Acid etching surface treatment of feldspathic, alumina and zirconia ceramics: a micromorphological SEM analysis. Int Dent South Afr. 2011;8.
124. Sorrentino, R et al. Effects of finish line design and fatigue cyclic loading on phase transformation of zirconia dental ceramics: a qualitative micro-Raman spectroscopic analysis. Materials. 2019;12(6):863.
125. Camposilvan, E et al. Aging resistance, mechanical properties and translucency of different yttria-stabilized zirconia ceramics for monolithic dental crown applications. Dent Mater. 2018;34(6):879–890.
126. Nakamura, K et al. Fracture resistance of monolithic zirconia molar crowns with reduced thickness. Acta Odontol Scand. 2015;73(8):602–608.
127. Sorrentino, R et al. In vitro analysis of the fracture resistance of CAD–CAM monolithic zirconia molar crowns with different occlusal thickness. J Mech Behav Biomed Mater. 2016;61:328–333.
128. Elsayed, A et al. Influence of the yttrium content on the fracture strength of monolithic zirconia crowns after artificial aging. Quintessence Int. 2019;50(5):344–348.
129. Papia, E et al. Bonding between oxide ceramics and adhesive cement systems: a systematic review. J Biomed Mater Res – Part B Appl Biomater. 2014;102:395–413.
130. Luthra, R, Kaur, P. An insight into current concepts and techniques in resin bonding to high strength ceramics. Australian Dent J. 2016;61:163–173.
131. Pilo, R et al. Effect of tribochemical treatments and silane reactivity on resin bonding to zirconia. Dent Mater. 2018;34(2):306–316.
132. Moon, JM et al. A comparative study of additive and subtractive manufacturing techniques for a zirconia dental product: an analysis of the manufacturing accuracy and the bond strength of porcelain to zirconia. Materials. 2022;15(15):5398.

3 Digital Technologies in Diagnosis and Treatment Planning in Prosthetic and Restorative Dentistry

Rizwan Jouhar, Muhammad Adeel Ahmed, Mohamad Syahrizal Halim, and Zohaib Khurshid

3.1 INTRODUCTION

In the eighteenth century, wax and plaster of Paris were used to make impressions, while hand-driven and subsequently water-driven turbines were utilized for powering dental devices [1]. For a simpler, quicker, more accurate, and more productive workflow, traditional dental treatments have been very effective for many years. But as dental technology has developed, contemporary ways of manufacturing have emerged, and prosthodontics and state-of-the-art dentistry are not exceptions. Digital applications have a lot of potential in prosthodontic dentistry. Digital dentistry is the practice of performing dental operations using dental technologies or instruments that have digital or computerized components [2].

A few of the many digital applications that are currently available include digital radiography, intraoral imaging, shade matching, digital smile designing, virtual articulators, digital face bows, lasers, occlusion and temporomandibular joint (TMJ) analysis, photography, CAD/CAM, and additive technology [2].

Today's market has become overrun with intraoral scanners, allowing dentists to design and mill materials in-office. After the impression is taken, the impression can be sent to a lab for fabrication. In fact, many dentists now routinely employ CAD/CAM to fabricate single crown and removable partial/complete dentures by taking intraoral digital impressions directly [2].

The advancement of additive manufacturing (AM) technology has made it possible for prosthetic applications to incorporate it into the digital process. CAM techniques such as additive manufacturing involve the construction of an object using layering building process [3].

Digital devices have drastically changed clinical procedures (e.g., optical impression, CAD/CAM technologies, stereolithography, 3D printers, etc.) as well as diagnostic procedures (e.g., computed tomography [CT], cone beam computed tomography [CBCT], nuclear magnetic resonance [NMR], ultrasonography, etc.) [4–6]. Intra-oral scanners (IOSs) and the incorporation of digital planning and previsualization software, in particular, have significantly improved interactions with patients, treatment planning clarification, improved procedural efficiency and patient comfort, specifically for surgical placement of implants, prosthodontics, and restorative dentistry [7, 8]. The advancements in digital imaging, CAD/CAM technology, and Internet connectivity have undoubtedly streamlined the diagnostic process and enhanced treatment outcomes.

The adoption of technology is influenced by a number of factors, including education, knowledge, cost, accuracy, and effectiveness. Adoption-related aspects are just as significant as innovation-related ones. The technology should eventually be able to fulfill the needs of today's practitioner and contribute to superior treatment outcomes. In order to preserve oral tissues with a timely diagnosis and to treat oral health conditions to achieve aesthetics and function with a high degree of predictability and even fewer sittings, research and progression in material science and associated fields are essential. Digital technology has a significant impact on dental research, practice administration, student training, patient motivation, laboratory processes, and clinical aspects. Modern dentist today has a wide range of alternatives, but in order to make use of them all, they must stay updated with emerging technologies. It is difficult to keep up with the growing body of research, yet it is urgently needed. The more current our knowledge, the better care we can give to our patients and so contribute to the advancement of the dental profession.

3.2 ROLE OF DIGITAL TECHNOLOGY IN DIAGNOSIS AND TREATMENT PLANNING IN PROSTHODONTICS

An appropriate diagnosis is crucial for effective treatment, and dental radiographs have been a vital diagnostic tool. Digital radiography has proven to be more effective than conventional radiography in detecting hard tooth tissue pathologies, including dental caries. A digital sensitivity of up to 1024 gray levels allows for better differentiation of initial changes, particularly in low-contrast areas like inter-proximal regions [9].

Digital impressions have transformed the procedure of taking impressions in prosthodontics, eliminating the use of materials and associated inaccuracies. This shift to digital impressions, often referred to as "bites to bytes," offers benefits such as reduced chairside time for CAD/CAM restorations, ease of cleaning, and improved comfort for patients with hypersensitive palates [10, 11].

 DOI: 10.1201/9781003428541-3

Digital technology has significantly revolutionized prosthetics and prosthodontics, offering advanced imaging techniques like CBCT and intraoral scanners. These tools provide high-resolution 3D images of oral structures, aiding in precise diagnosis and treatment planning. In prosthodontics, digital technology allows prosthodontists to create virtual treatment plans by simulating various prosthetic options and assessing potential outcomes. This enhances visualization and communication with patients about their treatment choices.

Furthermore, digital technology facilitates precise implant placement through guided surgery techniques, using CBCT scans, digital planning, and surgical guides. It ensures accurate implant positioning, reducing complications and improving implant-supported prosthodontic treatment success rates.

Digital dentistry is characterized by efficiency, accuracy, and superior treatment outcomes [12] by enabling remote consultations and teledentistry. This allows prosthodontists to communicate with patients, review treatment progress, and provide advice without in-person visits. This will benefits patients in remote areas or with limited mobility.

3.2.1 Digital Smile Design (DSD)

Digital smile design (DSD) is a state-of-the-art concept in dentistry that uses digital technology to create personalized and aesthetically pleasing smile designs for patients. The comprehensive approach of DSD considers various factors such as facial aesthetics, occlusal relationships, and individual patient preferences to achieve the best possible outcomes in terms of appearance, function, and patient satisfaction. Through the use of digital tools like intraoral scanners, facial analysis software, and DSD-specific software, dentists can design and simulate different treatment options, allowing patients to actively participate in the treatment planning process. This involvement enhances patient satisfaction, as they can visualize their potential smile transformations and provide feedback to fine-tune the final design.

DSD is a powerful tool that combines artistry with digital technology and comprehensive dental expertise. Through precise planning and meticulous attention to detail, DSD enables dentists to deliver highly customized and attractive smiles that align with the patients' facial features and individual preferences. This personalized approach not only enhances the aesthetics of the smile but also considers functional aspects and overall oral health, resulting in improved quality of life and increased patient confidence [11, 13]

The Steps for Understanding the Process of Digital Smile Design (DSD):

- *Data Collection*: The DSD process begins with the collection of complete data about the patient's facial features, dental structures, and occlusal relationships. This data is acquired using various digital tools, such as intraoral scanners, facial photographs, and videos.
- *Facial Analysis*: Advanced software is used to analyze the patient's facial aesthetics and facial proportions. This analysis helps in understanding the patient's unique facial characteristics, which play a significant role in designing a smile that harmonizes with their overall appearance.
- *Smile Design*: Based on the data and facial analysis, the dental team collaborates to design a new smile for the patient using specialized DSD software. They can visualize and simulate different treatment options, allowing for an interactive discussion with the patient.
- *Mock-up and Trial Smile*: Once the smile design is ready, a physical mock-up or a digital trial smile is created. This temporary version of the new smile allows the patient to see and feel how the final result will look before proceeding with the actual treatment.
- *Patient Feedback*: During the trial smile phase, the patient's feedback is crucial. They can provide input and make any necessary adjustments to ensure that they are satisfied with the proposed smile design.
- *Comprehensive Treatment Plan*: DSD is not just about improving the appearance of the teeth; it considers the overall function and oral health as well. The treatment plan may include various procedures such as teeth whitening, veneers, crowns, orthodontics, or implant-supported restorations, depending on the individual patient's needs.
- *Digital Communication*: DSD facilitates excellent communication between the dental team and the patient. The visual representation of the proposed smile design helps patients understand the treatment process and align their expectations with the result.
- *Precision and Predictability*: By using digital technology and meticulous planning, DSD offers a higher level of precision and predictability in achieving the desired aesthetic and functional outcomes.

- *Increased Patient Satisfaction*: DSD's patient-centric approach ensures that the final smile design is tailored to the patient's preferences and facial features, resulting in higher patient satisfaction with the treatment results [14].

3.2.2 Digital Radiography

Digital radiography provides instantaneous image viewing, which is very desirable for implant processes, intra-radicular post assessment, and patient education. It eliminate the use of chemicals and the need for. The user-friendly software can be used to improve images to make them easier to understand, diagnose, compare, and view subsequently. In addition to improving communication with other medical professionals, digital picture storage and distribution also results in less radiation exposure due to fewer retakes (since there are no processing inaccuracies) [15].

The benefits include the following:

- Less radiation.
- Significantly less time.
- Simpler organization and storage (no need for chemicals or dark room).
- Improvements to the images for simpler reading, assessment, and further viewing.

However, there are few drawbacks of digital radiography.

The application of computers in dental radiography must overcome software-related obstacles, and the high cost discourages many professionals. Additionally, it is challenging to prevent cross-contamination due to the fact that digital sensors and photostimulable phosphor (PSP) plates cannot be disinfected, necessitating plastic protection barriers.

3.2.2.1 Radiovisiography

In 1987, Dr. Francis Mouyen introduced the first digital radiography equipment, designated radiovisiography (RVG), the first digital radiography system, marking the beginning of the digital era in dental imaging. Scientist and engineer Paul Suni developed the charge coupled device (CCD) image sensor technology that enabled the creation of the RVG digital radiography system [16].

RVG is an array of components that enables a user to acquire colored photos with an intraoral camera from a patient's mouth and upload them to a computer. On the computer, these images can be zoomed, rotated, cropped, edited, and further modified by stretching the contrast, enhancing it, and reversing the images [17].

The most recent advancements in digital radiography are found in the RVG imaging system, which is frequently used in dentistry to take intraoral periapical radiographs and provides the highest image resolution (> 20 LP/mm). A detector, a display unit, and a microcontroller are the components that comprise an RVG. The detector's sensitive region measures 275 mm by 182 mm. A standard intraoral X-ray generator with a 200-mm cone and a 55-mm aperture is employed. It runs at 70 kV, 8 mA, and has a 2–3.2 second exposure period. Compared to the larger X-ray generator machines, the amount of radiation used will be drastically reduced. Without compromising the quality of the image, the outcomes are quicker and better [17].

3.2.2.2 Cone-Beam Computed Tomography (CBCT)

This imaging method uses divergent X-rays to create a cone-shaped beam of light. Apart from relevance in implant dentistry, there has not been much research done on immediate use in prosthodontics [18]. The cost, accessibility, and radiation dose factors have all restricted the use of complex CT imaging for the majority of specialty practitioners. CBCT has now been made available for the maxillofacial region, opening up a new window for demand for multiplanar imaging. The thin slice images are created not just in the axial plane by typical helical fan beam CTs but also in the coronal, sagittal, and even oblique or curved image planes in two dimensions (2D). This process is called multiplanar reformatting (MPR) [19, 20].

The primary benefit of CBCT is its accuracy in determining the true position of the condyle in the fossa, which frequently indicates the likelihood of a disk dislocation in the joint and the degree of translation of the condyle in the fossa. It is more effective because it makes it simple to measure the roof of the glenoid fossa and makes it possible to observe the condylar head and glenoid fossa relationship in three dimensions. [21]. Several benefits have led to CBCT becoming the preferred imaging method in situations involving trauma, discomfort, and temporomandibular joint dysfunction, such as fibrous or bony ankylosis, in addition to aiding in the diagnosis of condylar cortical and subcortical erosion, cysts, and other osseous abnormalities [22].

Applications of CBCT in prosthodontics are as follows:

- TMJ imaging.
- Implant prosthodontics.
- Maxillofacial prosthodontics.
- Craniofacial and airway assessments.
- Complete treatment planning for patients with overdentures [16, 23].

3.2.3 Optical Impression

3.2.3.1 Digital Impressions

Digital intraoral scanners have largely replaced traditional impression materials, making the process more comfortable and efficient for patients. Digital impressions provide accurate data for fabricating crowns, bridges, dentures, and other dental restorations, leading to better-fitting prosthetics. There are numerous oral scanner systems in the market. Two of these systems (CEREC AC and E4D Dentist) allow dental technicians to offer the option of in-office design and milling. The digital impressions created by two additional technologies (iTero and Lava Chairside Oral Scanner [C.O.S.]) must be designed and milled at a dental laboratory [24]. All these systems are capable of generating models from their digital data [25].

After the tissues have been pulled back to expose the tooth boundaries, the tooth is allowed to dry and is prepared for scanning in order to create a digital impression. In order to improve the scan quality and remove optical highlights from the surface of the preparation, several scanning systems allow for the application of an oxide powder to the tooth. The geometry of the tooth preparation is recorded by scanners using a sequence of static images [26].

The digital impression has the following advantages:

- Offers a cleaner and more effective impression technique without the intricacy of various materials necessary for conventional impressions with an elastomeric material.
- Offers enhanced accuracy and uniformity.
- Allows a dental professional to envision the process on a computer display from different viewpoints.
- Permits a practitioner to plan the restoration on a computer while depicting the opposing dentition.
- Provides fast feedback and display to allow for quick corrections.
- Lessens the negative environmental effects of discarding the material needed for traditional impressions.

3.2.4 Computer-Aided Design/Computer-Aided Manufacturing

3.2.4.1 Computer-Aided Design (CAD)

CAD software enables prosthodontists to design custom dental restorations with precise specifications based on the patient's anatomy and treatment requirements. CAD technology streamlines the design process, reducing errors and ensuring optimal outcomes.

3.2.4.2 Computer-Aided Manufacturing (CAM)

Once the prosthetic design is finalized using CAD, CAM technology comes into play. CAM systems use milling machines or 3D printers to fabricate dental restorations accurately and efficiently, often in a single visit. This quick turnaround benefits patients and improves overall treatment satisfaction.

In the 1980s, CAD/CAM was initially employed in dentistry. The first CAD/CAM machines were Procera (Nobel Biocare) and CEREC (Sirona).[27] When CEREC initially launched, it was only intended to be used as a chairside treatment for one-visit fixed restorations, particularly for inlays and onlays. A tiny intraoral camera is used by the dentist to take a digital image of the prepared tooth prior to making a chairside CAD/CAM filling. This computerized image includes 3D data regarding the tooth's dimensions and morphology, the defect that needs to be repaired, and the anatomy and relationships between the tooth and the neighboring teeth. The dentist uses CAD/CAM software to create the appropriate restoration in accordance with this digital image [28].

Benefits of chairside CAD/CAM technology include a one-visit fixed restorative procedure, reduced risk of error compared to conventional methods, assistance in preparation visualization, elimination of impression-taking and temporary restoration requirements, decreased risk of tooth sensitization, elimination of laboratory costs as no model or die pouring is necessary, and projection of a cutting-edge image.

Negative aspects of chairside soft tissue management using CAD/CAM techniques are more important than using conventional techniques; customization may be needed, there is a steep learning curve, and higher production levels are needed to make up for capital expenditures.

The "subtractive method" served as the foundation for CAD initially, while more current processes use "additive" methods like rapid prototyping, selective laser sintering, or a hybrid of the two [29, 30].

Based on their manufacturing processes, the advanced CAD/CAM systems that are currently available can be categorized into three distinct classes [31].

- *In-Office System*: A dentist prepares a tooth, digitally scans it, makes restorations at the chairside, and seats the tooth all in one visit.
- *In the Laboratory System*: Laboratories employ CAD/CAM to create restorations by scanning models created from physical impressions.
- *Centralized Production*: This method entails a dentist taking chairside digital impressions and sending the information to the lab through the internet.

3.2.5 Shade Matching

Automatic shade selection tools like colorimeters, spectrophotometers, and digital imaging tools are replacing visual shade matching in dentistry nowadays because they provide more uniform shade and a lifelike effect with the color coding of the chosen tooth. Digital imaging and color matching reduce inter- and intra-operator variability and make it simpler to communicate with the lab [32].

3.2.5.1 Colorimeters

Colorimeters calculate the tristimulus values by eliminating light from the red, green, and blue regions of the visual color spectrum. Colorimeters can be less precise than spectrophotometers since they do not record the whole visual light spectrum's reflectance. Two of these colorimeters are the ShadeEye NCC® (Shofu, Menlo Park, CA, USA) and ShadeVison® (X Rite, Grandville, MI, USA) [33].

3.2.5.2 Spectrophotometers

Spectrophotometers calculate and measure the quantity of visible radiant energy that an object reflects or transmits, one wavelength at a time, for every value, chroma, and hue that exists in the complete visible spectrum. Concerning color matching in dentistry, they might be the most precise tool [34]. Numerous clinical spectrophotometers of extremely high caliber and dependability are available on the market, such as the VITA EasyShade Compact® (Vita North America, Yorba Linda, CA, USA) and CrystalEye® (Olympus America, Center Valley, PA, USA). The VITA Easyshade, a compact spectrophotometer satisfies the most criteria for selecting shades in clinical environments. The tool can be used to assess the color of the tooth's entire surface as well as the shades of the cervical, middle, and incisal thirds of each tooth.

3.2.6 Virtual Articulators and Digital Face Bows

Virtual articulators and digital face bows are advanced digital technologies used in dentistry, particularly in prosthodontics, to enhance the accuracy and efficiency of treatment planning and dental restorations. They play a crucial role in creating precise and customized dental prosthetics for patients. The virtual face bow was created as a substitute for the traditional face bow when mounting casts to articulators [33]. The virtual articulator's function is to replicate jaw action so that it can be used to help create virtual crowns and other prostheses. By simulating centric relationship (CR), protrusion, and laterotrusion, a dental technician can minimize design error and create a high-quality prosthesis for the patient [34, 35]. Based on the technique used to simulate jaw action, there are two different types of virtual articulators available.

3.2.6.1 Virtual Articulators

Traditional articulators are mechanical instruments used by dentists to simulate the movement and occlusion (bite) of a patient's jaw. However, virtual articulators have taken this concept to the next level by digitizing the process.

Key features and benefits of virtual articulators include [36]:

- Software-based tools that simulate jaw movements digitally.
- Evaluate occlusal relationships and dental restoration function.

- Faster analysis and customization for better treatment planning.
- Facilitate communication with dental laboratories.

3.2.6.2 Digital Face Bow

A face bow is a dental instrument used to transfer the spatial relationship of a patient's maxillary arch (upper teeth) to the hinge axis of the jaw. This information is crucial for prosthodontists to design dental restorations that accurately fit the patient's bite and provide optimal occlusion.

Digital face bows, also known as electronic face bows, have replaced traditional mechanical face bows with digital technology. They use 3D scanning and digital measurements to record the patient's facial and jaw data accurately [36].

Benefits of digital face bows include:

- Replace traditional face bows with 3D scanning and digital measurements.
- Provide accurate facial and jaw data for restorations.
- Improve patient comfort and save time during data collection.
- Seamless integration with other digital technologies.

3.2.6.3 Mathematically Simulated Articulator

A mathematically simulated articulator is a virtual or computer-based system that replicates the movements and functions of a traditional dental articulator using mathematical algorithms and modeling techniques. This technology allows dentists and prosthodontists to simulate and analyze jaw movements and occlusal relationships without the need for physical articulator instruments [37].

Key features of mathematically simulated articulators include:

- *Digital Replication*: The system digitally replicates the movements of the TMJ and the jaw in a virtual environment.
- *Dynamic Analysis*: Dentists can analyze the dynamic occlusal relationships during various functional activities, such as chewing and speaking, to assess how dental restorations will interact.
- *Customization*: The system can be customized for each patient's unique occlusal patterns, improving the precision of treatment planning.
- *Real-Time Adjustments*: Dentists can make real-time adjustments to the virtual articulator to evaluate different treatment options and their impact on occlusion.
- *Integration with CAD/CAM*: Mathematically simulated articulators can be integrated with CAD/CAM systems for seamless fabrication of dental restorations.
- *Training and Education*: These virtual systems are valuable educational tools for dental students and professionals to learn and practice occlusal analysis and treatment planning.

The use of mathematically simulated articulators enhances the accuracy and efficiency of prosthodontic treatments, allowing for more precise evaluation and planning of dental restorations. These virtual systems represent a significant advancement in digital dentistry, offering dentists powerful tools to achieve optimal functional and aesthetic outcomes for their patients [38].

3.2.6.4 Completely Adjustable Articulators (Motion Analyzer)

Completely adjustable articulators, also known as motion analyzers, are sophisticated devices used in dentistry to replicate the complex movements of the jaw. They accurately simulate occlusal relationships during activities like chewing and speaking [39]. Dentists can customize them for each patient's unique jaw movements, making them valuable tools for treatment planning and occlusal adjustments. These articulators are essential in achieving optimal occlusion and function for dental restorations and serve as educational tools in dental schools and training centers [40].

Key features of completely adjustable articulators include [41]:

- *Replication of Jaw Movements*: Motion analyzers can mimic the natural movements of the patient's jaw, including hinge movements, lateral excursions, and protrusive movements. This replication enables dentists to evaluate the occlusal contacts during different functional activities like chewing and speaking.

- *Adjustability*: These articulators are fully adjustable, allowing for customization based on the patient's unique occlusal patterns. Dentists can modify the condylar paths, Bennett angles, and other parameters to match the patient's specific jaw movements.
- *Dynamic and Static Occlusion*: Completely adjustable articulators can replicate both dynamic and static occlusal relationships. Dynamic occlusion refers to the contact between teeth during jaw movements, while static occlusion refers to the contact when the jaw is at rest.
- *Mounting of Dental Casts*: Dentists mount the patient's dental casts on the articulator to create a replica of the patient's occlusal situation. This allows for precise analysis and planning of restorations without the patient being present.
- *Treatment Planning Tool*: Motion analyzers are essential tools in prosthodontics for planning complex restorative cases, full-mouth rehabilitations, and occlusal adjustments. They aid in achieving optimal occlusion and function for dental restorations.
- *Training and Education*: Completely adjustable articulators are used for educational purposes in dental schools and training centers to teach students and dentists about occlusion and treatment planning.

3.2.7 Laser

The use of lasers in different fields of prosthodontics, including frenectomy, vestibuloplasty, shaping of ridge structure, elimination of tori and hyperplastic or excessive soft tissue, and reduction of hard or soft tissue tuberosity, is becoming more and more common. In fixed prosthodontics, the use of a laser is beneficial for a variety of procedures, including crown lengthening, managing soft tissue around implant abutment, creating ovate pontic areas, preparing teeth for veneers and full coverage crowns and bridges, removing carious lesions and defective composite restorations before placing finished restorations, and more. In implantology, lasers are utilized for peri-implantitis and the second phase of uncovering [42].

Lasers are mostly used in maxillofacial prostheses for the initial analysis of 3D optical data collections of extra-oral abnormalities. Planning the form and placement of the prosthesis has proven to be a particularly effective application of laser technology [26]. The use of traditional impression procedures and their drawbacks, such as patient discomfort and soft tissue deformation, can be completely eliminated using lasers. As the patient is not subjected to a significant amount of radiation or any kind of pressure, lasers also eliminate the shortcomings of 3D CT and MRI reconstruction [26].

Rapid prototyping, direct laser metal sintering (DLMS), CAD-CAM, and other methods have all been utilized to fabricate prostheses using lasers. Pulsed laser deposition has been shown to be an effective method to generate pure, crystal-like, and adhesive hydroxy apatite (HA) coatings that show no degradation in a simulated bodily fluid when applied to titanium implants [43]. When compared with frequently employed acid etching procedures, the use of lasers for the surface preparation of titanium castings for ceramic bonding has demonstrated better bonding strength [44]. Additionally, lasers can also be used to fuse titanium prosthesis components.

One drawback of lasers is that they cannot be utilized for filling cavities between teeth or around previous fillings. They are also more costly than drilling and may still require typical drills to shape and polish fillings. Moreover, ocular injury, injury to tissues, respiratory risk, explosions and fires, and electric shock are a few other risks related to lasers [45].

3.2.8 Occlusion and Temporomandibular Joint Analysis and Diagnosis

Through the use of digital occlusion, the dentist's routine occlusion procedures are made easier and more predictable. Any dentist can concentrate on definitely troublesome occlusal contacts with the T Scan and create successful diagnostic and therapeutic strategies. [46] Dr. William Maness developed the T Scan in 1988 as an automated computerized sensor for analyzing the dental occlusion. It attempted to record the patient's bite instantly by means of the position, timing, and pressure of each tooth in contact by registering the patient's occlusion on a thin, disposable sensor with a 60 μ thickness. This data is shifted to a computer so that it may create an accurate simulation of the patient oclusion on a screen while assuming all of the numerous possibilities that could arise during eccentric, centric, and functional movement. This offers an evaluation of occlusion that is both qualitative and quantitative. It provides a significant instrument for training as well as a useful way for clinical evaluation and comprehension of the occlusal abnormalities [47].

The ease of use, dynamic occlusion viewing, timed force analysis during different tooth contact positions, and potential for permanent documentation and monitoring of the occlusal condition after completing various treatment regimens are the primary advantages of T Scan.

3.3 CHALLENGES IN DIGITAL DENTISTRY

Digital dentistry poses a number of challenges for dental professionals, dental technicians, and society as a whole. Cost is the primary barrier to the adoption of digital dentistry in most cases because new technology typically requires a higher capital investment [48]. The following are additional constraints.

3.3.1 Dental Technicians and Dentists Have a Significant Digital Gap

Regarding technological advancement, technicians are ahead of dentists. They get digital impressions, design the models in software, and transfer the digital data to milling machines that produce the prosthetic restorations. Many of them have had a fully digital workflow for years. However, many dentists continue to use traditional methods, such as molding impressions of their patients' teeth and physically delivering such impressions to dental labs [13].

3.3.2 High Digital Skills and Accuracy Are Required for Intraoral Scanner Use

Today, dental professionals are using intraoral scanners to streamline workflow, but doing so demands advanced digital skills and accuracy. For the dental laboratory to receive a correct digital file, an intraoral scanner is essential [23]. A digital impression does not allow for any errors at all, but a conventional impression allows for minor errors that can be corrected by the dental technician. The gap between dentists and technicians is being reduced as dentists' proficiency with the intraoral scanning technique improves, along with their comprehension of the entire digital dentistry process [24, 25].

3.3.3 Maintaining a Balance between Simplicity, Speed, and Reliability

Digitalization requires rapidity, ease of use, and dependability. Rapid technological advancement also causes manufacturing firms to expand too quickly to offer simplicity and quickness. In addition, they also need to stabilize their hardware and software to ensure the continued dependability of their digital processes. Consequently, it is the duty of manufacturing firms to guarantee the quality of their goods and support dental experts in streamlining workflow.

3.4 ARTIFICIAL INTELLIGENCE AND DIGITAL DENTISTRY

Artificial intelligence (AI) and digital dentistry are increasingly becoming interconnected, revolutionizing the way dental care is delivered [49]. AI, as a subset of computer science, enables machines to perform tasks that typically require human intelligence. When integrated into digital dentistry, AI brings numerous benefits and advancements to various aspects of dental practice [50, 51].

The transforming features of AI in digital dentistry [52]:

- *Image Analysis*: AI-powered algorithms can analyze dental images, such as dental radiographs and intraoral scans, with greater accuracy and efficiency. AI can assist to detect dental caries, periodontal diseases, and other oral conditions at an early stage, leading to more timely interventions and improved patient outcomes.
- *Treatment Planning*: AI assists in treatment planning by providing data-driven insights and recommendations based on a patient's specific oral condition. It assist dentists in selecting the most appropriate dental restorations and treatment options, considering factors like occlusal relationships and patient preferences.
- *Virtual Smile Design*: AI-driven virtual smile design tools can create highly personalized and aesthetically pleasing smile makeovers. By analyzing facial features and incorporating patient preferences, AI can generate smile designs that harmonize with the patient's unique characteristics.
- *Predictive Analytics*: AI algorithms can analyze patient data, including medical history, dental records, and lifestyle factors, to predict potential oral health issues and individualize preventive care plans. This proactive approach enhances oral health management and reduces the risk of complex dental problems.
- *Natural Language Processing (NLP)*: AI-powered NLP enables more efficient and accurate communication with patients through chatbots and voice recognition systems. Patients can receive immediate responses to common dental queries and schedule appointments seamlessly.
- *Virtual Consultations*: AI facilitates teledentistry by enabling sophisticated virtual consultations. Dentists can remotely diagnose and plan treatments for patients, making dental care more accessible to individuals in remote areas or with limited mobility.

- *Personalized Treatment Recommendations*: AI can analyze vast amounts of dental research and patient data to recommend personalized treatment protocols. This leads to better treatment outcomes tailored to individual patient needs.
- *Patient Management*: AI-powered software can streamline patient management tasks, including appointment scheduling, reminders, and electronic health records, optimizing the workflow of dental practices.

Despite these advancements, it is essential to address ethical considerations and ensure patient data privacy and security. As AI continues to evolve, its integration with digital dentistry holds great promise for improving the quality and accessibility of dental care, benefiting both dental professionals and patients alike.

3.5 SUMMARY AND FUTURE SCOPE OF DIGITAL DENTISTRY

Digital dentistry is a rapidly advancing field that leverages technology to enhance various aspects of dental care, including diagnosis, treatment planning, and the fabrication of dental restorations. Some key technologies in digital dentistry include digital radiography, intraoral scanners, CAD/CAM systems, virtual articulators, and digital face bows. These technologies have revolutionized prosthodontics by improving accuracy, efficiency, and patient satisfaction. Digital dentistry allows for better visualization, precise treatment planning, and reduced chairside time for restorations, leading to superior outcomes.

The future of digital dentistry holds immense potential for further advancements and innovations. Some potential areas of growth and development will be AI integration, AI can be integrated into digital dentistry to enhance image analysis, improve treatment planning algorithms, and facilitate more personalized patient care. The advancements in 3D printing technology could lead to more widespread use of in-office fabrication of dental restorations, reducing turnaround time and costs. Virtual reality (VR) and augmented reality (AR) could enhance patient education, allowing them to visualize treatment outcomes and participate more actively in the decision-making process. Teledentistry may further expand, enabling remote consultations, diagnostics, and treatment planning, making dental care more accessible to underserved areas.

The development of new biocompatible materials for additive manufacturing could lead to more durable and aesthetically pleasing dental restorations. Furthermore, the integrated digital workflow technologies could streamline the dental workflow, from diagnosis to treatment planning and execution, optimizing efficiency and accuracy. DSD advancements may evolve to incorporate even more precise facial analysis and AI-driven smile design for highly personalized aesthetic outcomes. As digital dentistry involves the collection and storage of sensitive patient data, future developments should also focus on strengthening data security and privacy measures.

Overall, the future of digital dentistry is promising, with continued advancements and innovations expected to revolutionize dental care, improving patient experience and treatment outcomes. Dentists, researchers, and technology developers will play critical roles in shaping the future of this exciting field.

FUNDING

This work was supported by the Deanship of Scientific Research, Vice Presidency for Graduate Studies and Scientific Research, King Faisal University, Saudi Arabia [Grant No. KFU253640].

REFERENCES

1. Bhambhani, R et al. Digitization and its futuristic approach in prosthodontics. J Indian Prosthodont Soc. 2013;13(3):165–174.
2. Gupta, C, Mittal, A. Role of digital technology in prosthodontics: a step toward improving dental care. Indian J Oral Health Res. 2018;4(2):35–41.
3. Revilla-Leon, M, Ozcan, M. Additive manufacturing technologies used for processing polymers: current status and potential application in prosthetic dentistry. J Prosthodont. 2019;28(2):146–158.
4. Colombo, M et al. Clinical applications and effectiveness of guided implant surgery: a critical review based on randomized controlled trials. BMC Oral Health. 2017;17(1):150.
5. Zhou, W et al. Clinical factors affecting the accuracy of guided implant surgery – a systematic review and meta-analysis. J. Evid. Based Dent. Pract. 2018;18(1):28–40.
6. Spagnuolo, G, Sorrentino, R. The role of digital devices in dentistry: clinical trends and scientific evidences. J Clin Med. 2020;9(6):1692.
7. Cervino, G et al. Dental restorative digital workflow: digital smile design from aesthetic to function. Dent J (Basel). 2019;7(2):30.
8. Moon, SY et al. Clinical problems of computer-guided implant surgery. Maxillofac. Plast. Reconstr. Surg. 2016;38(1):15.

9. Abesi, F et al. Diagnostic accuracy of digital and conventional radiography in the detection of non-cavitated approximal dental caries. Iran J Radiol. 2012;9(1):17–21.
10. Birnbaum, NS, Aaronson, HB. Dental impressions using 3D digital scanners: virtual becomes reality. Compend Contin Educ Dent. 2008;29(8):494–505.
11. Christensen, GJ. Impressions are changing: deciding on conventional, digital or digital plus in-office milling. J Am Dent Assoc. 2009;140(10):1301–1304.
12. Turkyilmaz, I, Lakhia, S. Challenges to digital dentistry in dental schools. J Contemp Dent Pract. 2019;20(12):1361.
13. Thomas, PA et al. Digital smile design. Journal of Pharmacy & Bioallied Sciences. 2022;14(Suppl 1):S43.
14. Lee, S, Kim, JE. Evaluating the precision of automatic segmentation of teeth, gingiva and facial landmarks for 2d digital smile design using real-time instance segmentation network. J Clin Med. 2022;11(3):852.
15. Jayachandran, S. Digital imaging in dentistry: a review. Contemp Clin Dent. 2017;8(2):193–194.
16. Mouyen, F et al. Presentation and physical evaluation of RadioVisioGraphy. Oral Surg Oral Med Oral Pathol. 1989;68(2):238–242.
17. John, GP et al. Applications of cone beam computed tomography for a prosthodontist. J Indian Prosthodont Soc. 2016;16(1):3–7.
18. Venkatesh, E, Elluru, SV. Cone beam computed tomography: basics and applications in dentistry. J Istanb Univ Fac Dent. 2017;51(3 Suppl 1):S102–S121.
19. Al-koshab, M et al. Assessment of condyle and glenoid fossa morphology using CBCT in South-East Asians. PLoS One. 2015;10(3):e0121682.
20. Alasmari, DS, Riyaz, MA. Role of imaging modalities in dental implantology. Int J Contemp Med Res. 2016;3(11):3224–3227.
21. Macleod, I, Heath, N. Cone-beam computed tomography (CBCT) in dental practice. Dent Update. 2008;35(9):590–594.
22. Logozzo, S et al. A comparative analysis of intraoral 3d digital scanners for restorative dentistry. Internet J Med Technol. 2008;5:1–18.
23. Mangano, F et al. Intraoral scanners in dentistry: a review of the current literature. BMC Oral Health. 2017;17(1):149.
24. Lecocq, G. Digital impression-taking: fundamentals and benefits in orthodontics. Int Orthod. 2016;14(2):184–194.
25. Duret, F et al. CAD-CAM in dentistry. J Am Dent Assoc. 1988;117(6):715–20.
26. Mörmann, WH. The evolution of the CEREC system. J Am Dent Assoc. 2006;137 Suppl:7S–13S.
27. Torabi, K et al. Rapid prototyping technologies and their applications in prosthodontics, a review of literature. J Dent (Shiraz). 2015;16(1):1–9.
28. Abduo, J et al. Trends in computer-aided manufacturing in prosthodontics: a review of the available streams. Int J Dent. 2014;2014:783948.
29. Miyazaki, T et al. A review of dental CAD/CAM: current status and future perspectives from 20 years of experience. Dent Mater J. 2009;28(1):44–56.
30. Tabatabaian, F et al. Visual and digital tooth shade selection methods, related effective factors and conditions, and their accuracy and precision: a literature review. J Esthet Restor Dent. 2021;33(8):1084–1104.
31. Brewer, JD et al. Advances in color matching. Dent Clin North Am. 2004;48(2):v, 341–358.
32. Cal, E et al. Comparison of digital and spectrophotometric measurements of colour shade guides. J Oral Rehabil. 2006;33(3):221–228.
33. Jafri, Z et al. Digital smile design-an innovative tool in aesthetic dentistry. J Oral Biol Craniofac Res. 2020;10(2):194–198.
34. Shetty, S. Virtual articulators and virtual facebow transfers: digital prosthodontics!!! J Indian Prosthodont Soc. 2015;15(4):291.
35. Yang, S et al. A novel technique to align the intraoral scans to the virtual articulator and set the patient-specific sagittal condylar inclination. J Prosthodontics. 2022;31(1):79–84.
36. Amezua, X et al. Analysis of the influence of the facial scanning method on the transfer accuracy of a maxillary digital scan to a 3D face scan for a virtual facebow technique: an in vitro study. J Prosthet Dent. 2022;128(5):1024–1031.
37. Lepidi, L et al. Digital fixed complete-arch rehabilitation: from virtual articulator mounting to clinical delivery. J Prosthet Dent. 2022;127(3):398–403.
38. Li, L et al. Design of occlusal wear facets of fixed dental prostheses driven by personalized mandibular movement. J Prosthet Dent. 2022;128(1):33–41.
39. Popat, H et al. Three-dimensional motion analysis – an exploratory study. Part 1: assessment of facial movement. Orthodont Craniofac Res. 2008;11(4):216–223.
40. Lin, YC et al. Assessment of occlusal vertical dimension change in mechanical and virtual articulation: a pilot study. Dentistry J. 2022;10(11):212.
41. Koralakunte, PR, Aljanakh, M. The role of virtual articulator in prosthetic and restorative dentistry. J Clin Diagn Res. 2014;8(7):ZE25–ZE28.
42. Gounder, R, Gounder, S. Laser science and its applications in prosthetic rehabilitation. J Lasers Med Sci. 2016;7(4):209–213.
43. Bose, S et al. Additive manufacturing of biomaterials. Prog Mater Sci. 2018;93:45–111.
44. Shilpa, P et al. Shear bond strength of ceramic bonded to different core materials and their pattern of failure: an in vitro study. Cureus. 2019;11(11):e6242.
45. Allen, EP. Use and abuse of lasers in periodontics. J Esthet Restor Dent. 2005;17(6):329–331.
46. Kerstein, RB. Current applications of computerized occlusal analysis in dental medicine. Gen Dent. 2001;49(5):521–530.
47. Maness, WL et al. Computerized occlusal analysis: a new technology. Quintessence Int. 1987;18(4):287–292.
48. Pang, M et al. Preliminary user evaluation of a new dental technology virtual simulation system: development and validation study. JMIR Serious Games. 2022;10(3):e36079.
49. Putra, RH et al. Current applications and development of artificial intelligence for digital dental radiography. Dentomaxillofac Radiol. 2022;51(1):20210197.
50. Kumar, PR et al. Analysis of advances in research trends in robotic and digital dentistry: an original research. J Pharmacy Bioallied Sci. 2022;14(Suppl 1):S185.
51. Fontenele, RC et al. Influence of dental fillings and tooth type on the performance of a novel artificial intelligence-driven tool for automatic tooth segmentation on CBCT images – a validation study. J Dent. 2022;119:104069.
52. Ma, J et al. Towards trustworthy AI in dentistry. J Dental Res. 2022;101(11):1263–1268.

4 Digital Workflow in Complete Denture Manufacturing

Artak Heboyan, Mario Alberto Alarcón-Sánchez, João Paulo Mendes Tribst, and Zohaib Khurshid

4.1 INTRODUCTION

The promotion of dental health care in older adults with edentulism has been a topic of considerable concern to the dental community [1–3]. Approximately 68% of older adults worldwide have lost their teeth because of a chronic infectious and inflammatory processes, such as dental caries or periodontal disease [4–6]. Furthermore, the number of older adults has been growing steadily [7], increasing the demand for the use of complete dentures (CDs) that not only functionally and aesthetically restore the patient, but are also sought to be biocompatible with the soft and hard tissues of the oral cavity [8–10]. In this sense, the digital workflow has revolutionized contemporary dentistry, significantly improving the quality of patient life [11–13]. Therefore, the purpose of this chapter is to present the current state of CDs fabrication using digital technology, its impact on the elderly patient with edentulism, and techniques and biomaterials used, as well as to highlight its advantages and limitations in the use of this type of technology restoration.

4.2 CONVENTIONAL AND DIGITAL METHODS IN THE FABRICATION OF A COMPLETE DENTURE

Complete dentures are removable dental prostheses that rehabilitate the entire dentition as well as the related structures of the maxilla and mandible [14, 15] (**Figure 4.1**). They can be manufactured by a conventional method or digitally [16, 17]. The classic or conventional method of constructing a complete denture consists of a series of sessions in the dental office along with a series of steps required for its fabrication in the dental laboratory, ongoing visits by the patient, and, in most cases, postoperative adjustments of the prosthesis [18–20].

From a clinical point of view, a proper and customized diagnosis should be associated with treatment planning for the success of prosthetic treatment [22–27]. It is important to take the patient's complete data to prepare their clinical record and to use the necessary biomaterials to limit the possible complications that may arise [28, 29].

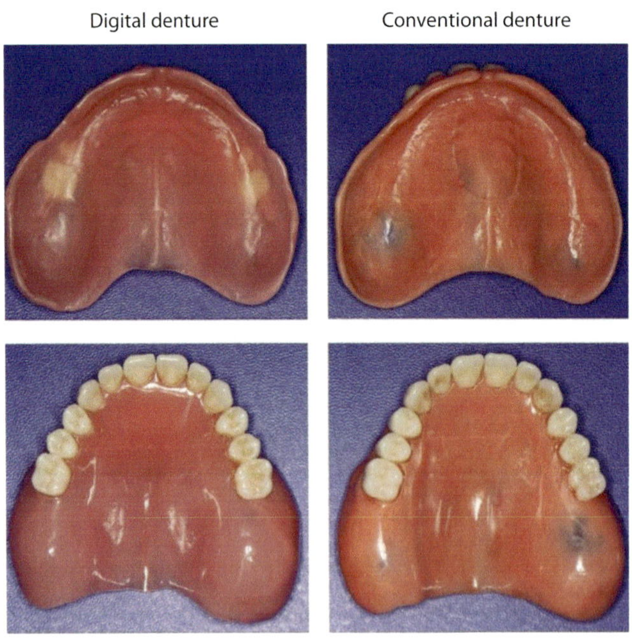

Figure 4.1 Types of conventionally and digitally fabricated complete dentures. (From Ref. [21] under Creative Commons Attribution license.)

 DOI: 10.1201/9781003428541-4

A complete digital denture corresponds to a complete prosthesis that is manufactured by automation using computer-aided design/computer-aided manufacturing (CAD/CAM) technology [30–32]. Digital techniques for the fabrication of complete dentures are expanding, and with this, current innovations and developments in digital dentistry have successfully led to the fabrication of this type of prosthesis [33–42].

4.3 TECHNOLOGY USED FOR THE CONSTRUCTION OF COMPLETE DENTURES

Over time, the technology implemented in the field of prosthodontics has advanced enormously [43, 44]. Digital design and fabrication have been used for the fabrication of removable complete dentures through versatile CAD software [45]. In most cases, the CAD algorithm recognizes the geometric shape of an object (mucosa, impression material, or wax), whereas CAM can be used for the fabrication of the prosthetic appliance [46].

After designing, the computer-designed complete dentures (CECD) are usually fabricated in two ways: First, through an additive manufacturing technique and second, through subtractive manufacturing [47]. Additive manufacturing is also referred to as layered, direct digital, three-dimensional (3D), or free-form solid manufacturing [48]. It is used to automatically create physical models from three-dimensional data; in fact, it has been used to create complex models in medicine since the early 1990s and has again become popular for the construction of removable prosthetic restorations [49, 50]. Additive 3D printing techniques include: Stereolithography, digital light projection, jet printing (PolyJet/ProJet), and direct laser metal sintering (DLMS)/selective laser sintering [51].

Subtractive manufacturing, on the other hand, is based on milling from a solid structure with a computer numerical control (CNC) system. In this case, the CAM software automatically transfers the CAD model to the CNC; this involves a calculation that targets the volume of material, including sequencing, milling tools, direction, and magnitude of the coordinate system [52, 53]. Milling accuracy must be equal to or less than 10 μm, plus approximately 90% of the initial block is removed to create the typical prosthetic restoration [54]. In addition, subtractive production methods also include spark erosion, which is a metal subtraction process that uses continuous sparks to erode the material from a metal block [55].

Both additive and subtractive systems have been used for many years for the fabrication of inlays, crowns, fixed partial dentures, abutments, and implant-supported prostheses, as well as in maxillofacial prostheses; however, few studies highlight their importance in the fabrication of removable complete dentures [56–59].

4.4 HYBRID DIGITAL WORKFLOW: STEP-BY-STEP PROCEDURES FOR THE FABRICATION OF CDs BY CAD/CAM TECHNOLOGY

Unlike conventional CDs, digital CDs follow a different set of steps that can be summarized as follows [60]:

First visit to the dental office:

1. Make impressions for the fabrication of custom casts and trays.
2. Make definitive impressions for the fabrication of definitive casts.
3. Make records of facebow and maxillomandibular relationship, determine smile line, canine and midline positions, and anterior teeth position for adequate lip support and optimal esthetics. Send the records to the dental laboratory so that the casts can be mounted in an articulator and for the virtual design of the complete prosthesis with the CAD software.

In a dental laboratory:

4. Scan the definitive casts. Import the data into the software for prosthetic design.
5. Virtual mounting of casts.
6. Adjust the occlusal plane. Marking of the anatomical landmarks. Positioning of teeth.
7. Customization of artificial teeth.
8. Design of the gingival anatomy.
9. Sending to the clinician for evaluation (optional).
10. Fabrication of CDs by milling in two steps. Milling of the teeth and denture base of the prostheses, including the position and adhesion of the teeth in the sockets (**Figure 4.2**).
11. Polishing and finishing.

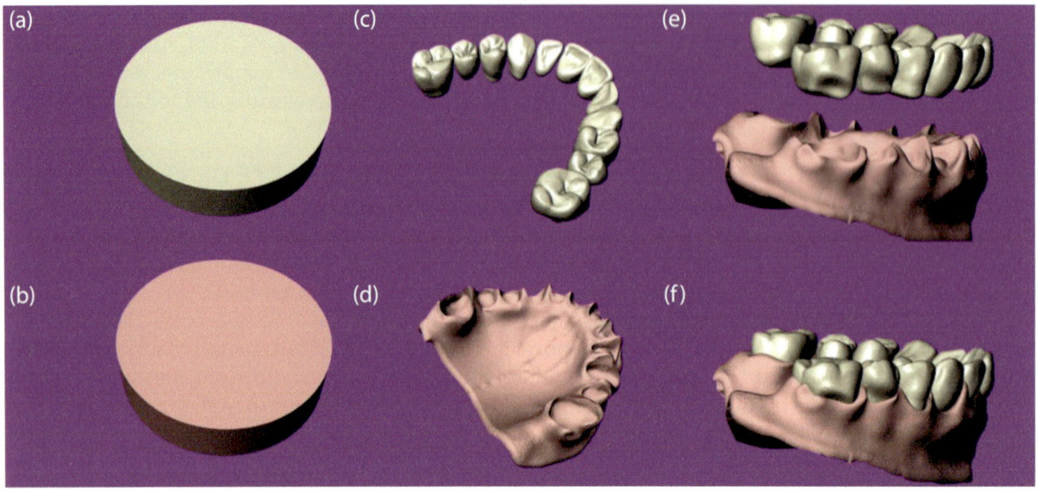

Figure 4.2 Two-step milled denture. (a) A PMMA tooth-colored disk is selected together with the counterpart (b), the pink PMMA. Then the teeth (c) and base (d) are milled in two steps and should be bonded together (e) to obtain the final prostheses (f).

Second visit in the dental office:

12. Evaluation of the trial CDs in the patient's mouth.
13. Deliver the finished CDs.

4.5 SIMPLIFIED WORKFLOW WITH ONE-PIECE DIGITAL PROSTHESES: USE OF THE IVOCLAR IVOTION DISK

The one-piece digital subtractive system has promising benefits. This technology offers excellent material quality with simple fabrication methods. The monoblock fabricated from Ivotion (Ivoclar, Schaan, Liechtenstein) offers greater stability compared to dentures fabricated from two components. The following is a summary of the steps for the fabrication of one-piece digital CDs [61].

Design of the prostheses with CAD software:

1. 3D facial scanning with and without the use of a transfer fork. The transfer fork allows the merging of intraoral and extraoral surface data and facilitates the correct occlusal plane orientation of the digitized models.
2. Alignment of the casts with the patient's face. Special attention is paid to the alignment of the prostheses about the skull in terms of orientation of planes and lines: Camper's plane, interpupillary line, and facial midline.
3. Alignment of the virtual disk by using "shell geometry" to achieve an optimal adaptation of the gingival contour concerning the dentition. This is necessary because the single Ivoclar Ivotion disc comprises a section for the denture base as well as a section for the teeth (**Figure 4.3**).

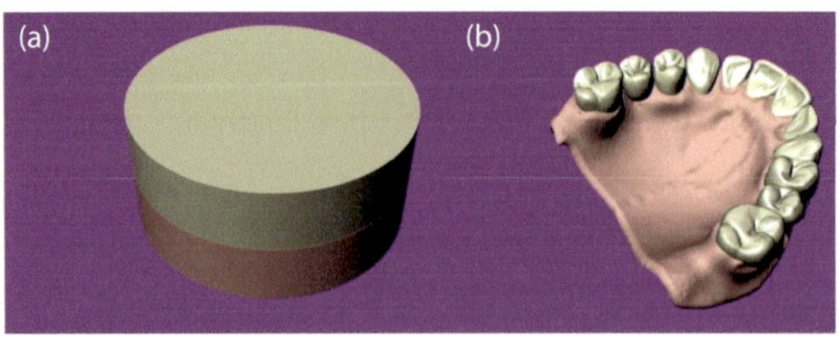

Figure 4.3 One-step milled denture. (a) A PMMA double-colored disk is selected to be milled in the shape of the final prosthesis (b).

4. Definition of the teeth. Teeth of a suitable size and shape for the CDs can be selected from a virtual library and correctly positioned.
5. Definition of the CD base. The modeling of the gingival areas is the final step in the design of the Ivoclar Ivotion prostheses.

Design of the prostheses with CAM software:

1. Creation of retaining pins on the outside of the base of the prosthesis to retain the disc.
2. Simulation of milling paths.
3. Generation of the CNC files for the PM7 (Ivoclar) milling machine.
4. Milling of the blocks for the construction of the prosthesis.
5. Final polishing.
6. Delivery of the prosthesis

Additive manufacturing technology has been categorized into different processes according to its printing method: Stereolithography (SLA), material jetting (MJ), material extrusion (ME) or fused deposition modelling (FDM), binder jetting, powder bed fusion (PBF), sheet lamination, and direct energy deposition (ASTM, 2009). **Figure 4.4** shows a schematic drawing of the commonly used 3D printing methods that can be used for the construction of complete dentures according to Arcila et al., 2020 [62].

4.6 IMPORTANCE OF COMPLETE DENTURES

Complete dentures have undergone a favorable development, benefiting from the introduction of new prosthetic biomaterials with greater biocompatibility and better mechanical properties for their fabrication [63]. The materials most frequently used in the fabrication of this type of prosthesis are polymethylmethacrylate (PMMA) and polyetheretherketone (PEEK), and ceramics (tooth) that exhibit excellent esthetics and a very good relationship with the soft tissues of the oral cavity [63, 64].

In this regard, the health of the soft and hard tissues is an important part of the placement of a complete denture [27, 62–64]. In removable prosthodontics, one of the most common oral diseases that affect patients wearing complete dentures is chronic candidiasis or prosthetic stomatitis [40, 64, 65], which is influenced by poor oral hygiene, long-term wear of dentures, poor fit, rough surface formation, and the porosity of acrylic resin in this type of prosthesis [66]. Additionally, among patients with complete edentulism, jaw atrophy is imminent, generating a loss of vertical occlusal dimension and leading to the development of fungal etiology angular cheilitis. Decreased cognitive independence and self-care due to dementia, delirium, and social isolation may further exacerbate the oral mucosa condition [67]. Thus, it is very important to choose the appropriate prosthetic biomaterials along with the effective fabrication method and to place great emphasis on oral and prosthetic hygiene to ensure better oral health care for the edentulous patient.

4.7 DIGITAL MANUFACTURING

Currently, there are a variety of systems for the fabrication of a CECD, such as AvaDent, Dentca, 3Shape Dental System, Wieland, Ceramil, Baltic Denture, and the Vita Vionic System [17, 68]. In this section, the fabrication of a CECD is described in general terms to avoid any conflict of interest with specific brands. During the design of a complete denture, 3D digital edentulous models are generated from intraoral scan impressions (IOS). IOS has become an increasingly popular technology to replace conventional impressions [69]. These digital impressions are divided into two types: Indirect digital technology or 2D scan-based technology, which uses non-contact optical scanners [70], and direct digital technology based on 3D scanning, which has been widely used in prosthodontics and, in recent years, in full arch impressions, despite the difficulty of obtaining accurate scans due to the dynamics of soft tissues [71, 72]. This is a controversial issue, as in vitro studies have shown that without soft tissue interference, the accuracy of certain digital scanning systems is comparable to the conventional impression technique [73]. Very similarly, conventional impressions have shown significantly higher accuracy compared to digital impressions made with IOS for implant-supported restoration of an edentulous arch [74]. Impressions obtained using IOS are a valid alternative to conventional impressions for partial-arch segments; however, they remain a challenge for this type of device [75]. In fact, some authors claim that the trueness and accuracy of IOS systems of single-unit preparations are equal or close to conventional impression [76]. Thus,

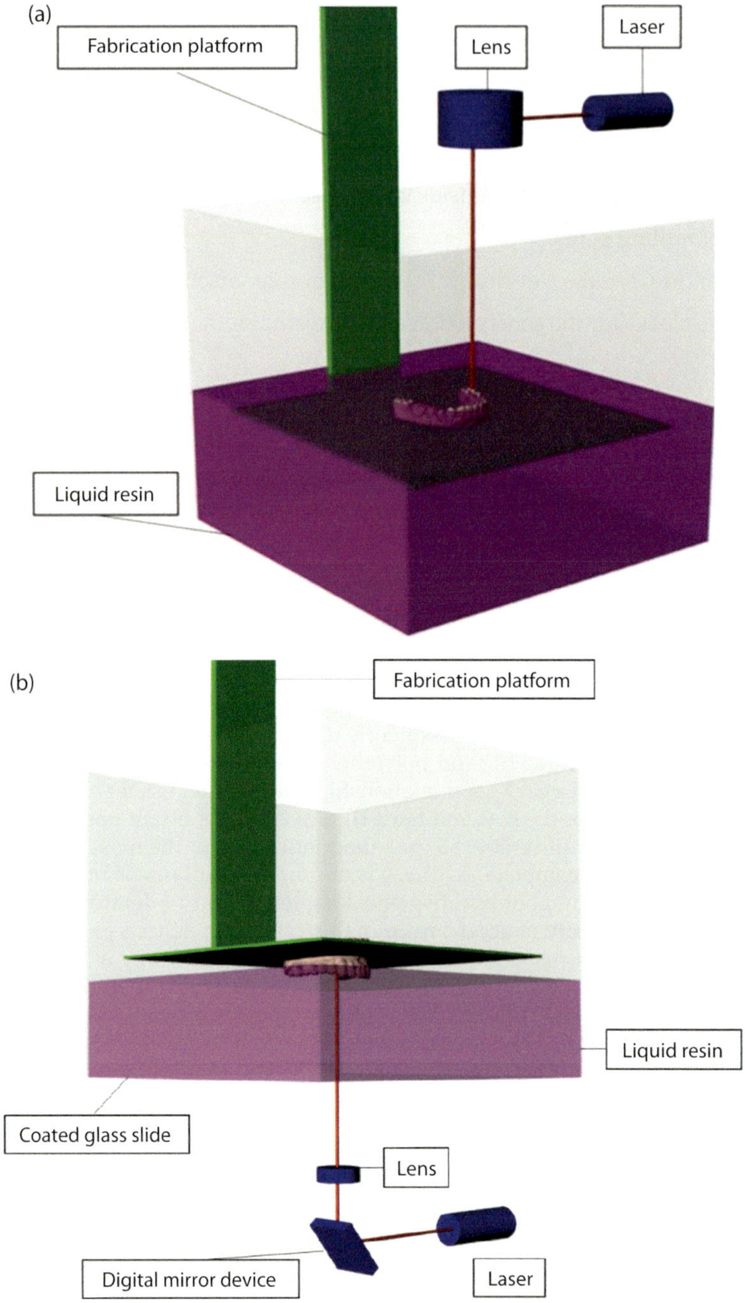

Figure 4.4 Two different approaches to stereolithography (SLA) printing. (a) The first approach is the bottom-up setup, where each new layer is printed on top of the previous one. (b) The second approach is the top-down setup, where each layer is printed underneath the previous one and the light-sensitive material is polymerized through irradiation from underneath.

compared to conventional printing, IOS systems can be reliably used for diagnostic and short-range scanning purposes. However, for full-arch scanning, IOS is susceptible to more deviations and/or errors. In summary, while the accuracy of IOS systems appears to be promising and comparable to conventional methods, they are still vulnerable to inaccuracies. To overcome this limitation, accuracy can be improved by reducing the scanning range and ensuring that scanned surfaces have minimal irregularities [77].

Digital impression technology is a viable option to reduce clinic visits and laboratory work, alleviate patient anxiety and stress, and improve patient comfort [78]. It was reported that IOS is generally preferred by patients over conventional impressions [79].

After obtaining the 3D models, the occlusal plane should be determined, followed by the features of the prosthesis, the margins for the base plates, the placement of the artificial dentitions, local defect fixing, esthetic analysis, and the occlusal relationship adjustment. The design is then saved and exported to the CAM software [80]. The dentitions and base plates are fabricated by milling, and finally, the bonding of the dentition to the base plate can be carried out when using two blocks (one for the pink base and one for the teeth) [81].

4.8 BIOMATERIALS USED FOR THE CONSTRUCTION OF COMPLETE DENTURES

There are several types of prosthetic designs and biomaterials for the rehabilitation of an older adult patient with edentulism. Depending on their type, they can be temporary or permanent [82]. In prosthodontics, temporary prosthetic restorations can be obtained from different types of biomaterials, which include those based on monomethacrylates or acrylic resins and dimethacrylates or bis-acryloyl/composite resins that are manufactured conventionally, as well as other modern materials, which are obtained by subtractive CAD/CAM technology, such as PMMA, or by additive technology, including 3D printed resins [83, 84]. The importance of provisional prosthetic restorations lies in testing different functional and biological parameters such as occlusal dynamics, vertical dimension, esthetics, and bone height maintenance [85]. Thus, the clinician must choose a biocompatible material for the fabrication of a provisional restoration with less negative effects on the tissues, which may compromise the patient's oral health [86].

Some other biomaterials, such as PEEK, can be used in the construction of temporary or definitive restorations (e.g., implant-supported restorations) due to their physical properties, chemical stability, esthetics, and favorable molecular interaction with the oral environment [87]. Finally, concerning dental ceramics, the introduction of monolithic zirconia has increased in recent years, becoming a promising material. This type of biomaterial presents better aesthetics, good mechanical behavior, and excellent biocompatibility with oral mucosal cells [88].

In dentistry, PMMA expanded its application scope, becoming one of the most widely used materials for the fabrication of restorations, due to its high clinical performance [89]. It corresponds to an acrylic-based resin, i.e., it is prepared using a liquid methyl methacrylate monomer (MMA) and a polymethyl methacrylate powder [90]. The reaction is shown in **Figure 4.5**. The advantages of using this type of material are durability, aesthetics, good marginal adaptation, and its low cost [91]. However, their interaction with the oral environment is complex [92]. Studies have shown that its use can have adverse effects and present toxicity at the cellular and tissue level, mainly in processes

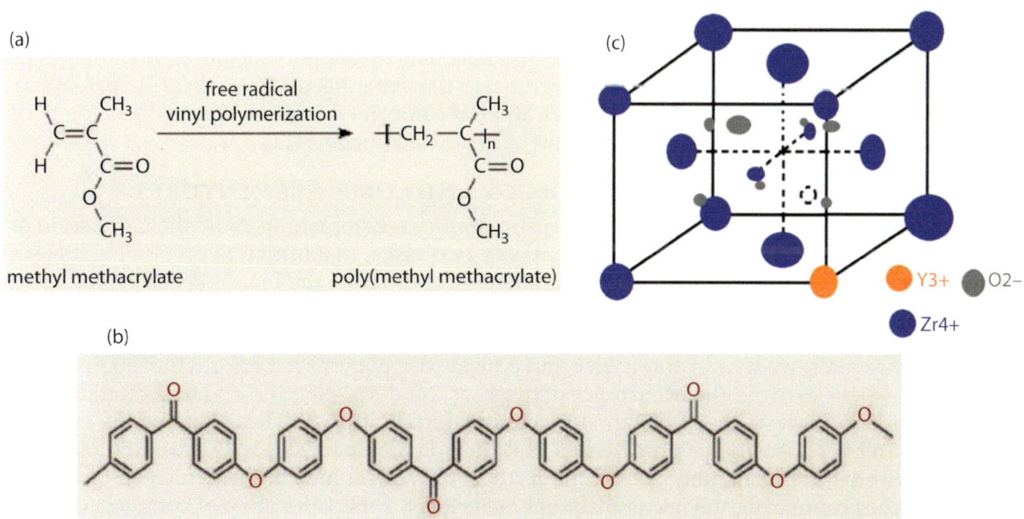

Figure 4.5 Chemical structure. (a) Polymethyl methacrylate (PMMA). (b) Polyetheretherketone (PEEK). (c) Yttria-stabilized zirconia (3Y-TZP). (From Ref. [29] under a Creative Commons Attribution licence.)

related to fibrosis, histiocytosis, and necrosis [93], as well as the release of residual monomers and influence on the salivary redox state [94]. It has rarely presented toxicity at the systemic level [95]. These elements become even more important when implant-supported complete dentures are fabricated, or other more extensive rehabilitation is performed [96].

In addition to being included in the composition of conventional temporary restorations, PMMA is used in the fabrication of digitally fabricated complete dentures. Based on its mechanical and topographical properties, the influence of the fabrication method is very important [97]. It has been shown that in complete dentures fabricated by CAD/CAM system, the hardness, strength and flexural modulus, dimensional stability, and the hydrophobicity of the blank are higher compared to conventionally fabricated prostheses, where restorations with poor physical characteristics have been observed, leading to prosthetic treatment failure in the short term [98]. Also, an important element is the surface properties of this type of restoration. It has been observed that conventionally fabricated complete dentures have a higher surface roughness compared to digitally fabricated dentures [99]. The fact that there are rougher surfaces on the prosthesis favors the creation of bacterial niches that are in contact with the keratinocytes of the buccal mucosa, initiating the immune response, which leads to tissue damage [100].

4.9 ADVANTAGES AND LIMITATIONS OF COMPLETE DENTURES MANUFACTURED BY CAD/CAM

CECDs have demonstrated high clinical performance, positive patient-related outcomes, and reasonable cost-effectiveness [101, 102]. CECDs offer several advantages over classic conventionally fabricated full dentures with reduced chair time and number of visits, which reduces stress on the part of the patient [103], digital archiving, i.e., easy reproduction of the prosthesis and thus fabrication of a complete denture using digital data stored in special software [104], shorter denture fabrication time [105], higher technical accuracy demonstrating increased bending and fracture resistance, more precise fit, better clinical retention, and thus minimal occurrence of wear-related traumatic injuries [106]. In addition, they provide better aesthetics and function, because users improve appearance, speech, and chewing ability, generating greater patient satisfaction [107]. A very interesting point is that it facilitates advances in the standardization of pilot testing for clinical research in removable prostheses [108], and to avoid bias, this technology promotes excellent quality control by clinicians and dental technicians [109]. Also, they offer several improved physical, topographical properties, i.e., this system reduces the formation of rough and irregular surfaces, creating smoother surfaces that greatly inhibit the retention and accumulation of microorganisms, especially bacteria and fungi, on the prosthesis [110] and consequent infection [21, 111, 112]. An update of studies comparatively evaluating digitally fabricated versus conventionally fabricated complete dentures is shown in **Table 4.1**.

On the other hand, digital technology has some drawbacks. For example, it has been reported that the greatest misalignment of digital complete dentures occurs in the posterior palatal seal area and border seal area [112]. Also, the inability to define the mandibular occlusal plane, the position of the incisal edge of the upper anterior teeth, and adequate lip support remain disadvantages [21]. The implementation of this technology is costly due to the materials used, which are expensive and require highly trained personnel for the fabrication of complete dentures. This justifies the necessary update in its management by the clinician or dental technician [113].

4.10 THE FUTURE OF DIGITAL TECHNOLOGY AND COMPLETE DENTURES

The advancement of digital technology in prosthodontics is astonishing. Now the fabrication of a complete digital denture can be carried out in only two visits, in addition to preserving its excellent biomechanical, esthetic, and tissue-compatible properties in the maxillofacial region. There is also a need to integrate this technology broadly in society, to decrease the problems related to its use, and to take advantage of all the tools that CAD/CAM systems can offer us. Also, as dental health professionals, we should emphasize and educate our patients to perform thorough oral and prosthetic hygiene to avoid the occurrence of diseases. Modern scientific research should include other aspects of interest: the application of nanomaterials in biomedical research is currently underway, and new prosthetic biomaterials that include nanoparticles with antimicrobial properties that inhibit the formation of biofilms in their polymeric matrix could also be developed. Further studies comparing the use of different materials for the fabrication of complete dentures using digital and conventional design on their chemical and physical properties, as well as at the tissue and cellular level, should be carried out to understand the oral biochemical interaction in total prosthodontics.

Table 4.1: An Update on the Comparative Evaluation of Digitally versus Conventionally Fabricated Complete Dentures

Authors/Year/ Type of Study	Country/Number of Visits	Subjects	Technique	Findings
Zupancic Cepic et al., 2023 Prospective randomized crossover study [21]	Austria/5 visits	10 adults, 8 males and 2 females with an average age of 53.6 years/ maxilla, mandible CDs	Conventional CD/ VDFP–Ceramill Mind and Ceramill Motion 2, CAD/ CAM	Found a trend towards better clinical efficiency of digital CDs compared to conventional CDs, while patient satisfaction was not affected by the type of fabrication.
Kang et al., 2022 Randomized, single-blind, crossover clinical study [113]	Republic of Korea/–	8 adults/maxilla, mandible CDs	Conventional/ VDFP– CAD-CAM	Digital CDs were inferior to conventional CDs in terms of masticatory efficiency, and pronunciation. However, internal adaptation and overall patient satisfaction were comparable between conventional and digital CDs.
Peroz et al., 2022 Randomized, blinded, controlled study [114]	Germany/2 visits	16 adults, 11 men and 5 women, mean age 66 years/maxilla, mandible CDs	Conventional/ VDFP– Baltic Denture System, CAD-CAM	From the patients' perspective, the method of CDs fabrication did not influence oral health-related quality of life. However, digital CDs required only 2 visits, 1 hour less time in the dental chair, and 5 hours less time for dental technicians.
Emera et al., 2022 Clinical crossover study [115]	Egypt/–	10 adults, aged 45–60 years/ maxilla, mandible-CDs	Conventional/ VDFP – Exocad Dental, Rasdent 3d printer y Dentca, CAD-CAM	3D printed CDs fabricated with dimethacrylate-based resin could be a promising alternative to conventionally fabricated CDs with satisfactory denture base adaptation and retention.
Arakawa et al. 2022 Retrospective study [116]	Switzerland/2 visits	32 adults, aged 35–85 years/ maxillary, mandible CDs	Conventional/ VDFP–AvaDent y Wieland, CAD/ CAM	For the fabrication of a CD, digital treatment was less costly overall, suggesting that in the future digital systems could replace conventional systems by reducing clinical treatment time and costs.
Otake et al., 2024 Retrospective study [117]	Japan/2 visits	44 edentulous adults, maxilla, mandible CDs	Conventional/ VDFP–Customized Disc Method – CAD/CAM	The custom disc method improved overall patient satisfaction. The labor and total costs of this method were significantly lower than the conventional method.
Clark et al., 2021 Retrospective cross-sectional study [118]	USA/–	314 adults, maxillary, mandible CDs	Conventional/ VDFP–CAD-CAM	When comparing both methods, digitally fabricated DCs required fewer patient appointments from start to finish and fewer postoperative appointments than conventional DCs. Fewer visits may be an important consideration for patients, especially those with limited access to dental health services.

(Continued)

Table 4.1 ***(Continued):*** **An Update on the Comparative Evaluation of Digitally versus Conventionally Fabricated Complete Dentures**

Authors/Year/ Type of Study	Country/Number of Visits	Subjects	Technique	Findings
Mai et al., 2020 Foundry model study [119]	Republic of Korea/2 visits	Maxilla, mandible CDs	VDFP/CAD-CAM	The base and tooth parts of the new dentures were designed efficiently and predictably. The digital protocol facilitated the design of the prosthesis in terms of edge sealing and tooth arrangement.
Srinivasan et al., 2019 Clinical case [120]	Switzerland/ 3 visits	Male, aged 65 years/CD maxilla and mandible Male, aged 75 years/Resin maxilla and mandible RPD	VDFP/Anatomical measuring device AvaDent/CAD-CAM	The digital denture protocol could prove to be very beneficial for older adult/edentulous patients as it could help decrease treatment burden by reducing clinical procedures, number of visits, time, and costs.
Lee et al., 2019 Clinical case [121]	Korea/ 2 visits	Male, aged 53 years/maxilla and mandible CDs	VFDP/CAD-CAM	Addition of conventional impression and maxillomandibular relationship with laboratory steps using CAD-CAM system. Minimized clinical time.

Abbreviations: CAD/CAM, computer-aided design/computer-aided manufacturing; CD, Complete denture; VDFP, virtual design and fabrication process.

4.11 CONCLUSION

Digital workflow reduces the processing time (clinical and laboratory time), which is convenient for both the clinician and the patient. The data stored in the digital record is very valuable for future appointments and follow-ups. The biomaterials for the construction of a prosthesis are predominantly PMMA due to their mechanical, esthetic, and biocompatible properties with the oral environment, but it is a field that still can be developed.

REFERENCES

1. Allen, F, Tsakos, G. Challenges in oral health research for older adults. Gerodontology. 2023;41(1):2–8.
2. Pazan, F, Wehling, M. Polypharmacy in older adults: a narrative review of definitions, epidemiology and consequences. Eur Geriatr Med. 2021;12(3):443–452.
3. Daniele, A et al. Oral frailty indicators to target major adverse health-related outcomes in older age: a systematic review. Geroscience. 2023;45(2):663–706.
4. Tahmasebi, E et al. Current infections of the orofacial region: treatment, diagnosis, and epidemiology. Life (Basel). 2023;13(2):269.
5. Janto, M et al. Oral health among elderly, impact on life quality, access of elderly patients to oral health services and methods to improve oral health: a narrative review. J Pers Med. 2022;12(3):372.
6. de Sam Lazaro, SL et al. Barriers and opportunities to support the oral health of older adults: a rapid review of health policy and systems. Int J Aging Hum Dev. 2023;96(1):51–62.
7. Mourelle, P et al. Global prevalence of edentulism and dental caries in middle-aged and elderly persons: a systematic review and meta-analysis. J Dent. 2022;127:104335.
8. Alarcón-Sánchez, MA et al. Potential impact of prosthetic biomaterials on the periodontium: a comprehensive review. Molecules. 2023;28(3):1075.
9. Marya, A et al. Biomolecular and biochemical aspects of the oral cavity. Molecules. 2022;27(24):8676.
10. Srimaneepong, V et al. Fixed prosthetic restorations and periodontal health: a narrative review. J Funct Biomater. 2022;13(1):15.
11. Tamimi, F, Hirayama, H. Digital Restorative Dentistry. A Guide to Materials, Equipment, and Clinical Procedures. 1, Springer Cham. 2019.
12. Ferencz, JL, Silva, NRFA. Fundamentals of CAD/CAM Dentistry. 1, American College of Prosthodontists. 2019.
13. Masri, R, Driscoll, CF. Clinical Applications of Digital Dental Technology. 1, Wiley Blackwell. 2015.
14. Friel, T, Waia, S. Removable partial dentures for older adults. Prim Dent J. 2020;9(3):34–39.
15. Auerbacher, M et al. Treatment plan and challenges in full-mouth rehabilitation of a quadriplegic patient: a clinical report. J Prosthodont. 2022;31(3):183–189.

16. Kopp, G et al. Long transmaxillary implants improve oral health-related quality of life of patients with atrophic jaws case series. Int J Implant Dent. 2021;7(1):29.
17. Mubaraki, MQ et al. Assessment of conventionally and digitally fabricated complete dentures: a comprehensive review. Materials (Basel). 2022;15(11):3868.
18. Alshammari, M et al. Oral health-related quality of life among elderly people with edentulous jaws in Hafar Al-Batin region, Saudi Arabia. J Int Soc Prev Community Dent. 2018;8(6):495–502.
19. Branchi, R et al. Can a prosthesis cause psychological disturbances? J Oral Rehabil. 2001;28(12):1133–1138.
20. The glossary of prosthodontic terms: ninth edn. J Prosthet Dent. 2017;117(5S):e1–e105.
21. Zupancic Cepic, LZ et al. Digital versus conventional dentures: a prospective, randomized cross-over study on clinical efficiency and patient satisfaction. J Clin Med. 2023;12(2):434.
22. Arantes, DC et al. Maxillofacial prosthetic rehabilitation of patients with resection of squamous cell carcinoma: a report of two cases. Contemp Clin Dent. 2020;11(3):294–297.
23. Sayed, ME et al. Linear dimensional change in acrylic denture teeth positions factored by different processing techniques and occlusal forms: an in vitro study. Appl Sci. 2022;12:7058.
24. Lee, H-J et al. Digital workflow to fabricate complete dentures for edentulous patients using a reversing and superimposing technique. Appl. Sci. 2021;11:5786.
25. Schmidt, MB et al. Combination of digital and conventional workflows in the CAD/CAM-fabrication of an implant-supported overdenture. Materials (Basel). 2020;13(17):3688.
26. Ashtiani, RE et al. The role of biomaterials and biocompatible materials in implant-supported dental prosthesis. Evidence-Based Complement Altern Med. 2021;2021:3349433.
27. Afshari, A et al. Biomaterials and biological parameters for fixed-prosthetic implant-supported restorations: a review study. Adv Mater Sci Eng. 2022;22:1–16.
28. Kharouf, N et al. Special issue, Recent advances in biomaterials and dental disease, part I. Bioengineering (Basel). 2023;10(1):55.
29. Ionescu, RN et al. Prosthetic materials used for implant-supported restorations and their biochemical oral interactions: a narrative review. Materials (Basel). 2022;15(3):1016.
30. Grant, GT et al. Glosario de términos dentales digitales: Colegio Americano de Prostodoncistas. J Prostodonte. 2016;25(Suppl 2):S2–S9.
31. Dimitriadis, K et al. Influence of heat treatment on the microstructure and the physical and mechanical properties of dental highly translucent zirconia. J Adv Prosthodont. 2022;14:96–107.
32. Heboyan, A et al. In vitro microscopic evaluation of metal- and zirconium-oxide-based crowns' marginal fit. Pesqui Bras Odontopediatria Clín Integr. 2022;22:e210144.
33. Watanabe, H, Fellows, C, An, H. Digital technologies for restorative dentistry. Dent Clin North Am. 2022;66(4):567–590.
34. Zitzmann, UN et al. Digital undergraduate education in dentistry: a systematic review. Int J Environ Res Public Health. 2020;17(9):3269.
35. Alghazzawi, TF. Advancements in CAD/CAM technology: options for practical implementation. J Prosthodont Res. 2016;60(2):72–84.
36. Janeva, NM et al. Advantages of CAD/CAM versus conventional complete dentures – a review. Open Access Maced J Med Sci. 2018;6(8):1498–1502.
37. Al-Humood, H et al. Marginal fit, mechanical properties, and esthetic outcomes of CAD/CAM interim fixed dental prostheses (FDPs): a systematic review. Materials (Basel). 2023;16(5):1996.
38. Heboyan, A et al. Bacteriological evaluation of gingival crevicular fluid in teeth restored using fixed dental prostheses: an in vivo study. Int J Mol Sci. 2021;22:5463.
39. Menini, M et al. Analysis of the subgingival microbiota in implant-supported full-arch rehabilitations. Dent J. 2020;5:104.
40. Abuhajar, E et al. Management of chronic atrophic candidiasis (denture stomatitis) – a narrative review. Int J Environ Res Public Health. 2023;20(4):3029.
41. Chávez, EM et al. Dental care for geriatric and special needs populations. Dent Clin North Am. 2018;62(2):245–267.
42. Gibson, G et al. Providing effective dental care for an ageing population. Int Dent J. 2022;72(4S):S39–S43.
43. Joda, T et al. The complete digital workflow in fixed prosthodontics: a systematic review. BMC Oral Health. 2017;17(1):124.
44. Baba, NZ et al. CAD/CAM complete denture systems and physical properties: a review of the literature. J Prosthodont. 2021;30(S2):113–124.
45. Chen, L et al. Duplicating complete dentures with conventional and digital methods: comparisons of trueness and efficiency. Dent J (Basel). 2022;10(3):35.
46. Kattadiyil, MT, AlHelal, A. An update on computer-engineered complete dentures: a systematic review on clinical outcomes. J Prosthet Dent. 2017;117(4):478–485.
47. Tosun, ON et al. Comparison of denture base adaptation between additive and conventional fabrication techniques. J Prosthodont. 2023;32(3):e64–e70.
48. Huang et al. Additive manufacturing technologies in the oral implant clinic: a review of current applications and progress. Front Bioeng Biotechnol. 2023;11:1100155.
49. Bilgin, MS et al. A review of computer-aided design/computer-aided manufacture techniques for removable denture fabrication. Eur J Dent. 2016;10(2):286–291.
50. Oh, KC et al. Accuracy of metal 3D printed frameworks for removable partial dentures evaluated by digital superimposition. Dent Mater. 2022;38(2):309–317.
51. Davis, R et al. A comprehensive review on metallic implant biomaterials and their subtractive manufacturing. Int J Adv Manuf Technol. 2022;120(3–4):1473–1530.
52. Sulaiman, TA. Materials in digital dentistry-a review. J Esthet Restor Dent. 2020;32(2):171–181.
53. Abduo, J et al. Trends in computer-aided manufacturing in prosthodontics: a review of the available streams. Int J Dent. 2014;2014:783948.
54. Presotto, AGC et al. Influence of spark erosion on the fit of screw-retained Co-Cr fixed complete denture frameworks veneered with different materials. J Prosthet Dent. 2018;119(5):797–803.
55. Pereira, RM et al. An engineering perspective of ceramics applied in dental reconstructions. J Appl Oral Sci. 2023;31:e20220421.

56. Heboyan, A et al. Insights into polymeric materials for prosthodontics and dental implantology. Materials (Basel). 2022;15(15):5383.
57. Heboyan, A et al. Insights and advancements in biomaterials for prosthodontics and implant dentistry. Molecules. 2022;27(16):5116.
58. Mirchandani, B et al. Biomechanical aspects of various attachments for implant overdentures: a review. Polymers (Basel). 2021;13(19):3248.
59. Faur, AB et al. Rescanning of digital impressions' mesh holes: in vivo and in vitro accuracy evaluation of three different scanning protocols. Appl Sci. 2023;13:2867.
60. Wimmer, T et al. Complete denture fabrication supported by CAD/CAM. J Prosthet Dent. 2016;115(5):541–546.
61. Edelhoff, D et al. CAD/CAM full-mouth rehabilitation of an elderly patient: one-piece digital complete denture meets multilayered zirconia with gradient technology. J Esthet Restor Dent. 2023;36(1):174–185.
62. Arcila, LVC et al. Indications, materials and properties of 3D printing in dentistry: a literature overview. Research Society Development. 2020;9(11):e80791110632.
63. Schweiger, J et al. 3D printing in digital prosthetic dentistry: an overview of recent developments in additive manufacturing. J Clin Med. 2021;10:2010.
64. Wajdan, N et al. Anti-fungal efficacy of miswak extract (Salvadora persica) and commercial cleaner against Candida albicans on heat cured polymethylmethacrylate denture base. J Appl Biomater Funct Mater. 2023;21:22808000231165666.
65. Avetisyan, A et al. Characteristics of periodontal tissues in prosthetic treatment with fixed dental prostheses. Molecules. 2021;2:1331.
66. Monteiro, DR et al. Oral prosthetic microbiology: aspects related to the oral microbiome, surface properties, and strategies for controlling biofilms. Biofouling. 2021;37(4):353–371.
67. Le Bars, P et al. Host's immunity and *Candida* species associated with denture stomatitis: a narrative review. Microorganisms. 2022;10(7):1437.
68. Lee, DJ, Saponaro, PC. Management of edentulous patients. Dent Clin North Am. 2019;63(2):249–261.
69. Suganna, M et al. Contemporary evidence of CAD-CAM in dentistry: a systematic review. Cureus. 2022;14(11):e31687.
70. Gracis, S et al. Digital workflow in implant prosthodontics: the critical aspects for reliable accuracy. J Esthet Restor Dent. 2023;35(1):250–261.
71. Marques, S et al. Digital impressions in implant dentistry: a literature review. Int J Environ Res Public Health. 2021; 18(3):1020.
72. Kihara, H et al. Accuracy and practicality of intraoral scanner in dentistry: a literature review. J Prosthodont Res. 2020;64(2):109–113.
73. Knechtle, N et al. Accuracy of digital complete-arch, multi-implant scans made in the edentulous jaw with gingival movement simulation: an in vitro study. J Prosthet Dent. 2022;128(3):468–478.
74. Shaikh, M et al. Do digital impressions have a greater accuracy for full-arch implant-supported reconstructions compared to conventional impressions? An *in vitro* study. J Indian Prosthodont Soc. 2022;22(4):398–404.
75. Ender, A et al. Accuracy of complete- and partial-arch impressions of actual intraoral scanning systems in vitro. Int J Comput Dent. 2019;22(1):11–19.
76. Zimmermann, M et al. Local accuracy of actual intraoral scanning systems for single-tooth preparations in vitro. J Am Dent Assoc. 2020;151(2):127–135.
77. Abduo, J, Elseyoufi, M. Accuracy of intraoral scanners: a systematic review of influencing factors. Eur J Prosthodont Restor Dent. 2018;26(3):101–121.
78. Srinivasan, M et al. CAD-CAM removable complete dentures: a systematic review and meta-analysis of trueness of fit, biocompatibility, mechanical properties, surface characteristics, color stability, time-cost analysis, clinical and patient-reported outcomes. J Dent. 2021;113:103777.
79. Siqueira, R et al. Intraoral scanning reduces procedure time and improves patient comfort in fixed prosthodontics and implant dentistry: a systematic review. Clin Oral Investig. 2021;25(12):6517–6531.
80. Ciocca, L et al. Analysis of the trueness and precision of complete denture bases manufactured using digital and analog technologies. J Adv Prosthodont. 2023;15(1):22–32.
81. Zhang, S et al. A fully digital 1-day technique for fabricating complete dentures based on an existing denture. J Prosthet Dent. 2023;133(1):48–56.
82. Saeed, F et al. Prosthodontics dental materials: from conventional to unconventional. Mater Sci Eng C Mater Biol Appl. 2020;106:110167.
83. Vieira, FR et al. Influence of different restoring materials on stress distribution in prosthesis on implants: a review of finite element studies. Eur J Dent. 2023;17(1):1–6.
84. Revilla-León, M et al. Artificial intelligence applications in implant dentistry: a systematic review. J Prosthet Dent. 2023;129(2):293–300.
85. Marin, E et al. Biomaterials and biocompatibility: an historical overview. J Biomed Mater Res A. 2020;108(8):1617–1633.
86. Wang, B et al. PEEK in fixed dental prostheses: application and adhesion improvement. Polymers (Basel). 2022; 14(12):2323.
87. Trzaskowski, M et al. Evaluation of mechanical properties of 3D-printed polymeric materials for possible application in mouthguards. Polymers (Basel). 2023;15(4):898.
88. Singer, L et al. Biomimetic approaches and materials in restorative and regenerative dentistry: review article. BMC Oral Health. 2023;23(1):105.
89. Al-Dwairi, ZN et al. A comparison of the surface properties of CAD/CAM and conventional polymethylmethacrylate (PMMA). J Prosthodont. 2019;28(4):452–457.
90. de Oliveira Limírio, JPJ et al. Mechanical properties of polymethyl methacrylate as a denture base: conventional versus CAD-CAM resin – a systematic review and meta-analysis of in vitro studies. J Prosthet Dent. 2022;128(6):1221–1229.
91. Jasiūnaitė, A et al. A comparison of mechanic properties regarding complete removable dentures, which were made from polymethylmethacrilate (PMMA) during conventional and CAD/CAM processes. Systemic literature review. Stomatologija. 2022;24(1):3–12.
92. Pantea, M et al. Biochemical interaction between materials used for interim prosthetic restorations and saliva. Materials (Basel). 2021;15(1):226.

93. Al-Dwairi, ZN et al. A comparison of the surface and mechanical properties of 3D printable denture-base resin material and conventional polymethylmethacrylate (PMMA). J Prosthodont. 2023;32(1):40–48.
94. Gad, MM et al. PMMA denture base material enhancement: a review of fiber, filler, and nanofiller addition. Int J Nanomedicine. 2017;12:3801–3812.
95. Polychronakis, N et al. Removal of denture adhesives from PMMA and polyamide denture base materials. J Appl Oral Sci. 2021;29:e20200448.
96. Díez-Pascual, AM. PMMA-based nanocomposites for odontology applications: a state-of-the-art. Int J Mol Sci. 2022; 23(18):10288.
97. Zidan, S et al. Assessing tensile bond strength between denture teeth and nano-zirconia impregnated PMMA denture base. Int J Nanomedicine. 20201;15:9611–9625.
98. Zafar, MS. Prosthodontic applications of polymethyl methacrylate (PMMA): an update. Polymers (Basel). 2020;12(10):2299.
99. Gad, MM, Abualsaud, R. Behavior of PMMA denture base materials containing titanium dioxide nanoparticles: a literature review. Int J Biomater. 2019;2019:6190610.
100. Luo, C et al. PEEK for Oral applications: recent advances in mechanical and adhesive properties. Polymers. 2023;15:386.
101. Schmutzler, A et al. Cleaning of removable dental prostheses. Evid Based Dent Pract. 2021;21(4):101644.
102. Jurado, CA et al. Digitally fabricated immediate complete dentures: case reports of milled and printed dentures. Int J Prosthodont. 2020;33(2):232–241.
103. Kattadiyil, MT et al. Clinical complications and quality assessments with computer-engineered complete dentures: a systematic review. J Prosthet Dent. 2017;117(6):721–728.
104. Alikhasi, M et al. Smile design: mechanical considerations. Dent Clin North Am. 2022;66(3):477–487.
105. Campbell, SD et al. Removable partial dentures: the clinical need for innovation. J Prosthet Dent. 2017;118(3):273–280.
106. Seals, RR Jr et al. Immediate complete dentures. Dent Clin North Am. 1996;40(1):151–167.
107. Matthes de Freitas Pontes, K et al. Clinical study of the biofilm of implant-supported complete dentures in healthy patients. Gerodontology. 2022;39(2):148–160.
108. Steinmassl, O et al. Influence of CAD/CAM fabrication on denture surface properties. J Oral Rehabil. 2018;45(5):406–413.
109. Janeva, N et al. Complete dentures fabricated with CAD/CAM technology and a traditional clinical recording method. Open Access Maced J Med Sci. 2017;5(6):785–789.
110. An, X et al. Digital workflow for computer-guided implant surgery in edentulous patients with an intraoral scanner and old complete denture. J Prosthodont. 2019;28(6):715–718.
111. Smith, PB et al. Economic and clinical impact of digitally produced dentures. J Prosthodont. 2021;30(S2):108–112.
112. Arai, K et al. Complete denture fabrication using digitally fabricated copy dentures for a patient with moderate dementia. Case Rep Dent. 2021;2021:9385095.
113. Kang, YJ et al. Comparative evaluation of digitally fabricated complete dentures versus conventional complete dentures: a randomized, single-blinded, cross-over clinical trial. J Prosthet Dent. 2022:S0022-3913(22)00339-0.
114. Peroz, S et al. Digital versus conventional complete dentures: a randomized, controlled, blinded study. J Prosthet Dent. 2022;128(5):956–963.
115. Emera, RMK et al. Comparison of retention and denture base adaptation between conventional and 3D-printed complete dentures. J Dent Res Dent Clin Dent Prospects. 2022;16(3):179–185.
116. Arakawa, I et al. Clinical outcomes and costs of conventional and digital complete dentures in a university clinic: a retrospective study. J Prosthet Dent. 2022;128(3):390–395.
117. Otake, R et al. Patient-reported outcome and cost-effectiveness analysis of milled and conventionally fabricated complete dentures in a university clinic: a retrospective study. J Prosthet Dent. 2024;131(2):227–232.
118. Clark, WA et al. A comparison of conventionally versus digitally fabricated denture outcomes in a university dental clinic. J Prosthodont. 2021;30(1):47–50.
119. Mai, HN, Lee, DH. A digital technique to replicate edentulous arches with functional borders and accurate maxillomandibular relationship for digital complete denture. J Prosthodont. 2020;29(4):356–359.
120. Srinivasan, M et al. CAD/CAM milled removable complete dentures: time and cost estimation study. J Dent. 2019;80:75–79.
121. Lee, Y et al. Rehabilitation of fully edentulous patient using Ceramill full denture system (FDS). J. Korean Acad. Prosthodont. 2019;57:232–237.

5 Digital Fixed Prosthodontics

Amir I. O. Ibrahim, Stephan Lampl, Marco Tudts, Deepa Gurunathan, Desigar Moodely, Mayson Salih, and Sompop Bencharit

5.1 INTRODUCTION

Fixed prosthodontics is the branch of prosthodontics dealing with the replacement of missing teeth or part of tooth with a restoration or prosthesis that is definitively fixed inside the oral cavity. The fixed prothesis often involves the complete or partial coverage of the abutment tooth in order to replace the missing tooth structure and/or retain the prosthesis. They include fixed partial dentures, crowns, inlays, onlays, and veneers. Conventional fixed prostheses require multiple clinical and laboratory steps that utilize different materials that are suitable for this purpose. With the advancement in material and equipment technology, this conventional process of fixed prosthetic fabrication has undergone rapid evolution, utilizing digital tools and materials in the diagnosis, prosthetic design, as well as manufacturing or fabrication.

5.2 WHY DIGITAL FIXED PROSTHODONTICS?

Conventionally, fixed prostheses are fabricated following a series of clinical and laboratory steps. However, with the advancement of digital dentistry and the introduction of several digital devices for the diagnosis and fabrication of fixed prosthodontics, the workflow and materials used in the fabrication of conventional fixed prostheses underwent a rapid evolution (**Figure 5.1**). One of the advantages of digital dentistry applications in fixed prosthodontics is optimal communication between the prosthodontist and the dental technician. A digital impression can be sent electronically to the dental technician immediately after the clinical procedure rather than sending the physical impression, which may take days, and thus allows impression dimensional change. Furthermore, other relevant information can be sent to the dental technician, including digital photography, diagnostics, and treatment plans, such as a new smile design using the different smile design software available, digital impressions, instruction for the dental technician, and the shade of the teeth [1].

Furthermore, the use of digital devices reduces the procedural errors that are encountered during the different stages of conventional prosthetic fabrication. For instance, when comparing the accuracy of digital impression using intra-oral scanner with the use of traditional impression materials, it was reported that digital impression produces prostheses with better marginal fit compared to restoration fabricated using traditional impression materials [2, 3]. On the other hand, some reports showed similar accuracy of restorations produced using digital impression and traditional impression materials [4, 5]. However, the use of digital impression is more convenient in term of simplicity and saves more time. In conclusion, digital impression can produce more accurate or comparable representation of the prepared natural abutment tooth compared to the use of traditional elastomeric impression materials.

The conventional laboratory techniques used for the fabrication of fixed prostheses are complex, as mentioned previously. These drawbacks are diminished in today for a digital fabricated prosthesis, when digital design and manufacturing of restorations are applied using different computer-aided design and computer-aided manufacturing (CAD/CAM) systems available in the market. The CAD/CAM systems work through a combination of three stages; data acquisition, data processing, and machining. The transferred digital impression is processed, and the restoration is designed virtually instead of via the conventional lost wax and porcelain application processes. The virtual design is then transferred to a milling machine to manufacture the definitive restoration. One advantage of using a CAM milling machine is that the machine can be located inside the dental office (chairside manufacturing); thus, it can reduce human error during impression-making, fabrication of gypsum models, die trimming, wax-pattern, investing procedures, and porcelain/ceramic applications. Furthermore, the chairside milling procedure reduces time and number of appointments for the patient (one-visit restoration) [1, 6].

The contemporary literature demonstrates that the use of digital technology in the fabrication of fixed restoration is comparable to the conventional technique in terms of accuracy with less time required and more cost effectiveness to fabricate the restoration [7, 8]. In the following sections, a more detailed review is provided in regard to the digital workflow in fixed prosthodontics, including diagnosis of fixed prosthodontics using digital tools, digital impressions, digital casts and dies, CAD/CAM systems, and CAD/CAM materials.

 DOI: 10.1201/9781003428541-5

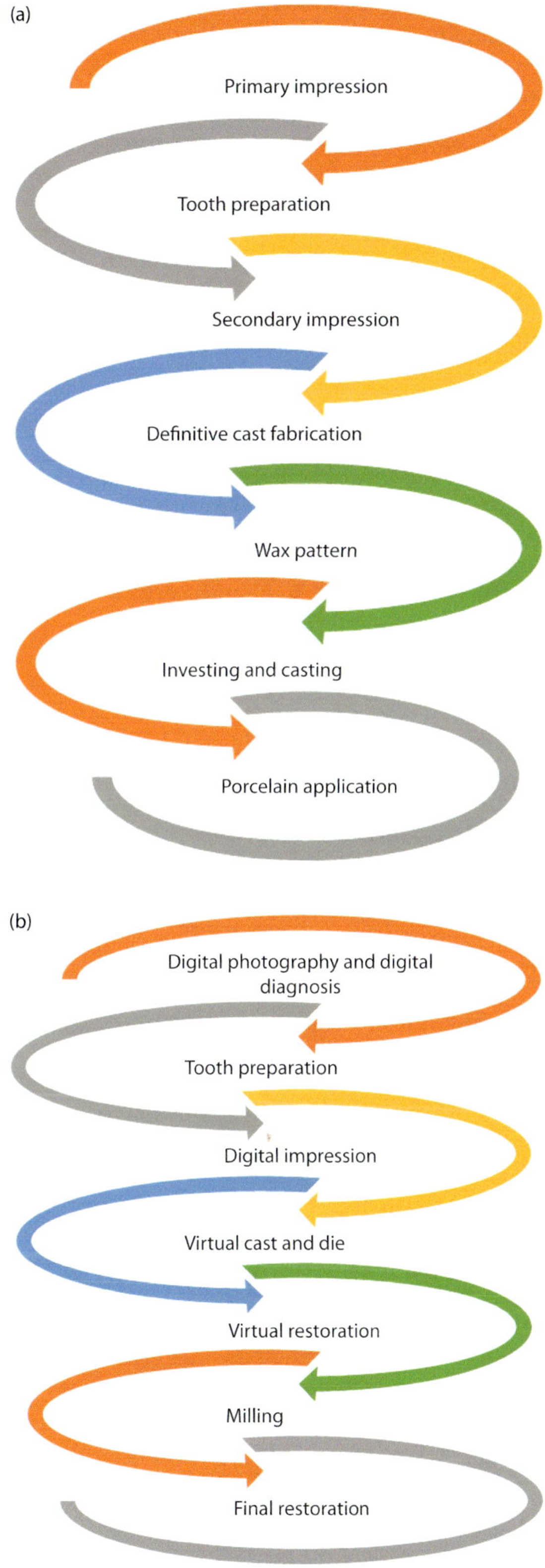

Figure 5.1 (a) Conventional fixed prosthodontic workflow. (b) Digital fixed prosthodontic workflow.

5.3 DIGITAL IMPRESSION AND 3D SCANNING

Dental impression plays an important role in a variety of procedures, such as general diagnosis, occlusion and tooth positional analysis, and prosthodontic fabrication techniques. Conventionally, in fixed prosthodontics, elastomeric impression materials have proven for decades their ability to capture sufficient details of the prepared abutment teeth for prosthetic fabrication [9]. However, the main shortcomings of traditional impression techniques include the time-dependent changeable physical properties of the material, the different consistency, which may affect the accuracy of the impression, and the unpleasant tastes and odors of the material, which may influence the patient experience [10]. As a result, clinicians have shifted their presence in recent years from conventional impressions to digital ones.

Nowadays, the possibility of digitally capturing prepared teeth with surrounding tissue (digital impression) is available as a result of introduction of dental scanners. Dental scanners are dental devices that capture a direct optical impression of the prepared tooth and its surrounding tissue by projecting a light source onto the target tissue. The light is captured by an image sensor and then processed digitally (by software) to create a 3D model for the scanned object [11]. Dental scanners are classified into two types: Extraoral laboratory scanners that scan cast models created by conventional impression, and intra-oral scanners (IOS) that can scan the oral cavity directly (**Figure 5.2**) [9, 12].

The use of intra-oral scanners enables the creation of a digital diagnostics setup, similar to a conventional diagnostic cast with wax up, allowing patients to almost immediately visualize the projected definitive prosthetic design [13]. Furthermore, digital impressions may allow chairside CAD/CAM systems to offer treatment protocol to be completed in a single clinical session, one-visit or same-day restoration [14]. Generally, intra-oral scanners were found to overcome many of the disadvantages of using traditional impression technique, such as:

a. Unpleasant impression material tastes and smells, and patient nausea and discomfort [15].
b. Dimensional change related to the different impression and die stone materials [16].
c. Cost-benefit ratio [17].
d. Storage space, time, and cost of transfer to the dental laboratory [18].
e. Risk of cross-contamination [19].
f. Problems and/or defects of the impression [20].
g. Electronic record-keeping and elimination of physical mailing of impressions or casts to the laboratory [21].

The following section will discuss the principles of digital impression systems, clinical procedures of intraoral scanning, and the factors that may affect the accuracy of 3D scanning.

5.3.1 The Principles of Digital Impression Systems

5.3.1.1 Extraoral Scanners

There are three types of extraoral scanner; contact, laser, and structured light. They differ in that contact scanners are based on capturing the surface of the teeth and oral tissue by means of mechanical

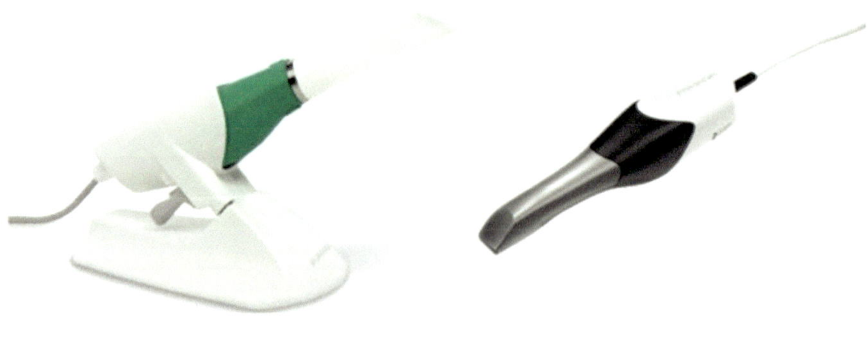

(a) (b)

Figure 5.2 (a) Planmeca Emerald. (With permission from Planmeca®.) (b) Primescan. (With permission from Dentsply Sirona.)

contact between a cast model and a detector unit. The laser and structure light scanners (non-contact scanners) are based on capturing the teeth and surrounding tissue by means of a light source such as laser or structure light technologies [22]. Furthermore, contact scanners are not affected by the optical properties of the object to be scanned, such as the brightness and shininess. The main advantage of the non-contact scanners is that they produce fast scanning and are not affected by the scanned object density [23–25]. Extraoral scanners of facial soft tissue are often used to help create a three-dimensional (3D) diagnosis of the patient's smile as well as other functions. They link virtual treatment planning to the intra-oral digital set up and thus enhance communications among clinicians and patients as well as laboratory technicians to achieve best aesthetic results [26].

5.3.1.2 Intraoral Digital Scanners

The number of intraoral scanners has increased recently with different types depending in the technology used and hence its clinical use. Intraoral scanners consist of cameras (hardware), computers, and software. Digital impression captured by intraoral scanners is created by a collection of information about projecting light recorded as video or individual images in a form of standard tessellation language (STL), locked STL, or polygon file format (PLY) files. The projecting light detects three points of interest (POI) on the surface of the scanned tooth surface. The similarity of the images captured by the intraoral scanner is determined by matching coinciding points of interest. The recorded images are compiled using specific software to reproduce natural-looking tissue displayed on the computer as a 3D images [27, 28].

Various intraoral scanners are available today in the market, differing in their technology used for data collection. Such technologies my include active wavefront used by LAVA C.O.S. (3M ESPE, St. Paul, MN, USA) and Lava True Definition scanner (3M ESPE), active triangulation, and optical microscopy used by CEREC AC Bluecam (Sirona Dental System GmBH, Bensheim, Germany) and CEREC AC Omnicam (Sirona Dental System GmBH); confocal technology used by iTero (Invisalign; Cadent Inc, Or-Yehuda, Israel) and 3Shape Trios (Copenhagen, Denmark); and projected pattern triangulation technology used by Planmeca Emerald (Helsinki, Finland) (**Figure 5.2**). The difference between these technologies is based on the distance-to-object technologies of each camera [28].

5.3.1.3 Software

Regardless of the technology used, all digital scanners produce a 3D cast by capturing and compiling multiple images from the oral cavity. The compiling process is created by a best-fit alignment in which a series of errors may arise and compromise accuracy [11]. Scanners generate a digital copy of the teeth and surrounding tissues in a standard tessellation language (STL) format, either open or locked, Wave-front Object file (OBJ), and Stanford Triangle format, or in the format language specially released by the developer company [29] (**Figure 5.3**).

5.3.2 Advantages of 3D Scanning and Digital Impressions

5.3.2.1 Immediate Visualization

Some of the errors that dental practitioners may encounter during the conventional impression are presence of defective impressions that failed to capture full details of the impression area. This drawback can be eliminated when using digital intraoral impression (scanning) instead of the conventional impression. A previsualization of the scanned area and the possibility of immediate rescanning provide a superior digital impression compared to conventional impression [10].

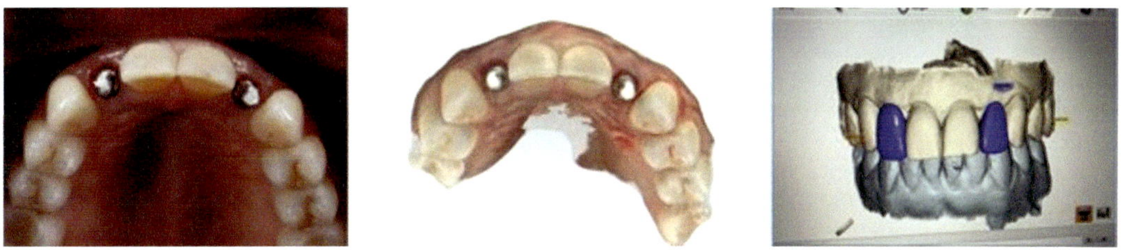

(a) (b) (c)

Figure 5.3 Prepared implant abutments (a), digitally scanned dental arch with the prepared abutment (b), and designed restorations using CAD/CAM software (c). (Courtesy of Prof. Sompop Bencharit.)

Furthermore, the possibility of immediate visualization of the definitive fixed prosthodontic design (digital wax-up or mock-up) is possible in the case of digital impression with a full chairside digital fixed prosthodontic workflow [13].

5.3.2.2 Time Required for the Impression

The time require to capture the final impression in fixed prosthodontics is critical. Digital impression showed that it is a faster technique compared to conventional impression. Usually, digital impression may take between 4–15 minutes to complete full arch scanning [28]. However, several variations were reported in the literature according to the type of intraoral scanning device used and the scan area. Overall, several factors may influence the time, such as operator skill, type and technology of the scanning machine used, the scan area, and scanning path [12].

Furthermore, digital impression was found to have a lower mean of reimpression (rescanning) time compared to conventional impression. However, the number of reimpressions was found to be higher in digital impression. This may be due to ability of the dental practitioners to easily rescan the missed area compared to complete redoing the entire conventional impression [10].

5.3.2.3 Comfort

According to several studies that evaluated the overall impression and discomfort, dentists and patients reported greater comfort and less difficulty with digital impression techniques than with conventional impression techniques [12, 30]. The frequent parameters reported by the patients that favor digital impression were: Bad taste resulting from conventional impression materials and more comfortable, less invasive impression techniques, especially in patients with a gag reflex or excessive salivation [27]. However, powdering of the scanned surface in the older intraoral scanning systems was found to be one factor that reduced patient comfort during digital impression [31].

5.3.2.4 Accuracy

The accuracy of impression is very critical in the success of fixed prosthodontic work as it will determine the final fit of the casted restoration in the prepared tooth/teeth. According to Aly and Mohsen [32], accuracy is defined as "the sum of the trueness and the precision in which trueness is defined as the closeness of agreement between the expectation of a test result or a measurement result and a true value"; whereas precision can be considered the "closeness of agreement between indications or measured quantity values obtained by replicate measurements on the same objects under specified conditions." The measurement becomes more predictable as the precision increases. Trueness, on the other hand, describes how close the measurements are to the true dimensions of the measured tooth surface [9].

In fixed prosthodontics, the trueness as for the restorative marginal accuracy is one of the important parameters that should be carefully evaluated before seating of final restoration into the prepared tooth, since any marginal discrepancy can result in a marginal gap, which in turn can lead to increased postoperative sensitivity, loss of luting cements, plaque retention, secondary caries, periodontal disease, and eventually loss of restoration [16]. The marginal discrepancies of digitally fabricated restoration such as crowns, fixed partial dentures, or veneers, showed superior accuracy compared to conventional fabricated restorations [16, 33]. Furthermore, there was no statistical difference in the marginal discrepancy of restoration fabricated using intraoral scanners compared to extraoral scanners [34].

5.4 DIGITAL CASTS AND DIES

Conventional gypsum casts and dies had in the past been considered the gold standard for the construction of fixed prostheses [35]. They have the advantages of being inexpensive, quick and easy to produce, and dimensionally accurate. However, they have many disadvantages, including poor abrasion resistance, the need for careful handling of the impressions, the need for storage space for resultant models, the cost of laboratory fabrication and transfer, and possible dimensional changes over time [36].

The application of digital technology in dentistry introduced the use of digital/virtual casts and dies [37]. Digital casts facilitate diagnosis, treatment planning, visualization, and fabrication of the final restoration without the need for conventional casts or dies [35]. The advantages of digital models include the ability to digitally manipulate the casts, the ability to share them easily with other dental professionals and laboratories, and no need for storage space. Moreover, digital casts or dies can be printed on demand to produce physical models. The 3D printed models are resilient and save time and laboratory costs compared to conventional models [36].

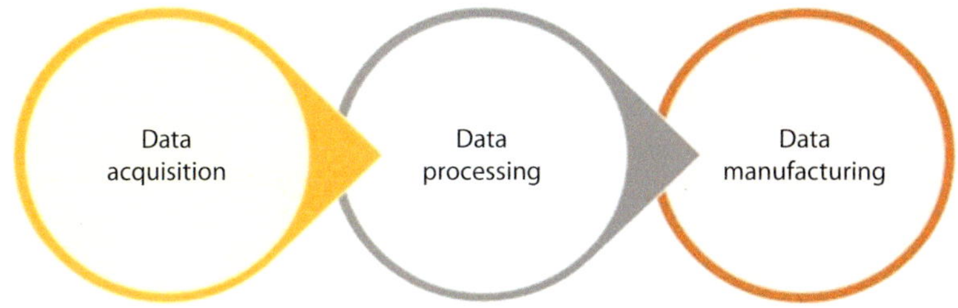

Figure 5.4 Flowchart showing the process of digital cast and die fabrication.

5.4.1 Fabrication of Digital Casts and Dies

The process of fabricating digital casts and dies involves data acquisition, data processing, and data manufacturing (**Figure 5.4**).

5.4.1.1 Data Acquisition

Different types of 3D image files are used to save direct and indirect scans. STL files are among the most commonly used within the field of digital dentistry [12]. They provides information regarding the geometry of the scanned object, but it does not include texture and/or shade [12].

5.4.1.2 Data Processing

After the acquisition, 3D image files can be imported into design software. The design software allows manipulating, editing, and designing for the virtual model and/or the final restorations [12]. Virtual models reproduce the shape and volume of the arches, as well as the occlusal contacts [38]. Moreover, they allow digitalizing the static and/or the dynamic jaw relation by replacing conventional articulators with virtual articulators [38, 39].

5.4.1.3 Data Manufacturing

The last step is manufacturing of a digital model (**Figure 5.5**). Despite the benefits of digital models, there is still a need to fabricate physical models for many clinical and laboratory procedures [40]. There are currently two methods to fabricate physical models from digital ones: Additive manufacturing (AM) and subtractive manufacturing (SM) [36, 40]. Although AM is widely used in dental model construction, both methods can produce models that possess high strength and good abrasion resistance.

Errors in printed models can affect the accuracy of occlusion evaluation and/or the final prosthesis. Previous studies investigated the accuracy of 3D printed dental models compared to the conventional and digital models and also investigated the accuracy of various 3D printing technologies [35, 40]. While the current 3D printed dental casts may have lower accuracy compared to conventional casts, additive manufacturing has rapidly evolved. Although there were some differences found regarding trueness and precision, the 3D printed models were within the clinically acceptable accuracy [36, 41, 42]. Other factors that may affect the accuracy of printed models include the type of resin used, printing angle, layer thickness, temperature, the shape of the printed model, and if the model is printed as filled or hollow [40].

5.4.1.4 Virtual Dental Patient

The development of digital procedures in dentistry is used to transfer patient data and construct the virtual dental patient. Digital data includes digital photography, intraoral and facial scanners, jaw motion analyzer, and cone beam computed tomography (CBCT). The virtual dental patient integrates all the patient's digital data into one software. The advantages of the application of the virtual dental patient include increased predictability and accuracy of treatment, simplifying the clinical evaluation and prosthesis adjustment, and improving aesthetic outcomes [43].

5.5 COMPUTER AIDED DESIGN AND COMPUTER AIDED MANUFACTURING (CAD/CAM) SYSTEM

In the early 1970s, the first CAD/CAM system was introduced by developing an instrument that uses an optical technology to develop an intraoral grid surface mapping system [44]. In 1971, Francois Duret developed the first CAD/CAM system (Sopha® system) [45], followed by Mormann, W. H, who developed the CEREC® system as the first chairside dental CAD/CAM system that uses an intraoral

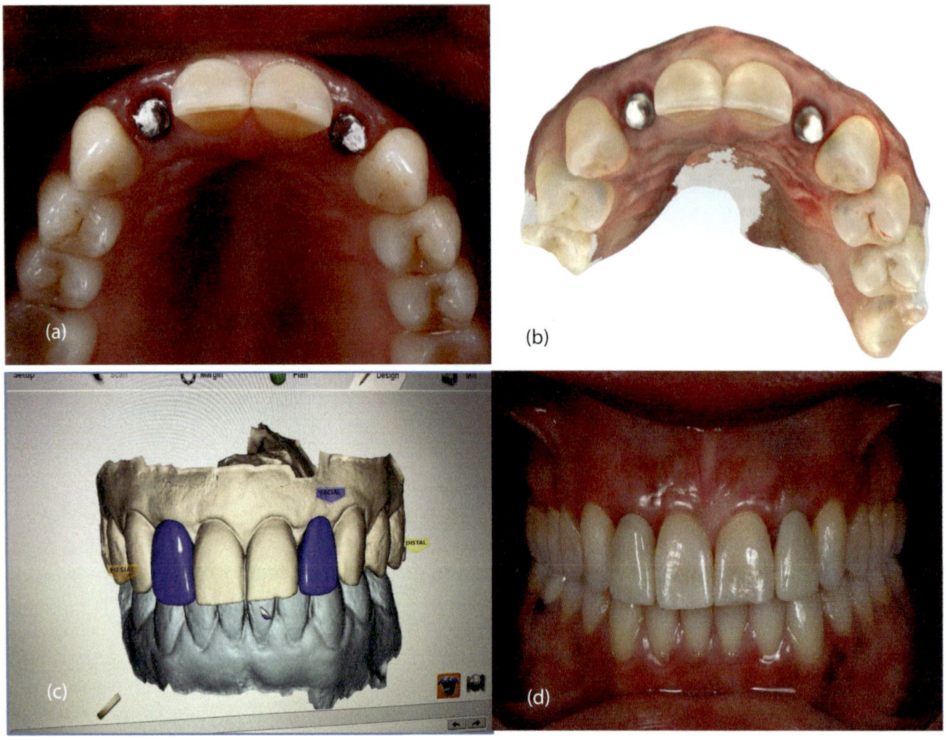

Figure 5.5 Workflow of CAD/CAM system, Prepared implant abutments (12 and 22) (a). Intraoral scanned prepared implant abutments showing a digital cast (b). Digitally designed definitive crowns (c). Definitive crowns in the mouth (d). (Courtesy of Prof. Sompop Bencharit.)

scanner, which provides the benefit of delivering the restoration on the same day as the tooth prepared [46]. Procera®, developed by Dr. Andersson, was the market's third developed system [47]. CAD/CAM systems are currently available in the dental market in a variety of configurations.

The CAD/CAM technology has revolutionized the field of dentistry, offering precise, efficient, and aesthetically pleasing solutions for dental restorations. CAD/CAM systems have become an integral part of the digital workflow in fixed prosthodontics, allowing dental professionals to create highly accurate and customized prosthetic restorations.

The CAD/CAM systems basic workflow (**Figure 5.5**) consists of three steps: Data capture, design, and manufacturing. Data capture is the first step in the CAD/CAM workflow. Using an intraoral or extraoral scanner, the prepared tooth is virtually scanned and captured, and the data is converted into digital numerical data. The numerical data is then processed to be displayed as a virtual tooth on a computer.

The second step is to design the desired restoration (full coverage crown, inlay, onlay, veneer, or fixed partial denture) virtually using specialized CAD software. This software enables virtual carving and shaping of the desired anatomical shape of the final restoration on a computer. Following the completion of the desired design, the restoration will be in the form of a virtual model, which can be transferred to a solid restoration under certain commands.

The final step is to manufacture the digitally CAM-designed restoration by sending the design to a milling machine (processing machine) (**Figure 5.6**) to carve the final design into a final restoration. Earlier milling machines used diamond burs to cut a prefabricated ceramic or zirconia block or discs into the designed shape.

The introduction of CAD/CAM technology provided several advantages in fixed prosthodontic fabrication compared to traditional method. These advantages include:

a. When compared to traditional impression techniques, this technique produces a faster impression with fewer technical errors.

b. Ability to design and fabricate a full coverage crown in few minutes.

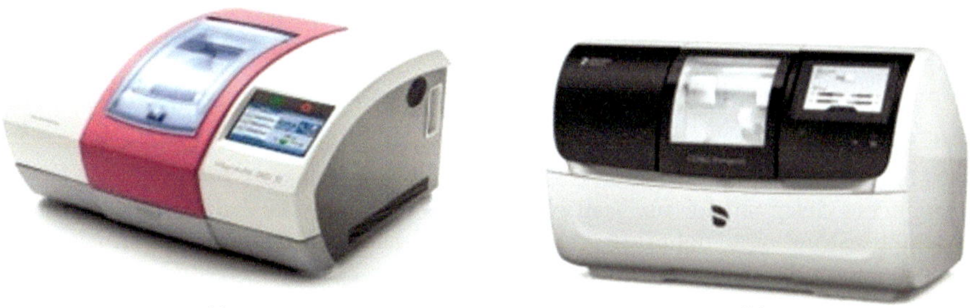

(a) (b)

Figure 5.6 CAD/CAM milling Systems: (a) PlanMill 30S. (By permission of Planmeca.) (b) CEREC Primemill. (By permission of Dentsply Serona.)

c. Reducing the number of appointments required by the patient to one to deliver the final restoration.
d. No need for provisional restoration.
e. Excellent accuracy, marginal adaptation, and marginal discrepancy.
f. Better aesthetic because CAD/CAM ceramic blocks provide superior translucency when compared to ceramic restorations fabricated using traditional techniques.

There are numerous CAD/CAM systems on the market today. As previously stated, CEREC® is one of the first chairside CAD/CAM systems, and it continues to improve its software and special ceramic blocks. According to the manufacturer, the most recent CEREC system comes with software that displays a virtual articulator and allows the practitioner to design the fixed restoration in static and dynamic positions to achieve optimal functional occlusion. It is supported by two types of intraoral scanners (Primescan and Omnicam), each with a different tip that allows for a full mouth scan as well as the ability to scan shiny surfaces and deep cavities for teeth prepared for inlays and onlays. The CEREC system, as one of the chairside CAD/CAM systems, is supported by a fast-milling machine (CEREC Primemill) that allows milling of zirconia and ceramic blocks in five minutes. This is due to the various burs used by this system, which range from milling to finishing burs. Also compatible with the CEREC system are dental ceramic material blocks such as glass ceramic blocks, zirconia ceramic blocks, feldspar ceramic blocks, and CEREC guide blocks.

The inLab CAD/CAM system (Dentsply Sirona, USA) is another CAD/CAM system that is based on an extraoral scanner. According to the manufacturer, the most recent version of this system has an extraoral scanner (inEos X5) that can scan impressions, dental casts, and multi-dies, both in arches and in occlusion, and provide detailed texture scans. The scanned surface is then transferred to inLab CAD software, which supports a variety of designs such as crown and bridge work, removable prosthodontic work, and implant prosthetics. The designed restoration is then transferred to a milling machine (MC X5) to mill and carve ceramic discs or blocks according to the designed restoration. There are also milling burs available in a variety of shapes and sizes to provide a final restoration.

Another CAD/CAM system on the market today is the Planmeca Romexis® CAD/CAM system (Planmeca OY, Finland). The prepared teeth are captured and scanned using an intraoral scanner (Planmeca Emerald® S), which is also available with different tip options and sizes. The captured and scanned tooth is transferred to Planmeca CAD/CAM software. The Planmeca Romexis CAD/CAM system includes three software packages. The first is Planmeca Romexis® CAD/CAM for scanning, analyzing digital impressions, and sharing scans with others. The second software is Planmeca PlanCAD Easy, which supports intraoral scanners and the design of various restorations. The third software is Planmeca PlanCAD premium, which supports advanced designs such as monolithic restorations, anatomical coping and coping restorations, wax-up designs, and telescopic crowns. Planmeca's CAD/CAM system includes three milling machines: The Planmeca PlanMill® 30 s, the Planmeca PlanMill® 35, and the Planmeca PlanMill® 60 s. This variety in milling machines enables both dry and wet milling, as well as simultaneous milling of multiple and complex units.

The iTero CAD/CAM system was introduced in 2007. Unlike other intraoral scanners that capture images through triangulation, the iTero system's intraoral scanner captures images through parallel confocal red laser light directed at the prepared teeth and converts the reflected light into digital data. According to the manufacturer, the iTero scanners support the design of various restorative and prosthodontic procedures because they are an open system, allowing them to work with different CAD/CAM software and milling machines from different companies.

5.6 CAD/CAM BLOCKS

CAD/CAM blocks play a pivotal role in this process. These blocks are prefabricated materials with specific properties designed for use with CAD/CAM systems. They are used to fabricate a wide range of dental restorations, including crowns, fixed partial dentures, inlays, onlays, and implant-supported prostheses. By utilizing CAD/CAM blocks, dental laboratories and clinicians can streamline the fabrication process and achieve consistent and reliable results.

The advantages of CAD/CAM blocks are numerous. They offer superior aesthetics, allowing for highly natural-looking dental restorations that closely resemble natural teeth. The ability to choose from a variety of shades and translucency levels allows for customized restorations that blend seamlessly with the patient's dentition. The blocks are available in a wide range of shades and translucency levels, enabling clinicians to closely match the color and optical properties of natural teeth. This results in restorations that seamlessly blend with the patient's dentition, enhancing overall aesthetics and patient satisfaction [48].

One of the key advantages of CAD/CAM blocks is their ability to provide a precise fit. The digital workflow ensures accurate intraoral scanning, eliminating the potential errors associated with traditional impression-taking. The CAD software enables clinicians to design restorations with exceptional marginal accuracy, resulting in minimal adjustments during the seating process. CAD/CAM blocks provide excellent marginal accuracy, ensuring a precise fit and reducing the need for adjustments during the seating process. This precise fit enhances restoration longevity, reduces the risk of microleakage, and promotes optimal oral health. This leads to improved patient satisfaction and reduces chairside time [49].

Another advantage of CAD/CAM blocks is the increased efficiency and productivity CAD/CAM technology offers. With traditional methods, the fabrication process involves multiple steps, including impression-taking, stone model preparation, and manual restoration creation. CAD/CAM technology eliminates many of these labor-intensive steps, resulting in faster turnaround times for both dental laboratories and clinicians [50].

CAD/CAM technology enables customization and patient-specific restorations. With the ability to digitally design and modify restorations, clinicians can create personalized solutions tailored to the unique anatomical characteristics and functional requirements of each patient. This customization extends beyond shape and size to include factors like occlusal anatomy, surface texture, and material selection. Patient-specific restorations lead to improved comfort, function, and overall treatment outcomes. Furthermore, CAD/CAM technology facilitates the storage and retrieval of digital records, enhancing communication and collaboration between dental professionals. Digital files can be easily shared, reviewed, and transferred, eliminating the need for physical transportation of models or restorations [1, 51].

The digital workflow eliminates the need for traditional model preparation, stone pouring, and manual waxing. Digital scanning and CAD software streamline the design process, reducing labor-intensive tasks. Additionally, the milling process for CAD/CAM blocks is automated and can be completed in a relatively short time. This improved efficiency allows for faster turnaround times, enabling dental laboratories to handle a higher volume of cases while maintaining high-quality standards. The streamlined communication process saves time and reduces the risk of errors or misplacements. Furthermore, digital records provide a valuable resource for long-term patient management and follow-up care [1].

However, this technology presents with some disadvantages. For instance, while CAD/CAM blocks offer a wide range of shade options, the available translucency levels may be limited compared to the variations found in natural teeth. This can affect the overall aesthetics of the restoration, particularly in cases where high translucency is desired. While manufacturers offer a variety of shades, achieving an exact match to the patient's adjacent teeth can sometimes be challenging, especially in cases requiring high translucency. This limitation may result in restorations that do not perfectly mimic the natural appearance of the surrounding dentition, which can be a concern for some patients [52].

Additionally, although CAD/CAM blocks have significantly improved in terms of strength and durability, certain materials may still present challenges in terms of wear resistance and long-term performance. With CAD/CAM there may exist a compromise in material strength, wear resistance, and long-term durability with certain types of blocks. For instance, while ceramic and hybrid blocks offer good mechanical strength and durability, other materials like resin or composite blocks may be more prone to wear and staining over time. Additionally, some CAD/CAM blocks may exhibit lower fracture resistance or compromised longevity compared to alternative materials used in conventional laboratory fabrication. Careful consideration is necessary when selecting the most suitable CAD/CAM block for each clinical scenario, taking into account functional requirements and long-term durability expectations [53].

It is important to note that the disadvantages of CAD/CAM blocks should be considered in the context of their overall benefits. Manufacturers continually strive to address these limitations by improving the materials and expanding the available options. Additionally, advancements in digital technology and materials research may lead to future innovations that mitigate or overcome these drawbacks.

The integration of CAD/CAM technology in dental practices requires dental professionals to develop new skills and undergo additional training. Proficiency in digital scanning, CAD software, and CAM milling techniques is essential for harnessing the full potential of CAD/CAM blocks. Dental professionals need to adapt their knowledge and workflows to accommodate the digital process. While technology offers efficiency gains, it necessitates an investment of time and resources to acquire and maintain the necessary skills. Continuous learning and staying updated with advancements in CAD/CAM technology are crucial for successful implementation.

The selection of a particular CAD/CAM block is important in relation to specific patient needs, restoration location, and aesthetic requirements. By understanding the limitations associated with CAD/CAM blocks, clinicians can make informed decisions, manage patient expectations, and select the most suitable materials and techniques for successful dental restorations.

5.7 CAD/CAM MATERIALS

Nowadays, a large number of CAD/CAM blocks are available and newer materials are introduced into the market at a rapid rate. Dental professionals are faced with a complex decision process when choosing a restorative material for a particular indication. The evolution of CAD/CAM materials mainly involves ceramics, resins and hybrid materials, resin-ceramic materials, or resin glass materials.

5.7.1 Ceramic Blocks

Ceramic CAD/CAM blocks are widely used in dentistry due to their excellent aesthetics and biocompatibility. They are composed of densely sintered ceramic materials, such as lithium disilicate or zirconia (**Figure 5.7**). Ceramic blocks offer high translucency, allowing for natural-looking restorations that closely mimic the optical properties of natural teeth. They exhibit good mechanical strength, durability, and resistance to wear [54]. Ceramic blocks find applications in various dental restorations, including single crowns, veneers, inlays, onlays, and short-span fixed partial dentures.

Generally, dental ceramics used in CAD/CAM technology can be divided into three classes, based on their microstructure namely, predominantly glassy ceramics, particle-filled glasses, and polycrystalline ceramics [55]. With predominately glassy ceramics, this glassy matrix permits the diffusion of light for translucency. However, mechanical properties decrease with the fragile glass phase [56]; hence, filler particles are added to the base glass to improve mechanical properties, such as strength, thermal expansion, and contraction behavior [57]. Within the glassy matrix, the nature of filler prevents the development of micro-fractures and is responsible for crack deflection, contact shielding and crack bridging.

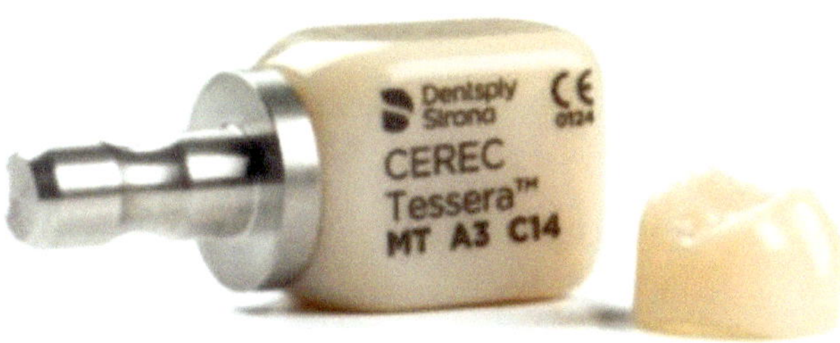

Figure 5.7 Lithium disilicate-based CAD/CAM blocks. (CEREC Tessera; by permission of Dentsply Sirona.)

While ceramics have overall superior mechanical and aesthetic properties, resin-composite materials offer advantages related to their ease of milling and the ability to repair defects or fractures intraorally. However, their main disadvantage is their inferior strength and aesthetic properties [58]. Ceramics on the other hand are stronger but more brittle and therefore, making them susceptible to chipping failure in the presence of any natural flaws within the material itself. Clinical durability of ceramics is highly related to their brittleness; most ceramic restorations fail because of crack propagation due to the material brittleness. Furthermore, microcracks can be introduced by the actual milling process as well, leading to long-term failure. Both natural flaws and machining flaws can act as failure origins [59]. Chipping of the veneering ceramic on zirconia restorations continues to be a problem [60].

Aesthetic properties of these CAD/CAM materials are largely defined by the glassy matrix [56], and predominantly glassy materials are best able to mimic the optical properties of enamel and dentine [55]. Since dental ceramics that best mimic the optical properties of enamel and dentin have a high glass content [57], it seems logical that technological advances in material science can advance the properties of a glassy matrix through the improvement of strength without compromising the aesthetic properties.

5.7.2 Resin Blocks

Resin CAD/CAM blocks, also known as composite blocks, are composed of a resin matrix filled with a mixture of ceramic or glass particles. They offer a good balance of strength, aesthetics, and ease of use. Resin blocks provide excellent color stability, allowing for long-lasting restorations with minimal discoloration over time. They are suitable for fabricating inlays, onlays, veneers, and provisional restorations. However, resin blocks may be more prone to wear and staining compared to ceramic blocks, making them less suitable for posterior load-bearing restorations [61, 62].

5.7.3 Zirconia Blocks

Zirconia CAD/CAM blocks are made from a crystalline form of zirconium dioxide (**Figure 5.8**). They are renowned for their exceptional mechanical properties, including high strength, fracture resistance, and biocompatibility. Zirconia blocks provide excellent durability, making them ideal for fabricating posterior crowns and bridges subjected to heavy occlusal forces. However, their potential high opacity may limit their aesthetic applications to nonvisible areas or cases where high strength is a priority over translucency [63]. Newer layered zirconia blocks with longer sintering time may provide better aesthetics.

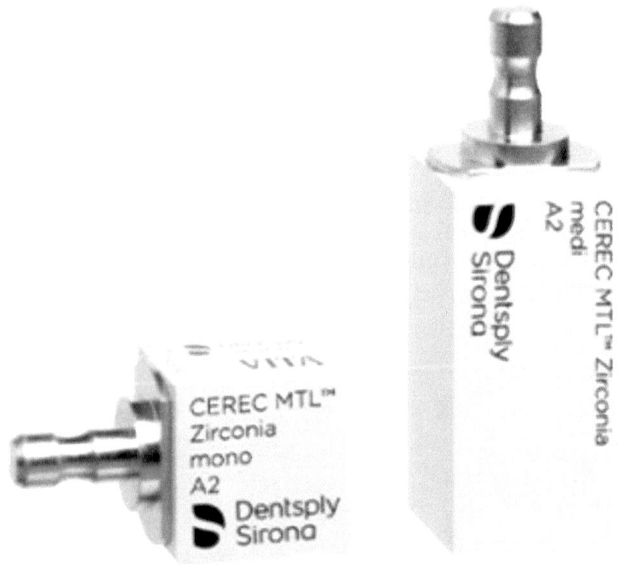

Figure 5.8 Zirconium base CAD/CAM blocks. (CEREC MTL Zirconia mono; by permission of Dentsply Sirona.)

5.7.4 Polymethyl Methacrylate (PMMA) CAD/CAM Blocks

Polymethyl methacrylate (PMMA) CAD/CAM blocks are temporary materials commonly used in dentistry. They are often employed for the fabrication of provisional restorations, temporary crowns, and diagnostic mock-ups. PMMA blocks offer ease of milling, good aesthetics, and satisfactory mechanical properties for short-term use. However, they lack the long-term durability and strength required for permanent restorations [64].

5.7.5 Hybrid Blocks

Hybrid CAD/CAM blocks combine the advantages of both ceramic and resin materials. They consist of a composite resin matrix infused with ceramic or glass fillers. Hybrid blocks offer improved mechanical properties compared to pure resin blocks, such as enhanced strength and fracture resistance. They provide excellent aesthetics and are commonly used for fabricating posterior restorations, including crowns and bridges. The hybrid composition allows for efficient milling while maintaining good color stability and wear resistance [65]. A variation of this hybrid type of block is from the manufacturer Edelweiss Dentistry (Wolfurt, Austria) that was recently introduced as a CAD/CAM block with a homogenous base material consisting of single glass phase (**Figure 5.9**). This is produced through a controlled laser sintering technology fusing the glass crystals. The finished glass product is characterized by a single-phase glass crystal that is embedded in a resin matrix. The Edelweiss CAD/CAM block is mainly composed of silica and barium glass with a very small portion. It also contains zinc oxide and fluoride for added antibacterial properties, a unique feature of the Edelweiss CAD/CAM material. According to the manufacturer, the optical properties are similar to those of predominately glass ceramics without the brittleness of the ceramics but maintain flexibility. This block belongs to a different class of materials, namely a hybrid glass block.

Thus, there is a wide variety of CAD/CAM blocks available on the dental market consisting of different types of materials that may vary in size, color, strength, and aesthetics with varying translucence and chromacity, and they may or may not require a post-milling treatment. Due to this large number of CAD/CAM materials available and the speed at which newer materials are being introduced, dental clinicians today face a difficult decision when choosing a CAD/CAM restorative material for a specific clinical indication. Nowadays, manufacturers suggest having more than 20 blocks available for chairside use [56] as both strength and aesthetics necessitate the need to have a variety of blocks in one's inventory. It may seem logical, therefore, to have blocks that can combine both strength and aesthetics into a single block. Edelweiss CAD/CAM blocks, for instance, through their latest laser sintered hybrid glass technology, make use of this concept of having a single translucent block that mimics the translucency of enamel while the underlying dentin shade can then be duplicated through the use of various resin composite/cement shades. Through this process of laser sintering, together with high temperature and pressure, the mechanical properties of the material have improved, giving the material a combination of resilience (principal property of the dentine) and resistance to wear (property attributed to the enamel). According to the manufacturer, its flexibility lies in its manufacturing process.

The composition of Edelweiss CAD/CAM blocks is mainly silicate glass, zinc oxide nanoparticles, aluminum oxide, and fluoride. According to the manufacturer, there is no need for any further silane/primer addition as the bond occurs with the silica present in the Edelweiss CAD/CAM material together with the Edelweiss composite, which acts as the luting cement. The addition of

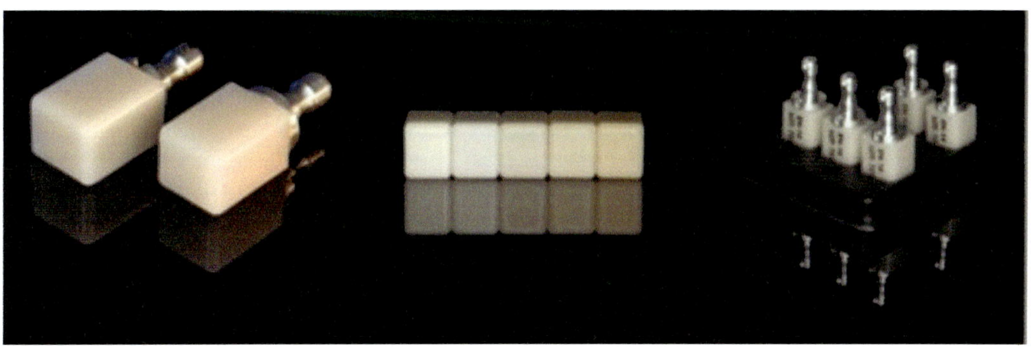

Figure 5.9 Hybrid CAD/CAM blocks. (By permission of Edelweiss Dentistry, Wolfurt, Austria.)

zinc oxide nanoparticles provides antibacterial properties, preventing any plaque accumulation on the surface of the material. Fluoride enables possible hydroxyapatite regeneration, if required. The addition of zinc oxide and fluoride is unique to the edelweiss CAD/CAM blocks. Aluminum oxide provides additional strength and improves the optical properties of the CAD/CAM block.

Color matching of a restoration to the adjacent teeth can at times be difficult due to the translucency of the ceramic and the visual exposure of the polymerized resin luting cement through the ceramic material [66]. Some hybrid CAD/CAM blocks, such as Edelweiss blocks, use luting cements similar to their composition, thus alleviating any visual exposure of the cement/restoration through the restoration or at the interface finish line. With such systems, resin composites of varying opacities can be used to color-match the restoration with adjacent teeth. In addition, some translucent blocks such as Edelweiss T Blocks (Translucent) mimic the enamel translucency. Different brightness effects of the tooth can be reproduced with the availability of opacity shades of the resin cement. Furthermore, clinicians are now in control of the final aesthetic outcome by being able to adjust both internal and external characterizations chairside according to the patient's needs, thereby eliminating any errors of miscommunication between the clinician and dental technician.

Partially sintered (no resin) CAD/CAM blocks have the disadvantage of ill-fitting final restoration because of the extensive sintering shrinkage that may occur during the post-sintering process [67]. Being of a homogenous crystalline glass phase, Edelweiss CAD/CAM blocks do not require any further post-sintering process, hence the advantage of a superior fit where no shrinkage is involved in the processing.

5.7.6 Comparison of CAD/CAM Materials

Understanding the composition and properties of these CAD/CAM blocks allows dental professionals to choose the most appropriate material for different clinical scenarios. Factors such as restoration location, functional requirements, and patient preferences should be considered when selecting the optimal block type for crowns, fixed partial dentures, and implant-supported prostheses. By selecting the right CAD/CAM block, clinicians can achieve restorations that offer a harmonious blend of aesthetics, functionality, and longevity, ultimately contributing to improved patient satisfaction and oral health outcomes.

Different CAD/CAM blocks exhibit variations in mechanical properties, such as strength, fracture resistance, and wear resistance. Ceramic and hybrid blocks, particularly those based on lithium disilicate or zirconia, offer excellent mechanical strength and durability. They are known for their high fracture resistance, making them suitable for posterior restorations subjected to heavy occlusal forces [68]. However, ceramics are brittle in thin sections and therefore need to be milled with at least 0.4 mm margins [69]. Ceramics also require extensive tooth preparations and need to incorporate resistance and retention forms into the preparation design. Zirconia blocks may be considered too strong and when used over implants may cause fracture of implant screws. Resin and composite blocks also possess satisfactory mechanical properties, but they may have comparatively lower wear resistance than ceramic-based blocks. Hybrid blocks like the edelweiss CAD/CAM blocks have strength similar to ceramics without the brittleness, making them ideal when used in minimal invasive preparations [53].

CAD/CAM blocks vary in their ability to provide natural-looking aesthetics. Ceramic blocks, such as lithium disilicate, offer superior aesthetics with high translucency and color-matching capabilities. They closely mimic the optical properties of natural teeth, resulting in restorations that blend seamlessly with the surrounding dentition. Zirconia blocks may appear to be opaque and hence may be used more in the posterior regions. Hybrid blocks, composed of a resin matrix infused with ceramic fillers, also provide good aesthetics while offering improved strength and fracture resistance. Resin and composite blocks offer satisfactory aesthetics but may exhibit limitations in terms of long-term color stability and staining resistance [70].

Studies comparing the performance of different CAD/CAM blocks have investigated various aspects of clinical outcomes. Fracture resistance is an important consideration, especially for posterior restorations. Research has shown that ceramic and hybrid blocks, particularly zirconia-based blocks, exhibit higher fracture resistance compared to resin and composite blocks [68, 71]. Marginal fit, which influences restoration longevity and the risk of microleakage, has also been evaluated. Ceramic and hybrid blocks tend to demonstrate better marginal fit compared to resin and composite blocks [72]. Surface finish, including smoothness and roughness, affects plaque accumulation and the overall aesthetics of restorations. Studies have shown that ceramic and hybrid blocks generally exhibit superior surface finish compared to resin and composite blocks. The hybrid glass blocks exhibit a gloss-like surface mainly because of their homogenous glass layers [73].

5.8 SELECTION OF CAD/CAM BLOCKS

The performance of CAD/CAM blocks can vary depending on multiple factors, including block material, milling technique, restoration design, and cementation protocol. Furthermore, the success of a CAD/CAM restoration depends not only on the block itself but also on the clinician's skill in designing and seating the restoration. To make informed decisions regarding CAD/CAM block selection, clinicians should consider the specific requirements of each case, including the location of the restoration, functional demands, aesthetic considerations, and patient factors. Keeping up with the latest research and clinical studies can provide valuable insights into the comparative performance of different CAD/CAM blocks and aid in the selection of the most suitable block for optimal clinical outcomes.

The location of the restoration is an important clinical factor when selecting CAD/CAM blocks. For posterior restorations exposed to higher occlusal forces, materials with excellent mechanical properties like ceramic or hybrid glass blocks, particularly zirconia-based blocks, are often preferred. These blocks offer enhanced strength and fracture resistance, making them suitable for load-bearing areas. In contrast, for anterior restorations where aesthetics play a crucial role, blocks with superior translucency and color-matching capabilities like ceramic blocks are typically chosen [74]. The magnitude and direction of occlusal forces exerted on the restoration should be considered when selecting CAD/CAM blocks. Restorations in areas with heavy occlusal forces require materials with high strength and durability, such as ceramic or hybrid glass blocks. These blocks can withstand the masticatory forces and minimize the risk of fracture or wear. On the other hand, restorations in areas with less occlusal forces may allow for the use of materials like resin or composite blocks, which offer satisfactory mechanical properties while providing acceptable aesthetics.

Each patient has unique needs and expectations that should be taken into account when selecting CAD/CAM blocks. Factors such as the patient's oral health, occlusal habits, aesthetic preferences, and financial considerations should be considered. Some patients may prioritize aesthetics, while others may prioritize durability or cost-effectiveness. Customization options offered by CAD/CAM blocks, such as shade matching and material selection, allow clinicians to tailor restorations to the individual patient's requirements. Hybrid glass blocks (Edelweiss Dentistry) can be milled to 0.2 mm margins, hence promoting gingival health and aesthetically superiority because margins are almost invisible.

Material selection is crucial for achieving optimal outcomes with CAD/CAM blocks. Different materials offer varying mechanical properties, aesthetics, and durability. Clinicians should carefully evaluate the advantages and disadvantages of each material, considering factors such as strength, wear resistance, fracture resistance, and aesthetic properties. The selection should be based on the specific clinical requirements, restoration location, and patient factors. It is important to stay updated with the latest research and clinical evidence regarding the performance of different materials to make informed decisions.

Achieving aesthetic harmony between CAD/CAM restorations and natural dentition requires careful shade matching and surface characterization. Clinicians should consider the color, translucency, and texture of the surrounding teeth when selecting CAD/CAM blocks. A comprehensive understanding of shade selection principles and techniques is essential to achieve seamless integration and natural aesthetics. Additionally, surface characterization techniques, such as staining, glazing, or polishing, can further enhance the aesthetic outcome by replicating the surface characteristics of natural teeth. The hybrid glass block offers superior aesthetics because of its glass-like nature and can easily be characterized.

By considering the restoration location, occlusal forces, patient-specific needs, material selection, shade matching, and surface characterization, clinicians can make informed decisions regarding the selection of CAD/CAM blocks. This comprehensive approach ensures that the chosen blocks are suitable for the clinical situation, provide the desired aesthetics, and deliver long-lasting, functional restorations that meet the specific needs of each patient.

5.9 DIGITAL WORKFLOW IN FIXED PROSTHODONTICS

A 40-year-old male patient (ASA 1) presented with discolored teeth and old defective restorations, and he felt that the old crowns looked too yellowish. The patient desired to restore his aesthetics. Clinically, he presented with defective restorations, insignificant loss of vertical dimension of occlusion (VDO) and compromised aesthetics (**Figure 5.10a**).

There were signs of loss of enamel on the labial surfaces of most of the teeth. The preoperative radiograph was within acceptable limits. In spite of the overall condition, the natural teeth were free

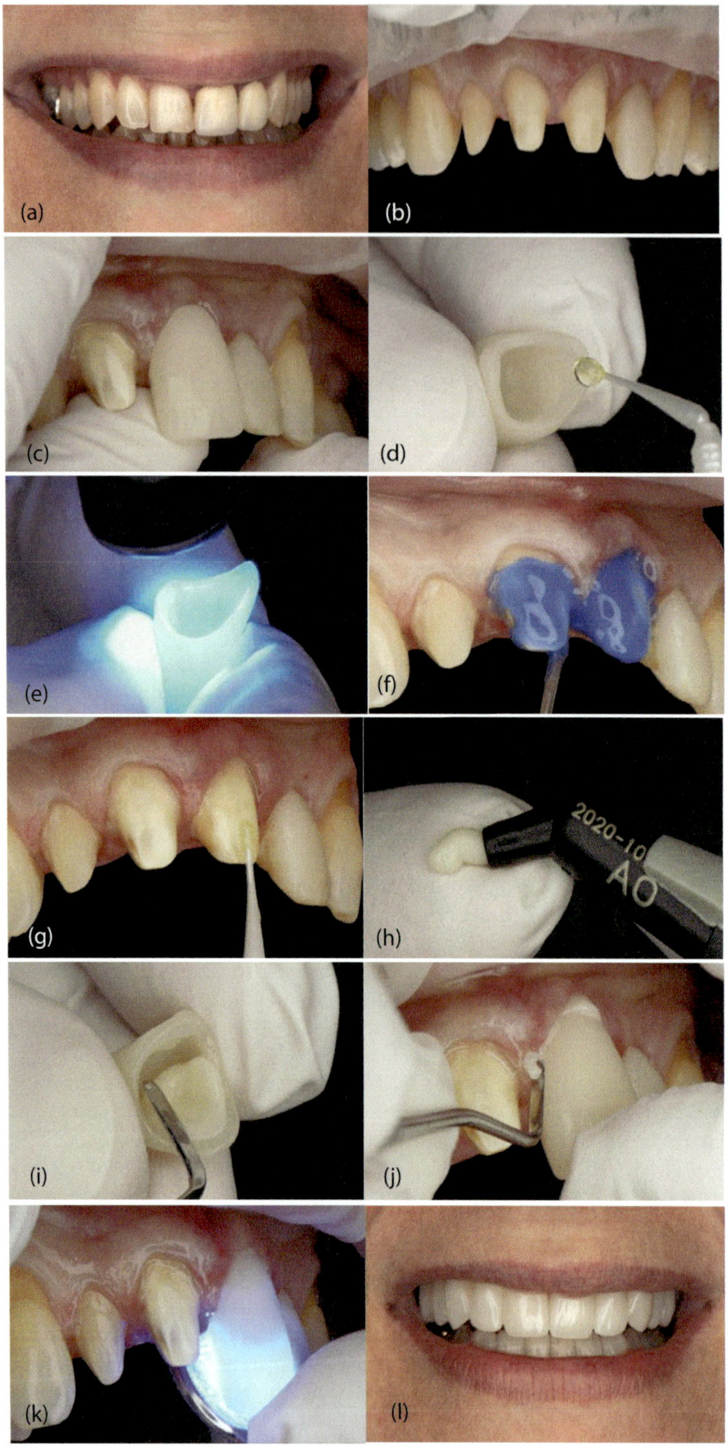

Figure 5.10 Preoperative frontal view revealing old crowns and unsightly buccal lesions (a). Teeth prepared with finish lines at gingival level (b). Try-in of the crown to assess the accuracy of the fit (c). Application of Edelweiss Bond to the inner surface of the crown (d). Light curing of Edelweiss Bond for 10 seconds (e). Teeth etched with 37% phosphoric acid for 15 seconds (f). Application of dentine bonding agent on to etched surfaces of teeth (g). Appropriate color of composite selected (h). Composite spread evenly onto the fitting surface crown (i). Crown inserted and excess composite removed along the margins (j). Light cured for 20 seconds in all directions (k). Postoperative view (l).

of active dental caries, and oral hygiene was good with good periodontal health. Occlusal examination revealed a stable intercuspal relation between maxillary and mandibular teeth position and no parafunctional habit was reported by the patient.

All old and defective crowns were removed, and the maxillary teeth were prepared according to the principles for full coverage crown restorations (**Figure 5.10b**). The finish line location was largely dictated by the finish lines of the existing crowns and where possible were prepared at the gingival level. The mandibular anterior teeth were prepared for more conservative veneer preparations. A light body polyvinylsiloxane material (President, Coltene Whaledent, USA) was carefully injected onto the tooth preparations, ensuring the material reached all teeth surfaces including the margins to be recorded. A stock tray loaded with putty material (President, Coltene Whaledent, USA) was seated over the dental arch to make the definitive impression. An interocclusal record at the patient's maximum intercuspation position was made using a polyvinylsiloxane bite registration material (Jet Blue Bite Fast, Coltene Whaledent, USA). The material was dispensed directly onto the occlusal surface of the lower teeth and mandible and was moved into patient's maximum intercuspation position. The shade was determined using a shade guide (Vitapan 3D Master, Vita, Lichenstein). The crowns and veneers were then manufactured by the dental laboratory team using Edelweiss CAD/CAM T (Translucent) Blocks (Edelweiss Dentistry, Austria). Once received, they were tried for accuracy of fit (**Figure 5.10c**).

The fitting surfaces of the restorations were prepared prior to cementation by applying a thin layer of Edelweiss Bond (Edelweiss Dentistry, Austria) (**Figure 5.10 [d and e]**), and were light cured for 10 seconds (Valo, Ultradent, USA). The prepared surfaces of the teeth were etched using 37% phosphoric acid (Untra-etch, Ultradent, USA) for 15 seconds (**Figure 5.10f**), then thoroughly rinsed off to remove all etchant. All-Bond Universal bonding agent (Bisco, USA) was applied liberally to the moist tooth surfaces (**Figure 5.10g**) and light cured for 20 seconds.

The appropriate shade of composite was selected, dispensed, and evenly spread on the inside of the crown, and then seated onto the prepared tooth. Excess composite was removed, light cured for 20 seconds on all surfaces, and the restoration margins were finished and polished using fine diamond burs, rubber finishers, and polishers (**Figure 5.10 [h–l]**).

Both the static and dynamic occlusion was checked, and after some minor adjustments and interferences were eliminated, the patient was dismissed with stable posterior contacts. At the first recall, the restorations were inspected and some minor modifications implemented. At this recall appointment, the patient expressed complete satisfaction with both the aesthetics and function.

REFERENCES

1. Rekow, ED. Digital dentistry: the new state of the art – is it disruptive or destructive? Dent Mater. 2020;36(1):9–24.
2. Syrek, A et al. Clinical evaluation of all-ceramic crowns fabricated from intraoral digital impressions based on the principle of active wavefront sampling. J Dent. 2010;38(7):553–559.
3. Ting-shu, S, Jian, S. Intraoral digital impression technique: a review. J Prosthodont. 2015;24(4):313–321.
4. Aswani, K et al. Accuracy of an intraoral digital impression: a review. J Indian Prosthodont Soc. 2020;20(1):27.
5. Seelbach, P et al. Accuracy of digital and conventional impression techniques and workflow. Clin Oral Investig. 2013;17:1759–1764.
6. Leu, MC et al. Digital design and fabrication in dentistry. In Bártolo, P, Bidanda B, eds. Bio-Materials and Prototyping Applications in Medicine. Springer; 2008:125–155.
7. Chochlidakis, KM et al. Digital versus conventional impressions for fixed prosthodontics: a systematic review and meta-analysis. J Prosthet Dent. 2016;116(2):184–190.e12.
8. Ng, J, Ruse, D, Wyatt, C. A comparison of the marginal fit of crowns fabricated with digital and conventional methods. J Prosthet Dent. 2014;112(3):555–560.
9. Husein, HA et al. Accuracy of conventional and digital methods of obtaining full-arch dental impression (in vitro study). Cureus. 2022;14(9):e29055.
10. Siqueira, R et al. Intraoral scanning reduces procedure time and improves patient comfort in fixed prosthodontics and implant dentistry: a systematic review. Clin Oral Investig. 2021;25(12):6517–6531.
11. Mangano, F et al. Intraoral scanners in dentistry: a review of the current literature. BMC Oral Health. 2017;17(1):1–11.
12. Takeuchi, Y et al. Use of digital impression systems with intraoral scanners for fabricating restorations and fixed dental prostheses. J Oral Sci. 2018;60(1):1–7.
13. Cicciù, M et al. 3D digital impression systems compared with traditional techniques in dentistry: a recent data systematic review. Materials. 2020;13(8):1982.
14. Bernauer, SA et al. Influence of preparation design, marginal gingiva location, and tooth morphology on the accuracy of digital impressions for full-crown restorations: an in vitro investigation. J Clin Med. 2020;9(12):3984.
15. Joda, T, Brägger, U. Patient-centered outcomes comparing digital and conventional implant impression procedures: a randomized crossover trial. Clin Oral Implants Res. 2016;27(12):e185–e189.
16. Ferrini, F et al. Influence of intra-oral scanner (IOS) on the marginal accuracy of CAD/CAM single crowns. Int J Environmental Res Public Health. 2019;16(4):544.
17. Arcas, LPB et al. Comparación de Precisión Dimensional de Modelos Físicos Generados por Métodos de Impresión Digital/Impresión 3D o Impresión Analógica/Yeso. Int J Odontostomatol. 2021;15(3):562–568.

18. Kim, J-H et al. In vitro analysis of intraoral digital impression of inlay preparation according to tooth location and cavity type. J Prosthodont Res. 2021;65(3):400–406.
19. Wezgowiec, J et al. Evaluation of antimicrobial efficacy of UVC radiation, gaseous ozone, and liquid chemicals used for disinfection of silicone dental impression materials. Materials. 2022;15(7):2553.
20. Berrendero, S et al. Comparative study of all-ceramic crowns obtained from conventional and digital impressions: clinical findings. Clin Oral Investig. 2019;23:1745–1751.
21. Bencharit, S et al. Recent Advancements in CAD/CAM Same-Day Dentistry in Practice and Education [internet]. Preprints, 2021: www.preprints.org/manuscript/202111.0490/v1.
22. de Villaumbrosia, PG et al. In vitro comparison of the accuracy (trueness and precision) of six extraoral dental scanners with different scanning technologies. J Prosthet Dent. 2016;116(4):543–550.e1.
23. Chan, D et al. The accuracy of optical scanning: influence of convergence and die preparation. Oper Dent. 2011; 36(5):486–491.
24. Persson, A et al. A three-dimensional evaluation of a laser scanner and a touch-probe scanner. J Prosthet Dent. 2006; 95(3):194–200.
25. Rudolph, H et al. Computer-aided analysis of the influence of digitizing and surfacing on the accuracy in dental CAD/CAM technology. Computers Biol Med. 2007;37(5):579–587.
26. Lee, SJ et al. Comparison of intraoral and extraoral digital scanners: evaluation of surface topography and precision. Dent J. 2020;8(2):52.
27. Ahlholm, P et al. Digital versus conventional impressions in fixed prosthodontics: a review. J Prosthodont. 2018; 27(1):35–41.
28. Richert, R et al. Intraoral scanner technologies: a review to make a successful impression. J Healthcare Engineer. 2017; 2017(1):8427595.
29. Özal, Ç, Ulusoy, M. In-vitro evaluation of marginal and internal fit of 3-unit monolithic zirconia restorations fabricated using digital scanning technologies. J Adv Prosthodont. 2021;13(6):373–384.
30. Gallardo, YR et al. Patient outcomes and procedure working time for digital versus conventional impressions: a systematic review. J Prosthet Dent. 2018;119(2):214–219.
31. Sailer, I et al. Randomized controlled clinical trial of digital and conventional workflows for the fabrication of zirconia-ceramic fixed partial dentures. Part I: time efficiency of complete-arch digital scans versus conventional impressions. J Prosthet Dent. 2019;121(1):69–75.
32. García-Gil, I et al. Comparative analysis of trueness between conventional and digital impression in dental-supported fixed dental prosthesis with vertical preparation. J Clin Exp Dent. 2020;12(9):e896–e901.
33. Svanborg, P, Hjalmarsson, L. A systematic review on the accuracy of manufacturing techniques for cobalt chromium fixed dental prostheses. Biomat Investigat Dent. 2020;7(1):31–40.
34. Shimizu, S et al. The accuracy of the CAD system using intraoral and extraoral scanners for designing of fixed dental prostheses. Dent Mater J. 2017;36(4):402–407.
35. Aly, P, Mohsen, C. Comparison of the accuracy of three-dimensional printed casts, digital, and conventional casts: an in vitro study. Eur J Dent. 2020;14(02):189–193.
36. Etemad-Shahidi, Y et al. Accuracy of 3-dimensionally printed full-arch dental models: a systematic review. J Clin Med. 2020;9(10):3357.
37. Dawood, A et al. 3D printing in dentistry. Br Dent J. 2015;219(11):521–529.
38. Lepidi, L et al. Virtual articulators and virtual mounting procedures: where do we stand? J Prosthodont. 2021;30(1):24–35.
39. Wu, Y et al. Optimum design of reference points distribution in three-dimensional reconstruction of dental model in intercuspal position. BMC Oral Health. 2021;21:1–8.
40. Shin, S-H et al. Evaluation of the 3D printing accuracy of a dental model according to its internal structure and cross-arch plate design: an in vitro study. Materials. 2020;13(23):5433.
41. Nulty, A. A comparison of trueness and precision of 12 3D printers used in dentistry. BDJ Open. 2022;8(1):14.
42. Yoo, S-Y et al. Dimensional accuracy of dental models for three-unit prostheses fabricated by various 3D printing technologies. Materials. 2021;14(6):1550.
43. Li, Q et al. The creation of a virtual dental patient with dynamic occlusion and its application in esthetic dentistry. J Prosthet Dent. 2021;126(1):14–18.
44. Young, JM, Altschuler, BR. Laser holography in dentistry. J Prosthet Dent. 1977;38(2):216–225.
45. Duret, F, Preston, J. CAD/CAM imaging in dentistry. Curr Opin Dent. 1991;1(2):150–154.
46. Mormann, W. Chairside computer-aided direct ceramic inlays. Quint Int. 1989;20:329–339.
47. Andersson, M, Odén, A. A new all-ceramic crown: a dense-sintered, high-purity alumina coping with porcelain. Acta Odontolog Scandin. 1993;51(1):59–64.
48. Shahmiri, R et al. Optical properties of zirconia ceramics for esthetic dental restorations: a systematic review. J Prosthet Dent. 2018;119(1):36–46.
49. Hamza, TA et al. Accuracy of ceramic restorations made with two CAD/CAM systems. J Prosthet Dent. 2013;109(2):83–87.
50. Touchstone, A et al. Digital transition: the collaboration between dentists and laboratory technicians on CAD/CAM restorations. J Am Dent Assoc. 2010;141:15S–19S.
51. Cooper, LF et al. Prospective assessment of CAD/CAM zirconia abutment and lithium disilicate crown restorations: 2.4 year results. J Prosthet Dent. 2016;116(1):33–39.
52. Bonfante, EA et al. Indirect restorative systems – A narrative review. J Esthet Restorat Dent. 2023;35(1):84–104.
53. Skorulska, A et al. Review on polymer, ceramic and composite materials for cad/cam indirect restorations in dentistry—Application, mechanical characteristics and comparison. Materials. 2021;14(7):1592.
54. Yin, R et al. Comparative evaluation of mechanical properties and wear ability of five CAD/CAM dental blocks. Materials. 2019;12(14):2252.
55. Kelly, JR. Dental ceramics: current thinking and trends. Dental Clin. 2004;48(2):513–530.
56. Lambert, H et al. Dental biomaterials for chairside CAD/CAM: state of the art. J Advanced Prosthodont. 2017;9(6):486–495.
57. Kelly, JR. Dental ceramics: what is this stuff anyway? J Am Dent Assoc. 2008;139:S4–S7.
58. Coldea, A et al. Mechanical properties of polymer-infiltrated-ceramic-network materials. Dent Mater. 2013;29(4):419–426.

59. Scherrer, SS et al. ADM Guidance – Ceramics: guidance to the use of fractography in failure analysis of brittle materials. Dent Mater. 2017;33(6):599–620.
60. Della Bona, A, Kelly, JR. The clinical success of all-ceramic restorations. J Am Dent Assoc. 2008;139:S8–S13.
61. Aydın, N et al. Investigating the color changes on resin-based CAD/CAM blocks. J Esthet Restorat Dent. 2020;32(2): 251–256.
62. Lauvahutanon, S et al. Mechanical properties of composite resin blocks for CAD/CAM. Dent Mater J. 2014;33(5):705–710.
63. Husain, NA-H et al. Mechanical stability of dental CAD-CAM restoration materials made of monolithic zirconia, lithium disilicate, and lithium disilicate–strengthened aluminosilicate glass-ceramic with and without fatigue conditions. J Prosthet Dent. 2022;128(1):73–78.
64. Perea-Lowery, L et al. Characterization of the mechanical properties of CAD/CAM polymers for interim fixed restorations. Dent Mater J. 2020;39(2):319–325.
65. Duarte, S et al. Ceramic-reinforced polymers: CAD/CAM hybrid restorative materials. Curr Oral Health Rep. 2016;3:198–202.
66. Mourouzis, P et al. Color match of luting composites and try-in pastes: the impact on the final color of CAD/CAM lithium disilicate restorations. Int J Esthet Dent. 2018;13(1):98–109.
67. Miyazaki, T et al. A review of dental CAD/CAM: current status and future perspectives from 20 years of experience. Dent Mater J. 2009;28(1):44–56.
68. Zarone, F et al. Current status on lithium disilicate and zirconia: a narrative review. BMC Oral Health. 2019;19:1–14.
69. Ellakwa, A et al. Influence of implant abutment angulations on the fracture resistance of overlaying CAM-milled zirconia single crowns. Austral Dent J. 2011;56(2):132–140.
70. Awad, D et al. Translucency of esthetic dental restorative CAD/CAM materials and composite resins with respect to thickness and surface roughness. J Prosthet Dent. 2015;113(6):534–540.
71. Miyazaki, T et al. Current status of zirconia restoration. J Prosthodon Res. 2013;57(4):236–261.
72. Goujat, A et al. Mechanical properties and internal fit of 4 CAD-CAM block materials. J Prosthet Dent. 2018;119(3): 384–389.
73. Mörmann, WH et al. Wear characteristics of current aesthetic dental restorative CAD/CAM materials: two-body wear, gloss retention, roughness and Martens hardness. J Mech Behav Biomed Mater. 2013;20:113–125.
74. Blatz, MB, Conejo, J. The current state of chairside digital dentistry and materials. Dent Clin. 2019;63(2):175–197.

6 Digital Dentistry in Implant Dentistry

Prashanthi Reddy and Raveena Makker

6.1 INTRODUCTION

Technology development has led to a significant shift in the field of implant dentistry over the course of dentistry's history. Gradually, advancements have been made in implant design, surgical technique materials, abutment design, and restorative materials. Nevertheless, digitization has provided practitioners with both challenges and helpful assistance over the years.

Digital technologies, artificial intelligence, and telemedicine have transformed medical science protocols as a result of technological and engineering advances, becoming integral components of many medical specialties. Computer-aided implant surgery (CAIS) has become the norm in both academic and private dental settings, making implant dentistry one of the first dental specialties to adopt widespread digital workflows. CAIS has grown in popularity due to benefits such as shorter surgery times, improved postoperative healing, anatomically safe implant placement, and fewer appointments [1]. It might even make up for a lack of surgical experience.

Cone beam computed tomography (CBCT) technology has made it possible to visualize bony structures in three dimensions while using less radiation. With a lower and safer radiation dose, CBCT can accurately measure 3D bone volume. Cross-sectional images of the bone are shown in relation to the location of the potential implant, and implant planning software can show 3D surface models. For the digital design of prostheses and/or the planning of osteotomy guides, dental surfaces are not sufficiently detailed in digital imaging and communication in medicine (DICOM) files. A number of references, including the tooth surface, can be used to achieve accurate registration and alignment [1]. Custom reference markers, also known as fiducial markers, are used when teeth are missing or when there are highly radio-opaque restorations present.

Aligning corresponding anatomical surface references is typically accomplished by artificial intelligence algorithms that are already present in the majority of software options. The most crucial information is that some implant planning software needs specific corresponding areas marked to enable (semi-automatic) registration and that clinicians frequently correct automated alignment and account for any potential inaccuracies. The following step is to gather information regarding the upcoming restoration (prosthetic plan). Modern implant planning systems are equipped with computer-assisted design (CAD)-based modules, which makes virtual prosthetic planning both practical and accessible. Older software versions demanded the use of a double-scan technique, in which two distinct model scans were obtained—one with the missing teeth and the other with a wax-up that included the location and style of the future prosthesis.

A different workflow involving two intraoral scans, one with the teeth prepared and the other with the temporary restoration in place, was also suggested. Planning and placement of implants that are driven by prosthetics remain the objective. Clinicians should be able to see where implants will be placed in relation to a future restoration, nearby teeth, the emergence profile, the incisal edge, the cervical region, etc., in the 3D bony environment.

Different datasets used in treatment planning for implant placement are revolutionized by the digital age. The various cutting-edge technologies include facial scanning, intraoral scanning, extraoral scanning, and CBCT imaging. After that, different software tools can be used to manipulate the digital data, and different datasets can then be incorporated to create a virtual reconstruction of the patient's maxillofacial anatomy.

For virtual implant planning, which incorporates numerous digital components, this digital dental technology is used. Taking digital images of the maxillofacial structures and using software to manipulate those images to perform virtual treatment planning or use computer-assisted design/computer-assisted manufacturing (CAD/CAM) technology are the two main components of this dataset [2].

Although CBCT can record the majority of orofacial structures, it is typically used to create digital replicas of structures with higher densities, like bone and teeth [2]. CBCT will generate a file in the standard format, which is widely used in the medical field. A surface scanner's intraoral surface (IOS) or extraoral surface (EOS) images are frequently combined with CBCT images. These scanners typically produce files in the STL file format (formerly known as Stereolithography format, now Standard Tessellation Language format). The stereolithography CAD software that 3D systems use natively produces STL files. Surface scanners create 3D models of an object's surface, as opposed to DICOM files.

 DOI: 10.1201/9781003428541-6

Table 6.1: An Overview of Digital Dentistry

In Clinics	Method
Patient record	A variety of software programs are available to store patient records, copies of which can be distributed to patients, other medical professionals, and labs
Diagnosis	Caries detection solution, Digital X-rays, CT scans, OPG, CBCT
Treatment	Air abrasion technology, soft tissue & hard tissue lasers, digital impression, electric hand pieces, digital matching, digital anesthesia system, and virtual drilling systems

Source: Modified from [4].
Abbreviations: CBCT, Cone Beam Computed Tomography; OPG, Orthopantomogram

This chapter elucidates the surface scanning, facial scanning, software used while implementing the digitization in implants and merging all datasets to obtain the output "digital dentistry" (**Table 6.1**) [3].

6.2 SURFACE SCANS

A precise duplicate of the teeth, implants, and surrounding tissues must be made while performing dental implant procedures in order to plan the therapy and permit the creation of the prosthesis.

Multiple undercut surfaces caused by variations in tooth morphology and axial inclination, the presence of fixed and movable soft tissues, frenal attachments, and the underlying muscles make exact duplication of the structures in the oral cavity difficult [2]. Additionally, errors may result from the varied characteristics of imprint materials, problems with the structure and rigidity of the tray, or patient compliance and movements.

CAD/CAM was introduced to replace traditional impression.

The initial step in the workflow is obtaining a digital representation of the tooth with the advent of CAD/CAM in dental prosthesis.

Surface scans are thought to be a simpler method than traditional impressions and may exhibit less variability when used to digitize the significant structures.

Analogue Imprints: For many years, dental implant locations have been recorded using conventional imprints. For these materials to faithfully reproduce the placements of the implants, a very high level of dimensional accuracy is needed.

The following factors could influence the accuracy of impression materials:

- Conditions of storage
- Errors in dosage, timing, and temperature
- Clinical approach, patient mobility, setting time, tray rigidity and location in the mouth, and ongoing chemical reaction after initial setting

Digitization of the Oral Cavity: The necessary intraoral structures must first be digitally documented in order to produce a CAD/CAM dental prosthesis. The computer-aided procedures can then use a digital or "virtual" working paradigm.

Instead of using the standard impression coping, while scanning dental implants, a scan body—a geometric item with defined dimensions—is attached to the implant. The scan body is often made of Polyetheretherketone (PEEK) material and has dimensions that the CAD program can identify. The clinical scenario is then surface scanned using specialized technology, creating a digital file that can be integrated into CAD/CAM software [2]. The STL file is the preferred file format for intraoral scanners.

The mouth cavity is digitally scanned, producing a "point cloud." This is a collection of data points in a 3D coordinate system, typically in the form of X, Y, and Z coordinates, used to depict an object's outside surface. In order to create the STL file, point clouds are typically transformed from polygon or triangular mesh models through a procedure known as surface reconstruction. The STL file production joins the little triangles' continuous geometry to create the desired shape.

Three distinct procedures can be used to digitize a complex intraoral morphology:

- Extraoral scanners that digitally scan and recreate a traditional stone model made using traditional imprint methods
- Extraoral scanners that digitally capture a traditional imprint through scanning
- Intraoral scanners, which use a light source to do non-contact optical scanning

Precision, Trueness, and Accuracy: When discussing the accuracy of digitizing the intraoral form, the terms trueness and precision are sometimes used interchangeably. Implant prostheses require a high level of accuracy to produce a prosthesis that passively fits the implants because dental implants are immobile things.

According to research by Abduo and Lyons [5], any mismatch in a framework for numerous implants can cause mechanical and biological issues. By minimizing human intervention and the accumulation of small fabrication errors common in analogue processes such as waxing, investing, casting, and polishing, CAD/CAM technology attempts to lower the possibility of misfits.

Requirement of Physical Models: Physical models are still sometimes required by dental technicians for specific stages of prosthesis completion. For the dental technician to perform the restoration in these cases, intraoral scanning might be employed to create models. When a model is required, it is typically a stereolithographic (SLA) polyurethane die or a 3D-printed model that includes a holder for a movable laboratory analogue.

6.2.1 Facial Scanning

CBCT and in-office digital IOS scanners have become more widely available, and this has been accompanied by an expansion of the software tools available to visualize, analyze, and combine the datasets produced by these scanners for use in routine clinical work. Since the invention of the so-called digital smile design (DSD), which offers the chance to assess the patient's aesthetics before taking into consideration the real dental repair, this technology has grown in popularity. Facial scanning technology is becoming increasingly popular in the disciplines of orthodontics and orthognathic maxillofacial surgery for use in planning complex and advanced situations [2].

Stereophotogrammetry: By supplying 3D coordinates, the collected pairs of photos are then merged to generate an image. A previous iteration of this technology, known as "analogue stereophotogrammetry," depended on processing traditional printed photos that were put into a device known as the "analytical stereo plotter," designed to produce a contour map depicting the 3D coordinates of various landmarks. This method was effective in mapping the maxillofacial area to examine facial asymmetry. This method is frequently used in dental laboratories for prosthetic dentistry to digitize dental imprints or dental casts, which serves as the foundation for creating CAD/CAM prostheses.

Similar trigonometric principles govern structured light scanning, or active stereophotogrammetry, but instead of using a laser, a safe (white or blue) light is thrown onto the object being scanned.

The camera records the distorted light pattern, and a 3D coordinate map of the face is created. A 3D surface representation of the face is then created using post-processing on this map. Digital 2D images of the patient are simultaneously taken, and the 3D surface data is then merged with this 2D texture image to create a colored 3D surface. Passive stereophotogrammetry is the last type of digital stereophotogrammetry. A dense 3D point cloud can be virtually recreated by taking just two high-resolution 2D digital photos and applying a sophisticated software technique. This method eliminates the requirement for a light pattern or any other kind of laser scanning.

Although CBCT can accurately depict the exterior soft-tissue profile, the quality of the 3D data is inextricably linked to the selected scanner system, scan parameters, and reconstruction methods.

The addition of facial scanning technology to the CBCT unit is a novel invention that enables accurate registration and seamless fusion. Some of the difficulties with post-processing registration may be resolved by such integration. However, compared to the conventional stereophotogrammetry setup, the method has longer scanning periods and lesser resolution.

Facial Scanners: The next significant step in developing the virtual patient is dynamic facial scanning, which involves capturing facial movement and translating the results to a lifelike computer animation of the human face. The establishment of a virtual patient and digital workflows could both be significantly impacted by its application in dentistry. To capture 3D face expressions, various methods can be used, such as 3D scanning, marker-based motion capture, structured-light systems, and image-based systems.

6.2.2 Software Packages

For digital workflows in implant dentistry to be successfully implemented, software packages are essential. As long as everyone on the team has access to the necessary tools, digital processes and solutions enable team members to easily communicate and exchange information regarding treatment proposals. Either an open or a closed software architecture is possible. The doctor has a great deal of freedom to work in the digital environment without being constrained by a single system, thanks to open software. It is possible to freely share information between several software platforms. All team members must have access to a specific software program in a closed software system, which may limit information sharing or disrupt the digital process [2].

Data Collection: Before beginning active treatment, the practitioner and the patient can preview treatment plans for the replacement and restoration of the dentition using digital smile design programs. Bringing in color images of the current clinical scenario simplifies the computer simulation of suggested modifications, giving the patient a clear picture of the ultimate prosthetic design. This can be a useful tool for clinicians and patients to communicate with one another. Traditionally, a diagnostic stone cast would be used to construct a wax-up of the prosthetic plan. A "virtual wax-up" on a "virtual model" in the CAD software program is possible because of the diagnostic feature in a software package. The ability to quickly develop a wide variety of design suggestions is one benefit of this digital technique over conventional processes.

Prosthetic and Surgical Planning: The surface scan of the intraoral situation can be combined with radiographic data from a CT or CBCT scan using implant planning software. The DICOM data format is the industry standard for radiography data. The two datasets must be properly merged and aligned within a software program as the initial stage in this process is to guarantee the highest level of planning accuracy. To align and integrate the CBCT scan data with the STL or surface scan data, the software must be able to find similarities between the two datasets.

Radiographic (fiducial) markers, such as prepared marker objects or radiopaque teeth placed within a trial setup, are necessary in cases of total edentulism to act as recognizable spots on the recorded pictures so that the data from CBCT and surface scan can be successfully combined. The size of the field that was chosen in the CBCT may also have an impact on how well the data is merged.

The planning procedure for dental implant therapy is always centered around restorative goals. The primary factor to take into account is where to place the required replacement teeth.

The program must let the import of the restoration plan with the replacement tooth and soft tissue form after the surface scan and CBCT dataset have been successfully aligned.

CAD: In cases of complete edentulism, radiographic (fiducial) markers, such as ready-made marker objects or radiopaque teeth placed within a trial setup, are required to act as recognized locations on the recorded images so that the surface scan and CBCT data can be successfully merged. The effectiveness of the data fusion may also depend on the size of the field that was selected for the CBCT.

Planning for dental implant therapy is always done with restorative objectives in mind. The key concern is deciding where the replacement teeth should be placed (**Table 6.2**).

Following the successful alignment of the surface scan with the CBCT dataset, the system must support loading the planned restorative design that incorporates the prosthetic tooth and the modeled soft-tissue architecture.

Final Prosthetic Design: The software's task is to precisely place the virtual dental implant inside the reconstructed surface scan, which can be an intraoral scan or a scan of a physical model made from an analogue imprint data set. To enable accurate and exact replication and meshing of the geometry, it is crucial that the relevant scan body library be referenced in the software setup. For the software to correctly locate the scan body, the entire contour of the scan body must be clearly visible in the surface scan. Deeply implanted or greatly divergent implants may affect the software's capacity to recognize the scanned body and, consequently, the actual implant position. Utilizing scan bodies that work with the software interface is crucial.

Table 6.2: CAD-CAM System

Systems	Various Parts	Data Processing
French system	• 3D probe system on electro-optical method • Surface modelling and screen display • Automatic milling	By shape recognition software
Minnesota system	• Optical impression • Photograph-based system using a 35-mm camera with magnifying lens • Milling	Data obtained in dental office sent to another location for processing and matching
Swiss system	• A desktop computer • Display monitor permitting visual verification of quality of data • Electronically controlled milling machine	By an interactive CAD unit

Source: Data from Ref. [6].

It is simple to customize the addition or removal of the layers of information on the screen for a clear visualization of the design parameters, and abutment curves and parallelism may be carefully regulated. To confirm that the required material thickness is met, cross-sectional views can be taken.

The software's capacity to quickly, accurately, and simply copy or match restorative shapes is one obvious benefit of the digital workflow for implant restoration in the aesthetic zone. The restoration's entire contour design is another benefit of using CAD design software for the creation of an implant-supported prosthesis. Full-arch restoration frameworks can be made to fully support the underlying restorative procedure [2].

Model-Building: Designing virtual models can be printed or milled using model-building functions. Any superfluous scan areas are removed from the surface scan. The software enables the creation of numerous implant analogue reproductions to be positioned virtually within the model. These digital analogues are movable in contrast to conventional implant copies, which are static when placed in dental stone.

Computer-Assisted Manufacturing: The milling procedure is the last step in creating the finished prosthesis.

Using the software's export feature, dental technicians can procure the services of a centralized milling facility. It is possible to configure the "export and share" function so that data is effortlessly transported to the milling facility. To assure the accuracy of the operation, the software packages provide certain milling tolerances that must be matched and calibrated with the chosen milling machine.

6.3 SHADE MATCHING

- Digital shade-matching systems help streamline discussions with the laboratory and cut down on the inconsistencies that can occur between or within operators [7].
- Colorimeters capture tristimulus data by filtering the light into RGB wavelengths, mirroring the primary colors of human vision.
- The Shade Vision and the Shade-Eye NCC are among the popular colorimeters available for clinical shade matching.
- Spectrophotometers work by measuring how much light an object reflects or transmits at each wavelength, allowing them to capture its value, chroma, and hue across the full visible spectrum. (Examples: VITA Easyshade compact, Crystal Eye.)
- Digital camera and imaging technologies typically operate on the RGB model, where individual red, green, and blue values are captured by the sensor. These primary color components are then processed and merged to produce the final-colored image. The system is intentionally designed to align with human color perception, allowing the captured images to appear natural to the viewer.

Advantages:

1. Cost benefit
2. Ease of use
3. Availability

6.4 DIGITAL SMILE DESIGN

- DSD is a comprehensive tool that aids the restorative team throughout the entire treatment process, enhancing planning, communication, and clinical outcomes [7].
- The use of reference lines and geometric guides on extra- and intraoral digital photographs broadens the diagnostic view for the dental team, allowing a more accurate evaluation of the case's aesthetic parameters, limitations, and associated risk factors.
- A variety of digital tools are available for smile design, including Smile Designer Pro, Digital Smile Design, 3Shape Smile Design, Smile Designer Rio, and Aesthetic Digital Smile Design, each offering features that enhance planning and visualization.

Advantages:

1. Aesthetic diagnosis
2. Communication
3. Feedback
4. Patient management
5. Education

Limitations:

1. DSD requires exact photographic and video records (**Figure 6.1**), and any deficiencies in these inputs can lead to inaccurate diagnostic interpretation and planning.

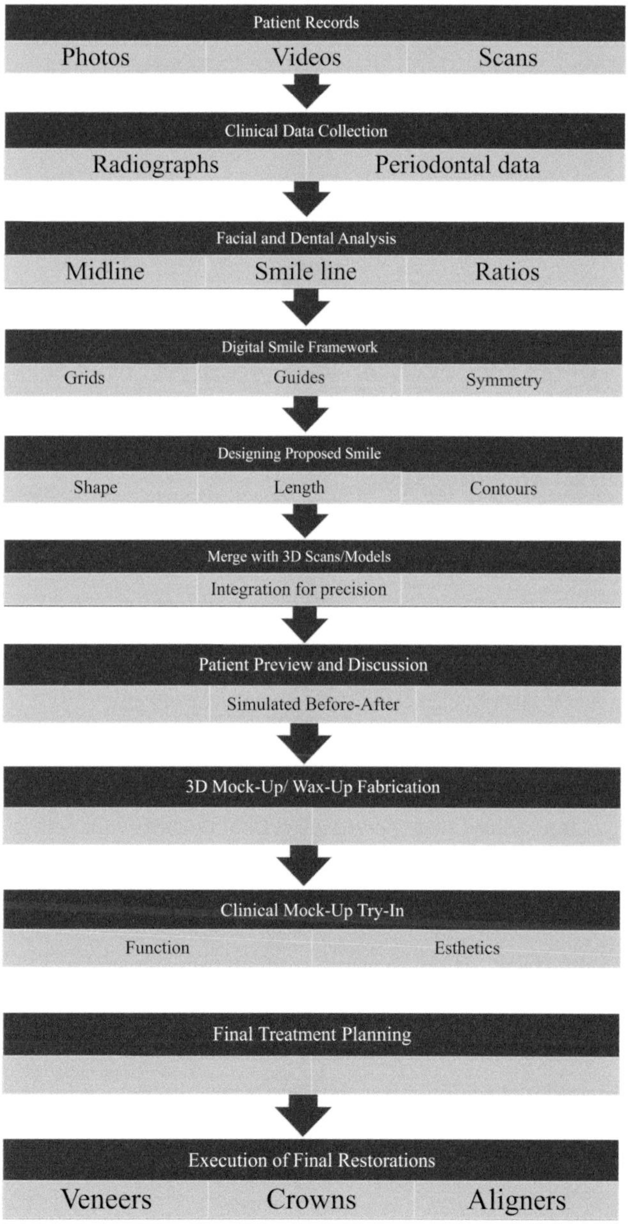

Figure 6.1 Protocol for DSD execution.

2. In addition, the reliance on specialized 3D technologies and software, together with the need for trained personnel, significantly elevates the overall time and financial investment.

6.5 VIRTUAL ARTICULATORS AND DIGITAL FACEBOWS

Virtual dental articulators work through digital "software articulators" that can mimic every movement of the mandible. By offering a clear visual simulation of how the jaws interact, they have strengthened the role of virtual reality in dentistry, especially for studying complex bite relationships. When paired with CAD/CAM technology, these systems create accurate virtual models that support both diagnosis and treatment planning, from simple single-crown cases to full-mouth rehabilitation, helping clinicians visualize the entire workflow from start to finish [8].

Advantages:

1. Virtual articulators give precise 3D simulations useful in prosthetics, orthodontics, and implant planning.
2. They help in jaw repositioning, tooth alignment, smile design, detecting occlusal interferences, and assessing wear or bruxism.
3. They allow clinicians to observe dynamic movements, including Temporomandibular Joint (TMJ) function.
4. They are valuable teaching tools for understanding jaw movements and occlusal relationships.

Limitations:

1. High cost of acquisition and upkeep, as they depend on supporting technologies like digital sensors, scanners, software, and multiple articulator models for different patient requirements
2. Demand for specialized knowledge, including precise data input, interpretation of scanner and motion data, and proficiency with mechanical articulators, CAD/CAM systems, and software

Method of Using Virtual Articulators [8]:

- A virtual cast of the patient's dentition is created.
- Three reference markers are placed on the patient's face—two over the TMJ region and one at the infraorbital point.
- The patient is then scanned using an optical scanner.
- The three most prominent cusps of the maxillary arch are identified by pressing articulating paper against the metal facebow fork positioned on the upper jaw.
- The pointer tip is aligned with each marked cusp, and each point is scanned.
- This procedure is repeated twice for accuracy.
- All collected data is transferred into the virtual articulator software, which then determines the precise spatial relationship of the maxilla between the articulator and the digital cast.

Virtual articulators can be divided into two types, depending on how they replicate the motion of the jaw [7].

1. **Mathematically stimulated articulator**: It reproduces the movements of a mechanical articulator using numerical data. Parameters such as Bennett angle, condylar inclination, protrusive, retrusive, and lateral excursions recorded from a conventional articulator or jaw-motion analyzer allow the system to simulate mandibular motion accurately.
2. **Completely adjustable articulator (motion analyzer)**: In this, mandibular motion is documented by an electronic jaw registration system, commonly referred to as a jaw motion analyzer, which records the true movement pathways of the lower jaw

6.6 MERGING DIGITAL DATASETS

The creation of a virtual patient requires the proper compiling and matching of several digital files, which necessitates the merging of files (digital data sets).

Table 6.3: Comparison of Conventional and Digital Approaches to Complete Dentures

	Conventional	Digital
Visit 1	Primary impression	Definitive impression and maxillomandibular record and selection of teeth
Visit 2	Definitive impression	Try-in (optional visit)
Visit 3	Maxillomandibular relation	Delivery
Visit 4	Try-in	
Visit 5	Delivery	

To ensure that no accuracy is lost when the transition from virtual to analogue is later carried out to build and deliver the prosthesis, the correctness of this matching procedure, which is described in detail in this chapter, is of utmost importance.

The operator will construct the surgical template for guided implant surgery, plan the implant position(s), design the prosthetic pieces for clinical delivery, and produce them in the virtual environment. However, the IOS scanner or EOS scanner digital data is used as positional references for the digitally generated guides or prosthetic components.

Importance of CBCT Scans: CBCT scans of the patient result in 2D image slices that can be seen separately or stacked to create a 3D image. Thus, it is necessary to match surface scanners with DICOM data produced from CBCT. CBCT DICOM files should be combined with files from surface scanners since the surface definition of CBCT scans is not as accurate as that acquired with a surface scanner image with volume from CBCT scans. Volumetric data of the region of interest's skeletal structure is produced using CBCT scans. CBCT data, as opposed to pixels (two-dimensional) data, contains voxels (3D data bits) [2].

Digital Workflow Application: A fully digital workflow consists of planning, prosthodontic, surgical, and diagnostic procedures [9]. Data files from an intraoral scanner (STL) and CBCT (DICOM) are the first step merging within the planning program. By using the desired prosthetic design as a guide, the implant placements are virtually planned within this software. A surgical guide is then digitally created and 3D printed to help install the implant. A functioning IOS, also known as a "digital impression," is taken following the osseointegration phase. The implant-borne prosthetic components are made using a CAD software program by manipulating the generated STL file [2].

6.7 DIGITILIZATION IN COMPLETE DENTURES

Digital Impression [10] *(Table 6.3)*

Advantages:

1. Chairside analysis
2. Cost saving of impression material
3. True mucostatic impression
4. Easy for patients with gag
5. Easy for patient with limited mouth opening
6. No need for disinfection
7. Ability to print or null master casts
8. Digital achievability

Disadvantages:

1. High initial cost
2. Steep learning curve

3. Often not possible for mandible
4. Often not possible for keratinized tissue
5. Must be done in one pass
6. Difficult to scan movable soft tissues
7. Capturing posterior palatal seal is difficult.

Prosthesis design:

- Denture design software offers a powerful tool that lets clinician select molds from a library of teeth to generate the teeth arrangement automatically.
- Proper positioning of denture teeth in terms of aesthetics, relationship to residual ridge, location of occlusal plane, and occlusal relationship is ensured.

6.8 MANUFACTURING TECHNOLOGIES

Since Poly methyl meth acrylate (PMMA) was developed by Wright in 1936, many issues were associated with conventional complete denture like polymerization shrinkage, tissue in fitting, strength, and release of monomer.

Two types of CAD/CAM fabrication methods are employed:

1. *Subtractive Manufacturing* (*Milling*): A block of material is milled by automated control of specialized cutting tools that receive information from computer.
2. *Additive Manufacturing* (*3D Printing*): Material is stacked layer by layer, one over the other to create a 3D structure. It reduces material waste by 40% and allows finer details compared to subtractive methods.

6.9 DIGITILIZATION IN REMOVABLE PARTIAL DENTURES (RPD)

The steps in RPD are set out in **Figure 6.2** [11,12].

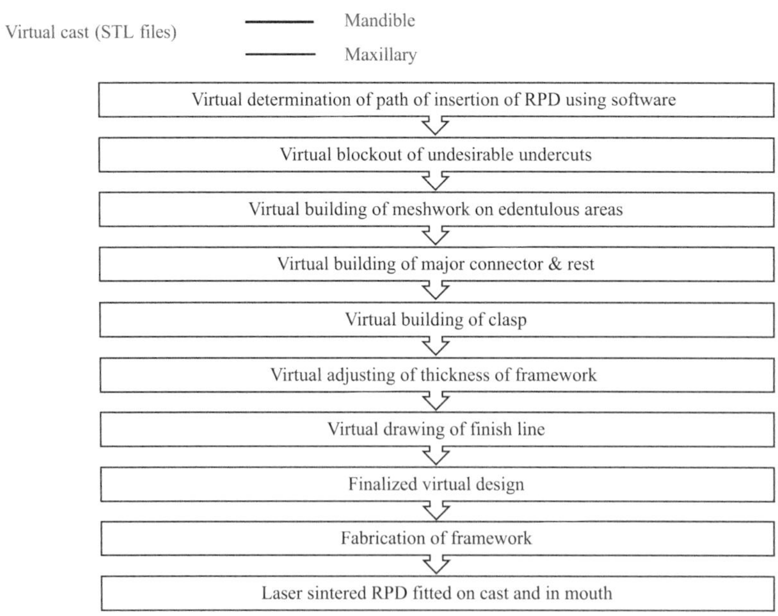

Figure 6.2 Steps in RPD procedure.

Advantages [13]:

1. Reduced maintenance costs for expensive furnaces and casting equipment
2. Less wasted alloy
3. No wasted wax
4. No wasted equipment material
5. Improved health and safety feature
6. Ability to recall, change design, and remanufacture without need to restart entire process
7. Shorter process workflow
8. Share design between technician and clinicians via internet

6.10 DIGITIZATION IN FIXED/IMPLANT PROSTHESIS

Comfort Control Syringe: An electronic, pre-programmed delivery system for local anesthetic dispenses the anesthetic in slower, more controlled, and more consistent manner than syringe and is virtually painless [14].

It has a special delivery system. The injection begins at a slow rate to minimize the discomfort associated with rapid injection.

The Wand: The Wand system comes in a small lightweight handpiece that resembles a pen.

The computer control allows an even flow of anesthetic in a comfortable and non-threatening manner.

Indications of virtual surgical guides [15]:

- Most cases of three or more implants in a row
- Any case with anatomic problems
- Problem related with proximity of adjacent teeth
- Patients with medical problems

Figure 6.3 shows the stages in the fabrication of a guide.

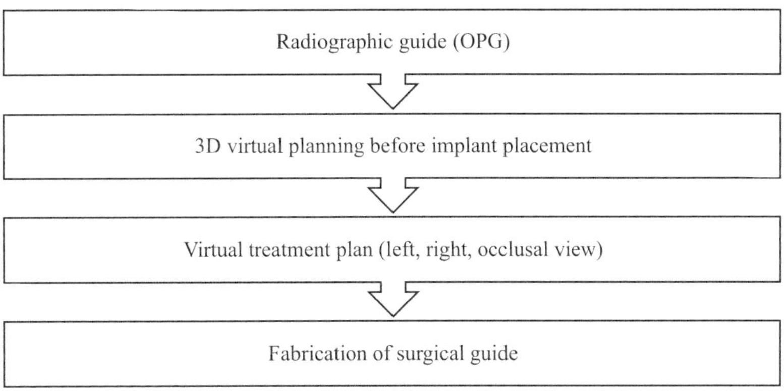

Figure 6.3 Fabrication of a guide.

REFERENCES

1. Masri R, Driscol CF, eds, Clinical Applications of Digital Dental Technology: Wiley; 2023.
2. Gallucchi GO et al. Digital Workflows in Implant Dentistry, ITI Treatment Guide Series, Vol 11: Quintessence; 2019.
3. Jain P, Gupta M, eds, Digitization in Dentistry: Springer; 2021.
4. Rathee M et al. Digitalization in prosthodontics: changing needs based on modern demands. Journal of the West Bengal University of Health Sciences. 2021;1(3):48–57.
5. Maiti N, Mahapatra N, Patel D, Chanchad J, Saurabhbhai Shah A, Mahboob Rahaman SK, Surana P. Application of CAD-CAM in Dentistry. Bioinformation. 2024 May 31;20(5):547–550. doi: 10.6026/973206300200547.
6. CAD/CAM restorations: Description of French, Swiss, and Minnesota systems. n.d.: www.scribd.com/doc/135837266/77562247-CAD-CAm.
7. Gupta C, Mittal A. Role of digital technology in prosthodontics: a step toward improving dental care. Indian journal of oral health and research. 2018;4:35–41.
8. Özdemir G et al. Virtual articulators, virtual occlusal records and virtual patients in dentistry. Journal of experimental and clinical medicine. 2021;38(3s):129–35.
9. Singh M et al. Digitization in prosthodontics. International journal of dental and health sciences. 2014;1(2):208–217.
10. Khurshid Z. Digital Dentistry: Transformation of Oral Health and Dental Education with Technology. Eur J Dent. 2023 Oct;17(4):943–944. doi: 10.1055/s-0043-1772674.
11. Tamini F, Hirayam H, eds, Digital Restorative Dentistry: A Guide to Materials, Equipment, and Clinical Procedures: Springer; 2019.
12. Tamimi F et al. Digital removable partial dentures. Clinical dentistry reviewed. 2020;4(9):1–12.
13. Mahrous A, Botsko DL, El-Gendy T, Elgreatly A. Enhancing digital workflows for removable partial dentures: A novel diagnostic surveyor and designer. J Prosthodont. 2026 Jan;35(1):102–107. doi: 10.1111/jopr.14059.
14. Galante JM, Rucio NA, Digital Dental Implantology: Springer; 2021.
15. Orentlicher G, Abboud M. Guided surgery for implant therapy. Oral and Maxillofacial Surgery Clinics of North America. 2011;23(2):239–256.

7 Applications of 3D Printing in Implant Dentistry*

Ahmed Yaseen Alqutaibi, Mohammed Ahmed Alghauli, and Muhammad Sohail Zafar

7.1 INTRODUCTION

In implant dentistry, incorporating digital tools such as computer-aided design and manufacturing (CAD/CAM) has brought about significant advancements, introducing novel clinical and technical approaches for performing surgical implant procedures and producing dental restorations [1]. Three-dimensional (3D) printing is a CAD/CAM system production technology known as additive manufacturing (AM), which seamlessly connects diagnostic assessments, treatment planning, and fabrication stages within a digital workflow [2]. Utilizing digital pathways enhances the safety of implant placements and restoration fabrication efficiency, reduces the workload on dental practitioners, and improves the overall patient care experience [3].

In the last decade, 3D printing has been increasingly adopted as a favored production method in dentistry, replacing the conventional computer numerical control (CNC) fabrication technology [3]. CNC machining or milling (subtractive manufacturing) typically involves shaping an object by removing material through turning, milling, or grinding processes. This method has long been established in dentistry due to its satisfactory precision and compatibility with a wide range of dental materials, making it suitable for large-scale production [3, 4]. However, despite its precision and versatility, CNC machining incurs high costs due to the considerable bulk of the raw material being wasted in the process, besides the inevitable wear of the cutting tools that imply their replacement after a limited number of milling cycles [5, 6]. Moreover, it faces challenges in producing intricate geometrical and hollow dental devices like custom-made root-form dental implants and customized titanium meshes, which might be more efficiently manufactured using 3D printing techniques [5, 7].

3D printing is a production method that constructs objects through the sequential layering of material, guided by a digital 3D model. This process involves translating the model into a series of two-dimensional (2D) layers, which are then meticulously stacked using a computer-controlled procedure to create the final product. The significant advantage of AM lies in its ability to overcome the limitations imposed by traditional subtractive machining, as it enables the rapid production of a wide array of intricate shapes. Additionally, AM is highly efficient regarding raw material consumption and has limited waste compared to CNC milling, as any surplus or unused raw material, such as resin or metal powder, can be recycled, leading to substantial cost reductions [3, 4, 8]. Moreover, the technology is more environmentally friendly and highly time and cost-efficient than CNC machining [4, 7–9].

When comparing AM to CNC milling, it becomes evident that each approach possesses distinct strengths and weaknesses; both methodologies often offer complementary advantages [3]. This chapter will thoroughly overview the latest developments in using AM or 3D printing technologies in oral implantology. It will analyze the current technologies and explain their applications in implant dentistry, highlighting the benefits for dental professionals and patients. Additionally, it will discuss the integration of AM into implant dentistry and its impact on clinical outcomes.

7.2 THE TECHNOLOGIES OF ADDITIVE MANUFACTURING

3D printing refers to a set of production techniques that involve gradually accumulating material layer by layer to construct objects. The additively manufactured implant components are physical analogs of digital 3D models generated by CAD software. Based on this data, the CAD designs are virtually cut into thin slices, and the manufacturing system constructs the part layer by layer. Consequently, AM is commonly referred to as layered manufacturing, physical free-form manufacturing, or direct digital manufacturing. The fundamental principle all 3D printing technologies share is the additive process; however, they vary in their forming techniques and the materials they employ. The selection of an appropriate 3D printing technology should be predicated on the specific requirements of the application [2, 3].

Additive manufacturing can be categorized into seven categories based on ISO/ASTM 52900:15 classification: 1. Vat photopolymerization (VP); 2. Material jetting (MJ) (inkjet printing [IJP]/direct ink printing [DIP]); 3. Powder bed fusion (PBF); 4. Directed energy deposition (DED); 5. Binder jetting (BJ); 6. Material extrusion (MEX) (robocasting [RC], or direct ink writing [DIW]); and 7. Sheet lamination

* This chapter builds on Alqutaibi, AY, Alghauli, MA, Aljohani, MHA, Zafar, MS. Advanced additive manufacturing in implant dentistry: 3D printing technologies, printable materials, current applications and future requirements. Bioprinting 2024;42:e00356.

DOI: 10.1201/9781003428541-7

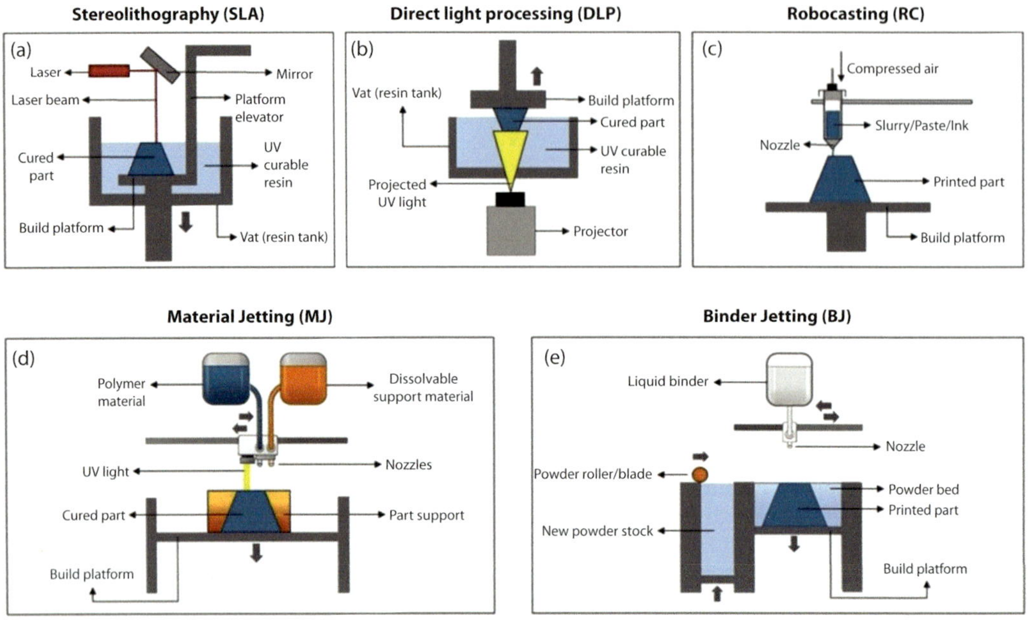

Figure 7.1 Five indirect ceramic and metal direct resin 3D-printing technologies commonly used in dentistry. (a) Stereolithography. (b) Direct light processing. (c) Robocasting. (d) Material jetting. (e) Binder jetting. (From Ref. [12] under Creative Commons Attribution licence.)

(SHL) (**Figure 7.1**). In the dental realm, particularly in implant dentistry, some approaches are more prominently used than others, due to their efficiency and ease in producing certain parts and working with certain materials. For example, VPP is the most commonly used technology to produce resin implant guides and other resinous dental parts, MJ is less commonly used, and PBF is mostly applied to produce the metal parts as denture frameworks and implant fixtures [2, 3].

7.2.1 Vat Photopolymerization (VPP)

This technique produces resin parts from photopolymerizable resins, applying UV light or UV laser (typically 380–405 nm) for photopolymerization of the resin liquid in a vat. The process builds up the object layer by layer on a platform until reaching the final desired form following the CAD design [2, 3]. Several daughter technologies of the VPP are described in **Table 7.1**, and the two most common technologies, stereolithography (SLA) and digital light processing (DLP), are represented in **Figure 7.1**. The difference between these daughter technologies is that they rely on light source and polymerization.

7.2.2 The Powder Bed Fusion (PBF) Technology

This technology is well known for metal printing, including in the dental field. Titanium and chrome-cobalt alloys are favored metals for biomedical applications due to their exceptional biocompatibility and mechanical properties. Additionally, these alloys exhibit remarkable heat resistance. PBF encompasses several methods, including selective laser sintering (SLS), direct metal laser sintering (DMLS), selective laser melting (SLM), and electron beam melting (EBM).

The printing process necessitates powerful lasers or electron beams to melt and fuse small particles of material, such as plastics, glass, ceramics, or metals in powder form. The process starts with preheating the powder to a temperature below the powder's melting point, and then the printing process starts. Once a layer is fused, the build platform moves by the thickness of one layer, allowing a fresh layer of powder to be evenly distributed over it for the subsequent layer to be printed [2, 3] (**Figure 7.2a**).

PBF printers can fabricate intricate 3D structures, rendering the technology extensively utilized for biomedical applications, including dental implantology and orthopedics. Furthermore, this technology enables the creation of customized titanium meshes and implant frameworks. The most notable factors limiting the speed of PBF are the regulation of the pre- and postprinting thermal cycle of the machine and the postprocessing procedures applied to the components [2, 3]. PBF includes

Table 7.1: VAT Photopolymerization Technologies

3 D Printing Technology	Description	Advantages	Disadvantages or Limitations	Materials Manufactured
Stereolithography (SLA)	Uses a UV laser directed by a mirror galvanometer to cure the resin layer by layer. The polymerization is intentionally left incomplete during UV exposure to enhance cohesion between layers. Additional light treatment finalizes the process (**Figure 7.1a**).	High accuracy and resolution, flawless surface finish, suitable for intricate geometric and hollow parts.	Manually detaching support structures; not suitable for ceramic and hard metals without additional steps like debinding and sintering.	Surgical guides, dental models, custom trays, temporary dental restoratives, high-strength ceramic parts. Metal printing is also possible, e.g., Lithoz, lithography-based metal manufacturing (LMM)
Digital light processing (DLP)	A digital micromirror device is used to cure the entire layers of resin at once. The technology reflects and focuses light on the printed object, controlling the curing process by adjusting UV light intensity (**Figure 7.1b**)	Faster printing speeds compared to SLA, economical for larger parts due to less slurry usage in bottom-up setups, and suitable for larger, intricate parts in top-down setups.	Generally, falls short in achieving the high-resolution details possible with SLA.	Dental models, larger objects with fewer intricate details. The technology showed good accuracy in producing such ceramic dental parts as zirconia crowns.
Lithography-based ceramic manufacturing (LCM)	Derived from DLP, LCM can produce a wide variety of ceramic-based materials. The systems are open, facilitating the production of various custom-specific ceramic materials.	Capable of producing a diverse range of ceramic-based materials. Used for restorative and prosthetic dental parts and medically for bone implants.	Specific to ceramic-based materials, they may not be as versatile as other types of materials.	Alumina, zirconia, silicon nitride, tricalcium phosphate, hydroxyapatite, bioglass, cermet, cordierite, porcelain, magnesium oxide.
Continuous liquid interface production (CLIP)	A subtype of DLP featuring a cylindrical resin reservoir with an oxygen-permeable window at the bottom, allowing UV light to solidify the resin. A "dead zone" of uncured resin created by oxygen interference prevents adhesion, enabling fast printing speeds.	Exceptionally fast printing speeds due to the continuous curing process and minimal adhesion issues thanks to the oxygen-permeable window.	Limited to specific uses where the balance of speed and detail is acceptable; may not achieve the highest resolution details.	Various resins are suitable for rapid prototyping and production.

Source: Refs. [2, 3].

several methods, such as SLS, DMLS, SLM, and EBM. **Table 7.2** summarizes the powder bed fusion technologies.

7.2.3 Direct Energy Deposition (DED)

This technology resembles PBF, but it does not direct the energy source to a powder bed; rather, it adds material and heat simultaneously through the melting of materials, deployed either as powder or wire. The material is deposited onto a surface by a moving nozzle head (**Figure 7.2b**). It allows for the repair or enhancement of existing components, and integration with CNC machining enhances finishing precision. This requires significant amounts of inert gas to maintain an inert environment, and the process can be inefficient due to the waste of unmelted material. Postprocessing is often required to achieve desired surface finishes. The technology can print titanium, aluminum, stainless steel, and copper. It is used mainly for repair or enhancement of parts. The technology can print hard ceramic objects from zirconia and alumina ceramic [2, 3].

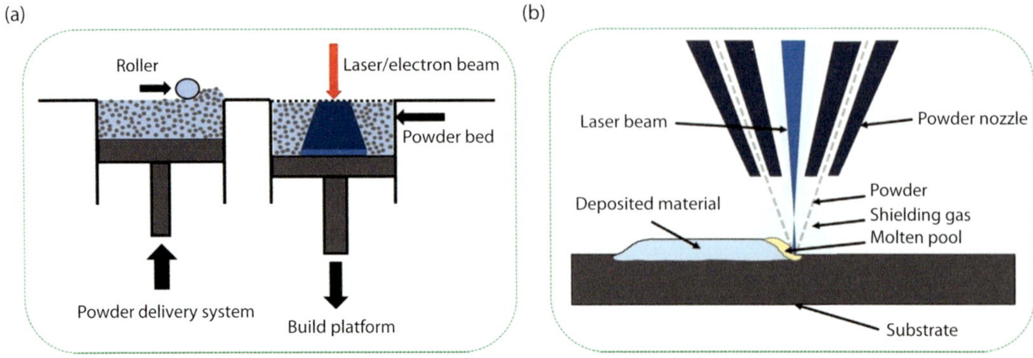

Figure 7.2 The two mostly commonly used ceramic and metal direct printing technologies: (a) powder bed fusion (PBF); (b) direct energy deposition (DED). (From Ref. [16] under Creative Commons Attribution licence.)

7.2.4 Material Extrusion (MEX) Technology

This technology is be known by other names that are applied in common life outside the medical and dental field, such as RC. DIW is another name that is applied medically. The process is characterized by using a stable slurry/ink/paste extrusion through a nozzle. The material is deposited layer by layer over the platform following the consecutive commands of the CAM program until the desired 3D object is manufactured [2, 3].

The MEX technology includes other daughter techniques before fused filament fabrication (FFF) or fused deposition modeling (FDM) [10]. The technique is used in filament in a coil that is heated until melted and injected through a nozzle with different sizes based on the desired layer of thickness. These injected filaments are deposited layer over layer until forming the final 3D object. FDM is the most utilized technique to produce medical and dental parts under the MEX umbrella. Nevertheless, the products should be expected to have lower accuracy than those produced with SLA [2, 3]. FDM can process materials including polylactic acid (PLA), polyamide (nylon), acrylonitrile butadiene styrene (ABS) plastic, metals with low melting points, ceramics, and foundry wax [11].

Table 7.2: Powder Bed Fusion 3D Printing Technologies

3D Printing Technology	Description	Advantages	Disadvantages or Limitations	Materials/or Part Manufactured
SLM	SLM involves using a high-powered laser to completely melt metal powders, allowing for the creation of dense and strong parts.	Produces parts with enhanced density and strength and allows for the manufacturing of complex geometries with precise dimensions.	It can develop significant internal stresses due to thermal gradients, often necessitating subsequent heat treatment to alleviate these stresses.	Dental implants, complex metal structures.
SLS	SLS fuses powders (metallic and non-metallic) by melting a binding agent or a metal with a lower melting point, rather than fully melting the powder.	Suitable for both metallic and non-metallic materials, provides versatility in manufacturing a range of products.	Parts generally have lower density and strength compared to those produced by SLM and may require postprocessing to improve mechanical properties.	Various products including plastics and metals, less structurally demanding components.
EBM	EBM uses an electron beam as its power source, which is different from laser-based methods. The technology is particularly suited for the production of implants due to its high-power concentration.	Offers superior energy utilization, absence of reflective issues (common in laser-based systems), and simplicity in beam focusing. High power concentration makes it ideal for dense and strong metal parts.	Despite its advantages, EBM generally operates at higher temperatures and may require specialized handling and material preparation. Also, the speed of manufacturing can be limited compared to other methods.	Mainly metals like titanium and cobalt-chrome alloys, ideal for medical implants

Source: Ref. [2, 3].

7.2.5 Material Jetting (MJ)

The technology is known as direct inkjet printing (DIP). The process started by heating the photocurable resin to 30–60°C to reach a printable viscosity, then depositing the viscous material's droplets on the platform. The droplets are deposited from a printing head that moves in X and Y directions; every droplet is polymerized by a UV light source [12]. The platform moves downward after every layer to build the next one, and the process is repeated until the final 3D object is formed. The technology is fast, efficient, and economical, allowing for accurate object production with minimum waste.

The PolyJet technology, a famous MJ technique, was innovated and patented by Objet in 2000. The method is integrated into Stratasys' portfolio. It relies on the precise ejection of a liquid photopolymer over a platform, with instant UV light polymerization. The PolyJet method emits a laser spot ranging from 0.06 to 0.10 mm, explaining its good printing accuracy compared to conventional SLA technology. These innovative devices can use multiple heads with different nozzle sizes and can deposit different materials or different colors, resulting in the efficient production of multicolor and multimaterial objects. Dental implant surgical guides from resin materials and high-strength zirconia ceramic for implant fixtures can be printed by this technology [2, 3].

7.2.6 Binder Jetting (Metal Binder Jetting)

The concept of this technology is very similar to material jetting. In BJ technology, the material is not ejected from a nozzle; rather, a recoating blade is used to deposit a thin layer of powder over the platform. A selective droplet of binding agent is deposited over the spread powder from the print head, and the binder joins the powder particles at selected printing sites. After completion of the first layer, the platform moves downward to build the next layer, and the process continues until the 3D object is completed.

The technology is simple, fast, and cheap; however, the initial investment in the device is higher compared with the VPP technology devices. Moreover, an important feature of this technology is that the produced part is free from any internal stresses due to polymerization or thermal management. Nevertheless, the mechanical properties of the BJ products might not be relatively high [2, 3]. The reputation of this technology might have played a role in that it is not primarily selected for printing implant parts or other dental parts. However, a study proposed this technology for dental implant fixtures manufacturing, such as the favorable mechanical properties owing to the approximated elastic modulus between the produced metal fixture and the alveolar bone compared with other technologies such as PBF [13].

The innovative and continuous development of BJ and its corresponding materials results in revolutionary enhancement and adoption of the technology in various industrial and medical realms. Numerous dental parts were produced successfully using BJ. A ceramic powder was developed by a study to assess the challenges facing the production of full ceramic prostheses when utilizing BJ technology [14]. Nevertheless, the metal frameworks, medical scaffolds, and maxillofacial prostheses produced by BJ are not as efficient as those produced by PBF and the conventional technique. The development of BJ printable materials continues, resulting in enhanced product accuracy [15].

7.3 MATERIALS USED FOR 3D-PRINTING IN IMPLANT DENTISTRY

7.3.1 Titanium and Titanium Alloys

Titanium and its alloys exhibit a high degree of chemical reactivity, characterized by forming a robust and tightly bonded oxide layer on their surfaces when exposed to air or various environmental conditions. These layers act as a protective barrier against corrosion. The outstanding strength, remarkable biocompatibility, and lightweight nature of titanium and its alloys render them extremely suitable for medical and dental applications and highly worthy to be provided as printable slurry/powder for additive manufacturing [17]. In the past 20 years, additive manufacturing, particularly PBF technologies, has emerged as a promising method for working with titanium and its alloys [2, 3]. These 3D printing methods are increasingly used to manufacture titanium-based medical implants and prosthetics. This rise in use is driven by their precision, ability to produce complex hollow structures efficiently, flexible design capabilities, cost- and time-effectiveness, and fine detail resolution [2, 3].

3D-printed titanium dental implants, such as the Tixos® system available before 2016, demonstrated successful clinical performance over three years in both upper and lower jaw single-tooth restorations [18]. Additively manufactured titanium scaffolds have also proven effective for periodontal ligament regeneration by enhancing connective tissue growth. DLMS-fabricated Ti-6Al-4V specimens exhibited biological properties comparable to conventionally machined implants [19]. More recent studies have reported favorable osseointegration outcomes for 3D-printed implants compared to traditional ones, along with similar biosafety profiles, indicating that 3D-printed implants could not only serve as alternatives but potentially surpass conventional fixtures [2, 3, 20].

Further improvements include hybrid titanium implants and surface coatings such as chitosan composites, which enhance bioactivity, support cell proliferation, and improve mechanical strength for bone regeneration [19]. Nonetheless, titanium and its alloys remain prone to corrosion after implantation, especially under mechanical forces and acidic oral conditions [21]. Additional limitations of 3D-printed titanium implants involve high manufacturing costs, wear, embrittlement, and toxicity concerns due to post-processing steps that may release harmful particles or chemicals [2, 3].

7.3.2 Biocompatible Photopolymers and Resins

7.3.2.1 Synthetic Polymers

Polymers are extensively utilized in 3D printing applications within the surgical and prosthetic phases of dental implantology, owing to their remarkable versatility. These materials are instrumental in the fabrication of various components, including surgical guides, customized trays, working models, provisional prosthetics supported by implants, as well as crowns and bridges. Recently, high-quality polymers have also been employed in the production of dental implant fixtures and superstructures [2, 3]. Noteworthy examples of polymers utilized in dental 3D printing encompass polycaprolactone (PCL), polymethyl methacrylate (PMMA), PLA, poly(lactic-co-glycolic acid) (PLGA), and ultraviolet (UV) curable resins, as elucidated in **Table 7.3**.

Table 7.3: 3D-Printed Synthetic Polymers

Material	Description	Applications	3D Printing Technology/ies Used
Polycaprolactone (PCL)	An aliphatic polyester known for its biocompatibility, adjustable degradation rate, and extensive applicability in biomedical science. It has a low melting point and is compatible with various fabricable substances.	Used in tissue engineering, as membranes for guided bone regeneration, and in enhancing biocompatibility with bioactive modifications.	Fused deposition modeling (FDM)
Polymethyl methacrylate (PMMA)	A polymer discovered in the 1930s, known for its ease of processing, affordability, and durability within the oral setting.	Utilized in the making of dentures, bone cement, temporary crowns and bridges, occlusal obturators, and orthodontic retainers.	Fused deposition modeling (FDM), stereolithography (SLA)
Polylactic acid (PLA)	An environmentally friendly, biodegradable aliphatic polyester with hydrophilic properties, suitable for future 3D printing applications.	Used in the creation of GTR/GBR membranes, drilling guides for dental implants, and bio-scaffolds for hard tissue engineering.	Fused deposition modeling (FDM)
Poly(lactic-co-glycolic acid) (PLGA)	A copolymer of PLA and PGA, recognized for its biodegradability and biocompatibility, suitable for various dental applications.	Employed in tissue engineering for creating scaffolds that facilitate cell growth and possess antibacterial properties.	Fused deposition modeling (FDM)
Ultraviolet (UV) Resin	Consists of polymer monomer, prepolymer, active diluent, photoinitiator, and photosensitizer, which polymerizes upon UV light exposure to form solid structures.	Used in producing dental crowns, bridges, surgical guides, and other dental prosthetics.	Digital light processing (DLP), stereolithography (SLA)
Polyaryletherketone (PEEK)	Part of the PAEK family, PEEK is a high-performance thermoplastic with excellent physical, chemical, and biological properties.	Increasingly used in dental biomedical applications where conventional materials like metals and ceramics are not suitable.	Not specifically mentioned but typically involves advanced thermoplastic 3D printing techniques.

Source: Ref. [2, 3].

7.3.2.2 *Natural Polymers*

Natural biopolymer-based composites are recognized for their superior biocompatibility and intrinsic biodegradability [22]. These materials are particularly advantageous for bioink formulation in 3D printing, as they can replicate critical characteristics of the extracellular matrix (ECM), including its architecture, self-assembling properties, and compatibility with tissue. As outlined in **Table 7.4**, several natural biopolymers, including collagen, hyaluronic acid (HA), chitosan, agarose, and alginate, have been effectively utilized in 3D bioprinting applications.

7.3.3 Dental Ceramics

Ceramics are traditionally defined as materials that are neither organic nor metallic. The materials in dentistry could be glassy, crystalline, or both, depending on their structure. Ceramics are chemically inert and typically rigid and can be melted to be shaped and densified into the desired form. Modern classification of dental ceramics comprises the glass-infiltrated, glass-matrix, and polycrystalline ceramic families; the latter is the most mechanically reliable material for several medical and dental parts [23]. A fourth classification arose in the last decade called polymer-infiltrated ceramic. Not all these materials are printable; glass-infiltrated and polymer-infiltrated ceramics are not printable yet. However, some showed auspicious outcomes as additively manufactured materials, such as polycrystalline ceramics, in particular zirconia ceramic crowns, bridges, and partial restorations, both in laboratory and clinical investigations [5, 7], considering that glass ceramics are difficult to print compared with polycrystalline ceramic, and all ceramic materials are difficult and complex to be printed compared with resin materials [5]. The composition of the final product depends mainly

Table 7.4: 3D Printed Natural Polymers

Material	Description	Applications	3D Printing Technology/ies Used
HA	A naturally occurring linear polymer that is a component of the ECM and typically derived from human or animal cartilage. HA-based hydrogels demonstrate superior mechanical properties and stability.	Used in tissue repair, wound healing, and the treatment of periodontitis and gingivitis. HA bioinks are also used in 4D printing for enhanced cell attachment and osteogenesis.	Commonly used in bioink formulations for 3D and 4D printing. Specific technologies are not mentioned but likely involve extrusion-based printing.
Collagen	An additional constituent of the ECM used for bioink formulation, either alone or in combination with other materials. Requires precise temperature and duration regulation for crosslinking or gelation.	Enhances cell adhesion and mechanical strength, useful in cartilage tissue engineering. Collagen combined with gelatin improves bioink flow characteristics and biological activity.	Typically used in extrusion-based 3D printing, specific technologies not detailed.
Chitosan	A biopolymer derived from natural sources, chitosan is not easily soluble in water but dissolves in acidic solutions. It exhibits excellent biocompatibility and regenerative capabilities.	Extensively used in prosthodontics, oral implantology, and endodontics. Its application in hard tissue regeneration is limited due to low mechanical strength, although this can be enhanced by incorporating calcium ions.	Extrusion-based 3D printing, specific technologies not detailed.
Alginate	A natural polysaccharide widely utilized in dentistry for traditional dental impressions. It's favorable for bioink development due to its water absorption properties.	Used to form 3D structures in bioinks, potentially enhanced by combining with other polymers like polycaprolactone (PCL) and gelatin.	Commonly used in extrusion-based 3D printing to create hydrogel-based structures.
Cellulose	Derived from plant fibers, cellulose is noted for its hydrophilic, insulating, and anti-static properties.	Used in fabricating tissue engineering scaffolds, wound dressings, and drug delivery systems. Enhanced viscosity of bioinks when combined with other polymers like alginate and PLA.	Frequently used in extrusion-based 3D printing, particularly in creating printable hydrogels and 3D scaffolds.

Source: Ref. [2, 3].

on the composition of the primary slurry/powder/paste. The hybridization in additive manufacturing is possible, although these printable materials are composite but not ceramic materials, referring to the composition by printing composite polymer materials containing the appropriate inorganic filler constituents, e.g., VarseoSmile from BEGO [2, 3].

3D-printed dental ceramic can be acquired in the hybrid form only before sintering, after the removal of the resin components through debinding and condensing of the green body, by sintering results in fully dense ceramic material free of resinous parts. It is important to understand the term "hybridization" in additive manufacturing, which refers to the production of certain parts using two different technologies, like the installation of additively manufactured parts on deep-drawn metal sheets. This could be of great advantage in implant dentistry, for example, by adding certain bioactive materials on machines, additively manufacturing dental implants, or integrating bioactive hydrogel in the porous dental implant structure. The other application of the term hybridization is the utilization of multicomponent printable material for the production of dental ceramic parts such as fixed dental prostheses from zirconia-toughened alumina material, the manufacturing of multimaterial through a multihead material jetting printer, or hybridization of two printing technologies [2, 3].

Glass-matrix ceramic materials production via 3D printing, including feldspathic and lithium disilicate ceramics, is feasible. The procedure is intricate, facing material purity and microstructural heterogeneity challenges to produce the same aesthetic material with good mechanical behavior as the prefabricated blocks supplied for CNC machining [2, 3, 5, 24]. Nevertheless, other laboratory studies reported highly dense additively manufactured lithium disilicate parts with over 400 MPa strength, clinically acceptable aesthetics, and promising accuracy and precision, rendering the material suitable for dental applications. Moreover, additive manufacturing of dental parts with thickness as low as 0.1 mm is feasible, but the material has not yet been fully adopted for clinical application [7].

The most successfully produced dental ceramic group utilizing the 3D printing technologies is polycrystalline ceramics (i.e., oxide ceramics), represented by alumina and zirconia dental parts, showing favorable cellular proliferation, biocompatible reaction, and acceptable cytotoxic effect [5, 7]. Alumina ceramic with high solid loading > 94% and 1600 °C postproduction sintering revealed satisfying structural features and fewer inter- and intralayer defects [24]. The addition of 10% aluminum powder to the printable silicate ceramic resulted in a uniform microstructure [24]. The produced inert alumina using DLP and INP can enhance cellular adhesion and induce differentiation of mesenchymal cells in human tissues [25, 26]. Moreover, the additive manufacturing of ceramic alumina/calcium phosphate structures by DLP 3D printing results in a biocomposite that mimics bone morphology, physical-chemical, and mechanical features [27]. The hybridization of inert alumina on the surface of zirconia dental implants might enhance the biological response of human alveolar bone to the zirconia dental implant and improve the osseointegration potential. Moreover, SLA printing of ATZ ceramic (20% alumina and 80% zirconia) results in a bi-layered alumina-toughened zirconia crown, with comparable strength as the 3D-printed 3Y-TZP crown [24].

The second polycrystalline ceramic material commonly used in the dental field as a 3D printable material is zirconia ceramic. This material has been studied for over eight years for clinical dental applications, and its 3D printing technology is now more advanced than other ceramics, including alumina. Zirconia has demonstrated favorable short-term clinical outcomes [5], with a high aesthetic match of molar crowns to adjacent teeth compared to CNC-milled zirconia crowns. Additionally, full-mouth rehabilitation cases have shown promising results with 3D-printed zirconia [3, 5]. The yttria content affects the mechanical-physical properties and transformation toughness of both machined and 3D-printed zirconia ceramics. Transformation toughness has been observed in 3D-printed zirconia dental implants, which exhibit a crystallographic phase similar to CNC-milled conventional zirconia used for dental implant production. Furthermore, the flexural and characteristic strength of 3D-printed zirconia dental implants is comparable to that of conventionally machined implant fixtures [28]. This transformation toughness may provide an advantage to zirconia dental implants over titanium implants, in addition to aesthetic benefits, as zirconia implants are less prone to deformation under load than titanium implants and superstructures [29, 30].

7.4 SELECTING THE RIGHT 3D PRINTING TECHNOLOGY

The selection of 3D printing technology depends on several factors, including the intended product, the material to be used, the cost of the printing device, and personal preferences. A summary of the product and material to be printed are summarized in **Table 7.5**.

Table 7.5: The Selection of the Proper Technology, the Dental Parts and Material Factors

Dental Product	Material	Preferable Printing Technology	Less-Used Printing Technology	Unused Technologies
Dental models	Resin	DLP SLA MSLA Typically named resin printers	FDM/FFF, CLIP, and LCD Expensive and relatively difficult to print resin	PBF and DED because of complexity to print resin SHL is not used in dentistry
Surgical guide	Resin	SLA, DLP Typically named resin printers	FFF PolyJet MJ Expensive, and relatively difficult to print resin	PBF DED SHL because of complexity to print resin using these technologies SHL is not used in dentistry
Dental implant fixture, prosthetic superstructures	Titanium and titanium alloy, cobalt-chromium alloy	PBF DED Most suitable to print metal	LMM specialized for metal production but need secondary binder MJ Expensive and need secondary binder	SLA, DLP, FFF Still in experimental stage SHL not applied in dentistry
	Zirconia, alumina, and glass ceramics	SLA, DLP, IJP, LCM Showed dependable accuracy and mechanical behavior	SLS, SLM Still experimental MEX, FFF still experimental, more specific for resins and polymers	EBM limited to metal SHL not applied in dentistry
	PEEK	FDM, need specialized high-tech devices SLS can print polymer MJF specialized for polymers	SLA, DLP, IJP, experimental stage	EBM limited to metal SHL not applied in dentistry
Provisional restorations and removable prostheses	Resin	SLA and DLP	MJ is expensive SLS very rarely FFF, still experimental	EBM limited to metal SHL not applied in dentistry

Source: Ref. [2, 3].

7.4.1 The Printing Device's Efficiency and Affordability

Among available 3D printing technologies, FDM printers offer low accuracy, while LCD printers are fast yet unreliable. DLP and SLA printers are quicker, more accurate, and more expensive. Print speed varies with the model type and largely depends on the specific device. For instance, modern SLA printers can produce orthodontic models in as little as nine minutes and high-accuracy restorative models in up to 110 minutes. The DLP Varseo XS by BEGO specializes in resin printing for dental applications like single restorations and denture teeth. The SLA Formlabs 4B model, launched in April 2024, features a platform more than twice the size of competitors, making it ideal for large or batch printing. It operates 1.6–3.4 times faster than brands like Akuretta, Asiga, and Sprintray, and 3.5 times faster than its predecessor, the 3B. Printing hollow models with a 2 mm shell is recommended to enhance speed and efficiency as a cost-effective and time-saving strategy. [31].

Expensive, high-efficiency printers like the multi-head PolyJet are not essential for producing simple dental implantology parts such as surgical guides. Consumer-level printers (DLP, SLA, FFF) have demonstrated comparable accuracy with significantly lower costs [32]. However, ultra-low-cost printers (under $700) may not ensure high-quality fit, especially in complex clinical cases, despite meeting accuracy thresholds in lab settings [33]. For anatomically demanding cases, higher-end devices are advisable to avoid procedural complications.

In situations with multiple printing options, such as zirconia ceramic 3D printing, using an integrated system – including a printer, software, and compatible materials – offers reliability. Lithoz's LCM technology is a prime example, capable of printing lithium disilicate glass restorations as thin as 0.1 mm [7]. Comprehensive CAD/CAM chairside systems like CEREC Primeprint and Planmeca

Cero also exist, offering data acquisition, design, and printing, but are limited to resin applications (e.g., models, guides, aligners). For advanced ceramic printing, Planmeca's Creo® C5 offers a full system, using materials developed by BEGO

7.4.2 Personal Preference

The choice of 3D printing devices and technologies ultimately depends on practitioner preference. One may invest in an all-in-one, high-cost system or opt for a more budget-friendly setup using standalone devices, third-party software, and materials. Alternatively, outsourcing to specialized companies offers access to a broader range of technologies and materials, allowing for the tailored production of diverse dental implantology components – from resin models and surgical guides to metallic implants, zirconia abutments, and high-quality ceramic restorations.

7.5 3D PRINTING APPLICATIONS IN THE SURGICAL PHASE

Integrating 3D printing into dental surgery, specifically for fabricating custom surgical guides, titanium meshes, bone grafts, dental implant fixtures, and root analogue dental implants (**Figure 7.3**), has significantly advanced presurgical planning and treatment outcomes.

7.5.1 Custom Surgical Guides

Surgical guides fabricated through 3D printing have been employed for more than a decade. The digital procedure for these guides comprises initial virtual planning and design utilizing computer software grounded on data obtained from 3D scans. The ensuing plans are executed using 3D-printed surgical guides [34–36]. SLA is currently the most employed technology due to its cost-effectiveness and rapidity. However, emerging technologies such as PolyJet are also being utilized for guide production [37, 38]. The guide fabrication process comprises a series of interconnected stages, including data gathering implant plan design, guide structure development, and subsequent manufacturing [39]. It has been acknowledged that errors made at any of these phases can have an accumulative effect on the final product. [34, 40] The factors affecting the precision of the guides can be divided into two categories: systematic errors that arise during CBCT scanning and data processing, which are beyond human control, and fabrication errors associated with the 3D printer [41], selection of printing materials, slicing techniques, and support structures [42–44]

7.5.2 Bone Grafts and Scaffolds

Bone tissue engineering, enhanced by 3D printing, enables effective treatment of bone defects through porous scaffolds with appropriate mechanical strength and macro/microstructures. These scaffolds, made from biomaterials, support cell attachment and guide tissue regeneration [45–47]. Scaffold performance depends on pore size, volume, mechanical strength, and chemical properties. Ideal biomaterials should offer structural stability, rapid curing, biocompatibility, biomimicry, and bone-like mechanical properties [48]. As bone properties vary by location and defect type, scaffold design must adapt accordingly [49]. Typical fabrication methods include chemical foaming, freeze drying, solvent casting, and foaming gel [50–53], using materials like gypsum, plastics, resins,

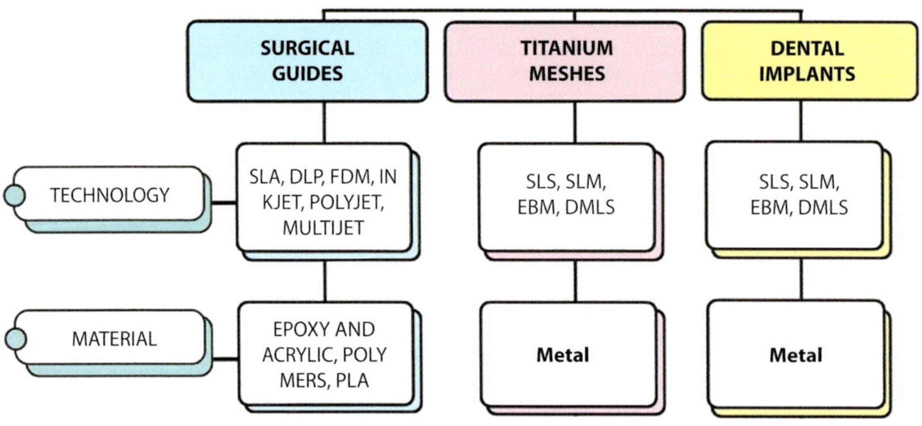

Figure 7.3 3D printing applications for the surgical phase of dental implantology.

ceramics, metal, polyetheretherketone (PEEK), and graphene [50]. Proper macro- and microarchitecture is critical to scaffold efficacy in bone tissue engineering [54].

7.5.3 Customized Titanium Mesh

3D printing of personalized titanium meshes has gained prominence in guided bone regeneration (GBR) for addressing the limitations of conventional meshes [55]. Using cone beam computed tomography (CBCT) to capture jawbone anatomy, an optimal alveolar bone model is digitally created with Computer-Aided Design (CAD) software, considering dental arch contours and implant positions [56]. The custom mesh is then fabricated via SLM or EBM [55, 57, 58].

These personalized meshes offer key advantages: they allow precise control over structure, pore size, and thickness for patient-specific fit [59]; they can be confined to defect areas, minimizing soft tissue disruption; and their design simplifies secondary removal through a minimal incision. Additionally, 3D-printed meshes shorten surgical time, reducing anesthesia exposure, blood loss, and wound exposure, and improving surgical efficiency and outcomes [58, 60].

7.5.4 3D Printing of Dental Implant Fixtures

Integrating interconnected pores into implant structures improves nutrient flow and surface roughness, both of which support bone regeneration and osseointegration [61, 62]. These pores also reduce implant stiffness, aligning the elastic modulus with that of jawbone and mitigating stress shielding over time [63]. Advances in 3D printing, particularly SLM and EBM, allow for precise fabrication of titanium implants with uniform microscale pores [64]. While titanium remains the dominant material, zirconia is gaining attention, and hybrid designs combining titanium roots with zirconia abutments are being explored to enhance both bone and soft tissue integration [65, 66].

Furthermore, 3D printing facilitates the production of complex, patient-specific implant geometries that mimic the shape of natural tooth roots. These custom designs enhance initial stability, match the contours of the extraction site, and replicate the natural stress distribution and gingival profile, improving both function and aesthetics in immediate implant placements [67, 68].

7.5.5 Root Analogue Dental Implant

This type of dental implant – also called an anatomical, custom, or truly anatomic implant – is a medical device designed to replace a tooth's root and superstructure immediately after extraction. It closely conforms to the shape of the alveolar socket, eliminating the need for invasive surgical modification. Implant design is based on data from a CT/CBCT scan of the original root or from a postextraction dental scan [69, 70], which is then processed using CAD software for fabrication through subtractive or, more recently, additive manufacturing methods [71]. The entire process, typically titanium or zirconia, can be completed within one to two days [70].

In 1997, the initial human trials involving tooth replica implants were commenced, documenting the replacement of upper lateral incisors. This methodology underscored its simplicity, the preservation of interdental papillae, and the potential for achieving aesthetic outcomes through implants designed to emulate natural tooth roots [72]. In 2008, Pirker successfully implanted a true anatomic zirconia implant to replace a lower first molar, reporting exceptional outcomes after a follow-up period of 2.5 years without any complications [73]. By 2012, technological advancements facilitated the utilization of CBCT data to generate 3D models, enabling the manufacturing of root analog implants via SLS printing [74]. Furthermore, a titanium-zirconia hybrid root analog implant was successfully implemented in the aesthetic zone, presenting a promising alternative to conventional threaded implants [75].

7.5.5.1 Planning and Designing

Based on insertion methods and data acquisition, root analog implant design can be categorized into two systems. The first method, direct scan with delayed placement, uses data from a direct scan of the tooth root after extraction. The second system, indirect data acquisition with immediate placement, utilizes CBCT to create a 3D model of the root for CAD design.

7.5.5.1.1 Direct Scan, Delayed Placement

i. The BioImplant™

   Introduced in 2007, this approach uses a direct laser scan of the extracted tooth root to create a CAD model of a zirconia implant [70]. A crown stump is designed alongside root replica. The buccal dimensions are minimized to reduce fracture risk of the thin buccal alveolar plate [70]. The technology was successfully applied in cases involving the upper lateral incisor [76], mandibular molar [73], and later, the first premolar and molar [75]. Clinical follow-ups reported positive outcomes, including minimal bone resorption after 18 months [77]. Modern CAD/CAM systems (e.g., Primemill) can produce crowns in under five minutes. Additive manufacturing, such as CEREC or Planmeca systems, now enables transitioning from a four-day postextraction timeline to a single-visit procedure [71, 78].

7.5.5.1.2 Indirect Data Acquisition, Immediate Placement

i. Direct Laser Metal Sintered (DLMS) Implant

First implemented in 2014, this technique uses CBCT imaging to construct a 3D model of a tooth root. Various tools – including reconstruction, reverse engineering, and Pro/Engineering CAD – are employed to finalize the design of the titanium alloy implant [79]. The CAD file is converted into microlayers and fabricated via DLMS using Ti-6Al-4V alloy [80]. To ensure cleanliness, the implant undergoes ultrasonic cleaning and chemical treatment in NaOH and hydrogen peroxide solutions [77]. Studies confirm the implant's primary stability through palpation and percussion, reporting a 100% success rate after one year [75, 79].

This option is particularly suitable for uncomplicated extractions. Conventional implants are advised in cases involving bone loss or intricate root anatomy [79]. The option was applied successfully in 2019 for maxillary anterior tooth replacement [81] and validated after 10 years with stable soft tissue and no bone resorption [82].

ii. The Replicate™ Tooth System

This method combines CBCT scans with either impressions or digital scans to fabricate a hybrid implant – a titanium root replica joined with a milled zirconia crown [83]. Both parts are sintered to eliminate microgaps that may promote bacterial growth and tissue inflammation. Micro-CT scanning confirms a precise fit, and surface treatments (polishing and corundum abrasion) ensure a high-quality finish [84]. A temporary, resin-bonded prosthesis is provided postplacement. Due to potential titanium hypersensitivity, full-zirconia root replicas have been explored. In 2017, Moin et al. used DLP additive manufacturing to produce zirconia root analogue implants (RAIs) with acceptable accuracy compared to the original CAD model [78].

7.5.5.2 Pros of Root Analog Dental Implant

- Simple and practical.
- No expertise required.
- Simple tools for application within a minute.
- No need for drilling, graft, or complex surgical procedures as sinus left is needed.
- Implant is placed directly following the extraction.
- It easily and perfectly fits the root socket, replicating the natural tooth.
- It mimics a natural tooth's hard and soft tissue profile, which adds to the aesthetic value.
- No gap between the abutment and fixture, so no periimplantitis or soft or bony issue loss.
- No altered anatomy or structure, so there are no consequences to the implant procedure.

7.5.5.3 Cons of Root Analog Dental Implant

- The option has not been thoroughly investigated in clinical studies, with the majority of available research consisting of case reports.
- This approach is not suitable for already-extracted teeth or existing edentulous regions.
- In certain pathological cases, modifications to the implant fixture design may be necessary; thus, the placement of implants should be performed exclusively by operators with advanced knowledge and skills.
- The macroretentive mechanisms are insufficient for adequate stress distribution across the alveolus.
- The stability of these implants may not be comparable to conventional fixtures.

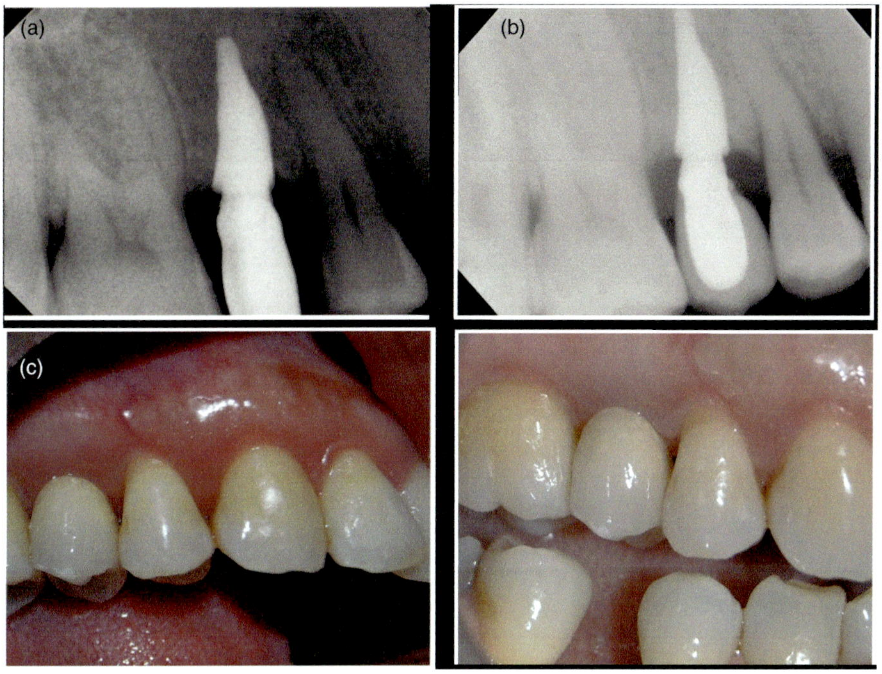

Figure 7.4 (a) Radiograph displays the first clinical root-analogue implant (five-year follow-up), (b) this radiograph demonstrates ten-year follow-up for the same implant (osseointegrated successfully). (c) Clinical images revealed healthy soft tissues with no signs of inflammation. (From Ref. [82] under Creative Commons Attribution license.)

- There is a relatively higher failure rate associated with these implants compared to traditional implant fixtures.
- The indirect scanning and immediate placement necessitate a CBCT scan, thereby exposing them to radiation risks.

7.5.5.4 *Future Perspectives*

Root analog dental implants have emerged as a promising treatment option, offering the flexibility of immediate placement or insertion within two days after extraction. Multiple fabrication methods exist, including sending digital data to specialized manufacturing centers. However, with the rapid advancements in dentistry, especially the advent of additive manufacturing, it is increasingly feasible to complete the entire process chairside. By integrating essential tools such as intraoral scanners, CAD software, and ceramic 3D printers, clinicians can potentially complete implant fabrication and placement within a matter of hours. This approach is further supported by the growing integration of artificial intelligence into dental technologies, which enhances the efficiency and precision of both scanning and design workflows. Implementing such chairside systems could eliminate the need for CBCT imaging required in indirect scanning protocols and reduce reliance on the guided implant placement methods typical of conventional procedures (**Figure 7.4**).

With the integration of current technologies, scanning the extracted tooth root, designing the implant, and fabricating it within a few hours is feasible. The concept of hybrid root analog implants – typically involving a titanium root form combined with a zirconia crown – can evolve further. A next-generation approach could involve the direct 3D printing of both zirconia and titanium components, followed by surface hybridization using highly bioactive materials. This advancement would significantly enhance the implant's bioactivity, promote more effective interaction with the alveolus, and improve overall osseointegration [85, 86].

7.6 3D PRINTING APPLICATIONS IN THE PROSTHODONTIC

Advances in CAD/CAM and 3D printing technologies have led to substantial improvements in multiple facets of prosthetics utilized in dental implants (**Figure 7.5**).

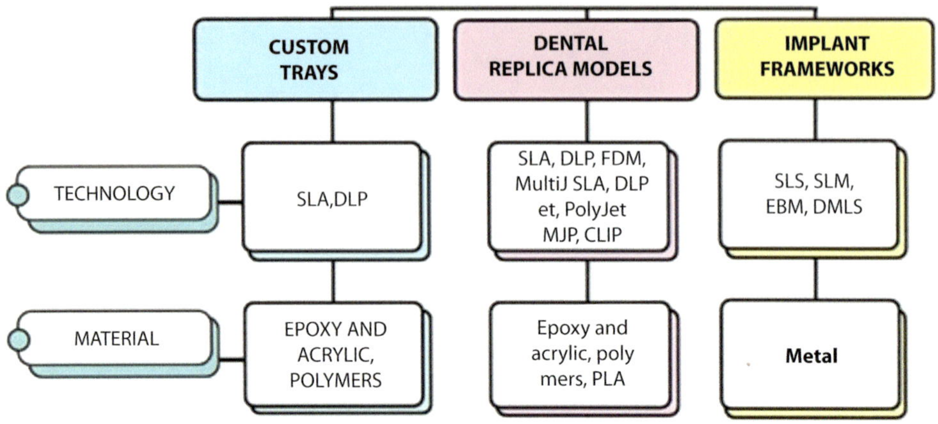

Figure 7.5 Applications of 3D printing in the prosthodontic stage of implant therapy.

7.6.1 Custom Abutments and Frameworks

CAD/CAM is extensively applied in designing and fabricating implant-retained prosthetic frameworks [87]. Once the CAD is complete, the frameworks are manufactured using additive or subtractive methods [88]. Subtractive manufacturing offers simple clinical workflows and reduced human error than conventional casting, but it also leads to material waste and may not accurately reproduce fine structural details [89]. AM techniques, such as SLM and EBM, offer a material-efficient alternative [90], producing frameworks with mechanical properties comparable to or superior to those of conventionally cast versions [91]. Moreover, the framework retainers can be customized to improve resin bonding.

Laser sintering is a common approach for producing cobalt-chromium crowns and bridges [88]. With optimized postprocessing, this method yields stress-free, accurate frameworks, even for long-span bridges. Its ability to fabricate multiple units simultaneously enhances efficiency, making it a cost-effective and standard method for creating fixed prostheses with nonprecious alloys.

7.6.2 Provisional and Final Prostheses

3D printing has significantly transformed dental prosthetics, advancing the fabrication of temporary and permanent devices like crowns, bridges, and overdentures. This technology enables highly precise, efficient, and patient-specific prostheses using digital scans for accurate fitting and minimal adjustments [92]. Rapid production of temporary prostheses also reduces patients' time without teeth, improving aesthetics and function. As the technology evolves, it continues to streamline workflows, shorten turnaround times, and expand possibilities in dental restoration and rehabilitation [93].

7.6.3 Custom Trays Fabrication

The introduction of 3D printing led to the fabrication of customized trays for implant restorations [94]. Revilla-León et al. and Piedra et al. described digital workflows for full-arch impressions using digitally designed metal splints and custom trays produced through DMLS and DLP, respectively [95–97]. These metal splints fit precisely with impression copings, simplifying intraoral placement. 3D-printed versions offer significant advantages compared to manually fabricated trays. They provide a more uniform and spacious area for impression material between the splint and tray, enhancing the accuracy of tissue capture [98]. Additionally, they shorten clinical time by reducing the need for resin-based fixation of impression posts, thereby minimizing errors from resin polymerization shrinkage [95, 99].

7.6.4 Models of Dental Implants

The earliest uses of 3D printing in dentistry were fabricating physical models from digital scans [4, 95]. These models must accurately reflect implant positioning and orientation relative to adjacent teeth. Unlike traditional plaster casts, 3D-printed models are lighter and stronger, have a superior finish, enhance abrasion resistance, and avoid implant analog misalignment [100, 101]. They also offer a tangible reference for assessing occlusion and interproximal contact, which digital models alone cannot provide [102]. Inaccuracies stem from distortions during scanning, design software settings, and printing processes [101]. Factors like the scanner type and digitization method may affect such inaccuracies. The maximum deviation for implant restorations should be below 100 micrometers and not more than 150 micrometers [103].

7.7 CONCLUSION

3D printing has become a transformative tool in implantology through a flexible manufacturing approach for various biomaterials, including ceramics, polymers, metals, and composites. This approach enhances production speed, accuracy, and consistency while minimizing waste and reducing reliance on skilled manual labor. Integrating digital scanning, visualization, and computer-aided design with 3D printing has fostered innovation in developing implant fixtures and prostheses such as temporary crowns and bridges.

Despite its promise, the continued adoption of 3D printing in dentistry faces several challenges. Although it is progressing toward replacing conventional porcelain, metal, and ceramic restorations, critical issues remain, most notably ensuring printed materials' biocompatibility and functional reliability. Issues about using uncertified materials and the growing trend of do-it-yourself applications that bypass regulatory standards have also arisen. Additionally, the incompatibility of metallic implants with MRI highlights the need for alternative materials. Moving forward, the success of 3D printing depends upon addressing limitations while exploring biofunctional, tissue-engineered solutions that could redefine restorative treatment. Ongoing research and innovation in additive manufacturing will be key to shaping the future of dental restorations.

REFERENCES

1. Alqutaibi, AY et al. Digital fabrication of complete dentures, compared to conventional methods, may offer a more cost-effective approach with improved patient outcomes. J Evid Based Dent Pract. 2024;24(2):101986.
2. Alqutaibi, AY et al. Advanced additive manufacturing in implant dentistry: 3D printing technologies, printable materials, current applications and future requirements. Bioprinting. 2024;42:e00356.
3. Alghauli, MA et al. Evolution of medical 3D printing, printable biomaterials, prosthetic and regenerative dental applications. Bioprinting. 2025;46:e00395.
4. Alghauli, MA et al. Impact of 3D printing orientation on accuracy, properties, cost, and time efficiency of additively manufactured dental models: a systematic review. BMC Oral Health. 2024;24(1):1550.
5. Alghauli, M et al. 3D-printed versus conventionally milled zirconia for dental clinical applications: trueness, precision, accuracy, biological and esthetic aspects. J Dent. 2024;144:104925.
6. Alghauli, MA et al. Advanced subtractive manufacturing, micromilling, and laser micromachinery in dentistry: current applications, limitations, and future perspectives. Biomaterials Connect. 2025;2(1):1–10.
7. Alghauli, MA, Alqutaibi, AY. 3D-printed intracoronal restorations, occlusal and laminate veneers: clinical relevance, properties, and behavior compared to milled restorations: a systematic review and meta-analysis. J Esthet Restor Dent. 2024;36(8):1153–1170.
8. Alghauli, MA et al. Influence of different print orientations on properties and behavior of additively manufactured resin dental devices: a systematic review and meta-analysis. J Prosthet Dent. 2025;133(3):736.e1–736.e12.
9. Alqutaibi, AY et al. Physical–mechanical properties and accuracy of additively manufactured resin denture bases: impact of printing orientation. J Prosthodont Res. 2025;24:00263.
10. Bozkurt, Y, Karayel, E. 3D printing technology; Methods, biomedical applications, future opportunities and trends. J Mat Res Technol. 2021;14:1430–1450.
11. Gielisch, M et al. Steam-sterilized and degradable fused filament fabrication-printed polylactide/polyhydroxyalkanoate surgical guides for dental implants: Are they accurate enough for static navigation? Int J Bioprint. 2023;9(2):655.
12. Branco, AC et al. Recent Advances on 3D-Printed Zirconia-Based Dental Materials: A Review, Materials (Basel) 2023;16(5):1860.
13. Xiong, Y et al. Fabrication of porous titanium implants by three-dimensional printing and sintering at different temperatures. Dent Mater J. 2012;31(5):815–20.
14. Miyanaji, H et al. Process development of porcelain ceramic material with binder jetting process for dental applications. JOM. 2016;68:831–841.
15. Janzen, K et al. Influence of different powder conditioning strategies on metal binder jetting with Ti-6Al-4V, Materials (Basel) 2024;17(3):750.
16. Yang, X et al. A physically-based structure-property model for additively manufactured Ti-6Al-4V. Mater Des. 2021;205:109709.
17. Hatamleh, MM et al. Surface characteristics and biocompatibility of cranioplasty titanium implants following different surface treatments. Dent Mater. 2018;34(4):676–683.
18. Tunchel, S et al. 3D printing/additive manufacturing single titanium dental implants: a prospective multicenter study with 3 years of follow-up. Int J Dent. 2016;2016:8590971.
19. Kim, JH et al. Mechanophysical and biological properties of a 3D-printed titanium alloy for dental applications. Dent Mater. 2020;36(7):945–958.
20. Lang, NP et al. Sequential osseointegration of a novel implant system based on 3D printing in comparison with conventional titanium implants. Clin Oral Implants Res. 2023;34(6):627–638.
21. Sarao, TP et al. Enhancing biocompatibility and corrosion resistance of Ti-6Al-4V alloy by surface modification route. J Thermal Spray Technol. 2018;27(8):1388–1400.

22. Park, S et al. Biopolymer-based composite materials prepared using ionic liquids, Applicat Ionic Liquids Biotechnol 2019;2019:133–176.
23. Spitznagel, FA et al. Clinical outcomes of all-ceramic single crowns and fixed dental prostheses supported by ceramic implants: A systematic review and meta-analyses. Clin Oral Implants Res. 2022;33(1):1–20.
24. Alghauli, MA et al. Influence of 3D printing orientations on physico-mechanical properties and accuracy of additively manufactured dental ceramics. J Prosthodont Res. 2025;69(2):181–202.
25. Lauria, I et al. Inkjet printed periodical micropatterns made of inert alumina ceramics induce contact guidance and stimulate osteogenic differentiation of mesenchymal stromal cells. Acta Biomater. 2016;44:85–96.
26. Lei, H et al. Rational design and additive manufacturing of alumina-based lattice structures for bone implant. Mater Des. 2022;221:111003.
27. Esteves, AV et al. Additive manufacturing of ceramic alumina/calcium phosphate structures by DLP 3D printing. Mater Chem Phys. 2022;276:125417.
28. Alghauli, MA et al. The physical-mechanical properties of 3D-printed versus conventional milled zirconia for dental clinical applications: A systematic review with meta-analysis. J Mech Behav Biomed Mater. 2024;156:106601.
29. Tribst, JPM et al. Failed Dental Implant: When Titanium Fractures, Diagnostics (Basel). 2023;13(12):2123.
30. Leo, SJ et al. Rotational load fatigue performance of titanium vs titanium-zirconium implant-abutment connections. Int J Oral Maxillofac Implants. 2022;37(4):740–747.
31. Bennett, GW, DiGiovanni, T. Effect of wall thickness of 3D-printed models on resisting deformation from thermal forming in-office aligners. Clin Exp Dent Res. 2024;10(1):e827.
32. Wegmüller, L et al. Consumer vs. high-end 3d printers for guided implant surgery –an in vitro accuracy assessment study of different 3d printing technologies, J Clin Med 2021;10(21):4894.
33. Bennett, GW, Kim, SK. Comparison of the fit of surgical guides manufactured with low-cost 3D printers. Gen Dent. 2022;70(1):18–21.
34. l'Alzit, FR et al. Accuracy of commercial 3D printers for the fabrication of surgical guides in dental implantology. J Dent. 2022;117:103909.
35. Unsal, GS et al. Advantages and limitations of implant surgery with CAD/CAM surgical guides: A literature review. J Clin Experiment Dent. 2020;12(4):e409.
36. Zhang, F et al. The clinical accuracy of the implant digital surgical guide: A meta-analysis. Am J Dent. 2020;33(6):296–304.
37. Henprasert, P et al. Comparison of the accuracy of implant position using surgical guides fabricated by additive and subtractive techniques. J Prosthodont. 2020;29(6):534–541.
38. Sedov, YG et al. A classification of surgical guides application for dental implantation. Stomatologiia. 2021;100(1):84–88.
39. Alqutaibi, AY. CAD-CAM surgically-guided oral implant site expansion and implant placement in severely atrophic maxilla. J Taibah University Med Sci. 2020;15(2):153–159.
40. Putra, RH et al. The accuracy of implant placement with computer-guided surgery in partially edentulous patients and possible influencing factors: A systematic review and meta-analysis. J Prosthodont Res. 2022;66(1):29–39.
41. Zhang, C et al. Material extrusion based fabrication of surgical implant template and accuracy analysis. Materials. 2022;15(5):1738.
42. Cho, JY et al. The accuracy of a partially guided system using an in-office 3D-printed surgical guide for implant placement. Int J Computerized Dent 2021;24(1):19–27.
43. Elliott, T et al. Additively manufactured surgical implant guides: A review. J Prosthodont. 2022;31(S1):38–46.
44. Rubayo, DD et al. Influences of build angle on the accuracy, printing time, and material consumption of additively manufactured surgical templates. J Prosthet Dent. 2021;126(5):658–663.
45. Abdalla, RIB et al. Does the adjunctive use of platelet-rich plasma to bone graft during sinus augmentation reduce implant failure and complication? Systematic review and meta-analysis. Quintessence Int 2018;49(2):139–146.
46. Ali, RMM et al. Effect of submerged vs nonsubmerged implant placement protocols on implant failure and marginal bone loss: a systematic review and meta-analysis. Int J Prosthot. 2018;31(1):15–22.
47. Alqutaibi, AY, Altaib, F. Short dental implant is considered as a reliable treatment option for patients with atrophic posterior maxilla. J Evidence Based Dent Pract. 2016;16(3):173–175.
48. Whitehouse, MR, Blom, AW. The use of ceramics as bone substitutes in revision hip arthroplasty. Materials. 2009;2(4):1895–1907.
49. Koons, GL et al. Materials design for bone-tissue engineering. Nat Rev Mater. 2020;5(8):584–603.
50. Haleem, A et al. 3D printing applications in bone tissue engineering. J Clin Orthopaed Trauma. 2020;11:S118–S124.
51. Bose, S et al. Effect of chemistry on osteogenesis and angiogenesis towards bone tissue engineering using 3D printed scaffolds. Ann Biomed Engineer. 2017;45:261–272.
52. Vaishya, R et al. Computed tomography based 3D printed patient specific blocks for total knee replacement. J Clin Orthopaed Trauma. 2018;9(3):254–259.
53. De Witte, TM et al. Bone tissue engineering via growth factor delivery: from scaffolds to complex matrices. Regen Biomater. 2018;5(4):197–211.
54. Tarafder, S et al. 3D printed tricalcium phosphate bone tissue engineering scaffolds: effect of SrO and MgO doping on in vivo osteogenesis in a rat distal femoral defect model. Biomater Sci. 2013;1(12):1250–1259.
55. Xie, Y et al. Titanium mesh for bone augmentation in oral implantology: current application and progress. Int J Oral Sci. 2020;12(1):37.
56. Romero, PM et al. Customized surgical protocols for guided bone regeneration using 3D printing technology: A retrospective clinical trial. J Craniofac Surg. 2021;32(2):e198–e202.
57. Cucchi, A et al. Custom-made titanium mesh for maxillary bone augmentation with immediate implants and delayed loading. J Oral Implantol. 2019;45(1):59–64.
58. Seiler, M et al. Customized lattice structure in reconstruction of three-dimensional alveolar defects. Int J Comput Dent. 2018;21(3):261–267.
59. Jung, GU et al. Preliminary evaluation of a three-dimensional, customized, and preformed titanium mesh in peri-implant alveolar bone regeneration. J Korean Assoc Oral Maxillofac Surg. 2014;40(4):181.
60. Hartmann, A et al. Evaluation of risk parameters in bone regeneration using a customized titanium mesh: results of a clinical study. Implant Dent. 2019;28(6):543–550.

61. Chen, J et al. Production of inter-connective porous dental implants by computer-aided design and metal three-dimensional printing. J Biomater Applic. 2020;34(9):1227–1238.
62. Yu, T et al. Effects of immediately static loading on osteointegration and osteogenesis around 3D-printed porous implant: A histological and biomechanical study. Mater Sci Eng C. 2020;108:110406.
63. Wally, ZJ et al. Selective laser melting processed Ti6Al4V lattices with graded porosities for dental applications. J Mech Behav Biomed Mater. 2019;90:20–29.
64. Mangano, F et al. Maxillary overdentures supported by four splinted direct metal laser sintering implants: a 3-year prospective clinical study. Int J Dent 2014;2014:252343.
65. Pillai, S et al. Dental 3D-printing: transferring art from the laboratories to the clinics. Polymers. 2021;13(1):157.
66. Westover, B. Three-dimensional custom-root replicate tooth dental implants. Oral Maxillofac Surg Clin. 2019;31(3):489–496.
67. Figliuzzi, M et al. A novel root analogue dental implant using CT scan and CAD/CAM: selective laser melting technology. Int J Oral Maxillofac Surg. 2012;41(7):858–862.
68. Moin, DA et al. Designing a novel dental root analogue implant using cone beam computed tomography and CAD/CAM technology. Clinical Oral Implants Res. 2013;24:25–27.
69. Evans, ZP et al. Anatomic customization of root-analog dental implants with cone-beam CT and CAD/CAM fabrication: a cadaver-based pilot evaluation. J Oral Implantol. 2018;44(1):15–26.
70. Pirker, W, Kocher, A. Immediate, non-submerged, root-analogue zirconia implants placed into single-rooted extraction sockets: 2-year follow-up of a clinical study. Int J Oral Maxillofac Surg. 2009;38(11):1127–1132.
71. Aldesoki, M, Keilig, L, Dörsam, I, Evers-Dietze, B, Elshazly, TM, Bourauel, C. Trueness and precision of milled and 3D printed root-analogue implants: A comparative in vitro study. J Dent. 2023;130:104425.
72. Heydecke, G, Kohal, R, Gläser, R. Optimal esthetics in single-tooth replacement with the Re-Implant system: a case report. Int J Prosthodont. 1999;12(2):184–189.
73. Pirker, W, Wiedemann, D, Lidauer, A, Kocher, AA. Immediate, single stage, truly anatomic zirconia implant in lower molar replacement: a case report with 2.5 years follow-up. Int J Oral Maxillofac Surg. 2011;40(2):212–216.
74. Mangano, FG et al. Custom-made, root-analogue direct laser metal forming implant: a case report. Lasers Med Sci. 2012;27(6):1241–1245.
75. Saeidi Pour, K et al. Innovative single-tooth replacement with an individual root-analog hybrid implant in the esthetic zone: case report. Int J Oral Maxillofac Implants. 2017;32(3):e153–e160.
76. Pirker, W, Kocher, A. True anatomic immediate dental implant method. Implants. 2009;10:10–14.
77. Patankar, A et al. Immediate, non submerged root analog zirconia implant in single rooted tooth replacement: case report with 2 years follow up. J Maxillofac Oral Surg. 2016;15(Suppl 2):270–273.
78. Anssari Moin, S et al. A novel approach for custom three-dimensional printing of a zirconia root analogue implant by digital light processing. Clin Oral Implants Res. 2017;28(6):668–670.
79. Mangano, FG et al. Immediate, non-submerged, root-analogue direct laser metal sintering (DLMS) implants: a 1-year prospective study on 15 patients. Lasers Med Sci. 2104;29(4):1321–1328.
80. Mangan, C et al. Stereo imaging and cytocompatibility of a model dental implant surface formed by direct laser fabrication. J Biomed Mater Res A. 2009;88(3):823–831.
81. Figliuzzi, M et al. A direct metal laser sintering (DMLS) root analogue implant placed in the anterior maxilla. Case report, Ann Ital Chir 2019;8:S2239253X19030044.
82. Figliuzzi, MM et al. 10-year evaluation of the first root analogue implant on humans, made using a CT scan, CAD/CAM and DMLS. Biomimetics (Basel). 2022;7(1):2022.
83. Pour, R et al. Innovative single-tooth replacement with an individual root-analog hybrid implant in the esthetic zone: case report. Int J Oral Maxillofac Implant. 2017;32(3):e153–e160.
84. Happe, A et al. Effects of different polishing protocols on the surface roughness of Y-TZP surfaces used for custom-made implant abutments: a controlled morphologic SEM and profilometric pilot study. J Prosthet Dent. 2015;113(5):440–447.
85. Zhong, W et al. 3D-printed titanium implant-coated polydopamine for repairing femoral condyle defects in rabbits. J Orthop Surg Res. 2020;15(1):102.
86. Li, J et al. Hybrid fabrication of photo-clickable vascular hydrogels with additive manufactured titanium implants for enhanced osseointegration and vascularized bone formation. Biofabrication 2022;14(3). doi: 10.1088/1758-5090/ac6051.
87. Kapos, T, Evans, C, CAD/CAM technology for implant abutments, crowns, and superstructures. Int J Oral Maxillofac Implants 2014;29(Suppl):117–136.
88. Revilla-León, M et al. Metal additive manufacturing technologies: literature review of current status and prosthodontic applications. Int J Comput Dent. 2019;22(1):55–67.
89. Svanborg, P et al. Additively manufactured titanium and cobalt-chromium implant frameworks: fit and effect of ceramic veneering. Int J Oral Maxillofac Implants 2018;33(3):590–596.
90. Barbin, T et al. 3D metal printing in dentistry: An in vitro biomechanical comparative study of two additive manufacturing technologies for full-arch implant-supported prostheses. J Mechanical Behavior Biomed Mater. 2020;108:103821.
91. Revilla-León, M et al. Discrepancy at the implant abutment-prosthesis interface of complete-arch cobalt-chromium implant frameworks fabricated by additive and subtractive technologies before and after ceramic veneering. J Prosthet Dent 2021;125(5):795–803.
92. Alghauli, MA et al. Properties and behavior of additively manufactured provisional fixed dental prostheses: a systematic review on 3D printing orientations relative to applied materials and postprocessing. J Esthet Restor Dent. 2025;37(6):1407–1418.
93. Alghazzawi, TF et al. Advancements in CAD/CAM technology: Options for practical implementation. J Prosthodont Res. 2016;60(2):72–84.
94. Kim, JE et al. Computer-based implant planning involving a prefabricated custom tray with alumina landmark structures. J Prosthet Dent. 2019;121(3):373–377.
95. Revilla-León, M, Özcan, M. Additive manufacturing technologies used for processing polymers: current status and potential application in prosthetic dentistry. J Prosthod. 2019;28:146–158.
96. Cascón, WP, Revilla-León, M. Digital workflow for the design and additively manufacture of a splinted framework and custom tray for the impression of multiple implants: a dental technique. J Prosthet Dent. 2018;120(6):805–811.

97. Alnazzawi, AA et al. The accuracy of custom-made metal posts manufactured using selective laser sintering versus conventional casting techniques: a laboratory study. BMC Res Notes. 2024;17(1):349.
98. Sun, Y et al. Clinical evaluation of final impressions from three-dimensional printed custom trays. Sci Rep. 2017;7(1):14958.
99. Kim, JE et al. A digital implant custom tray fabrication method using the design process for simulating the position of the impression copings and 3D printing technology. J Prosthet Dent. 2019;121(4):566–570.
100. Monaco, C et al. The prototype concept in a full digital implant workflow. J Am Dent Assoc. 2018;149(10):918–923.
101. Tian, Y et al. A review of 3D printing in dentistry: Technologies, affecting factors, and applications. Scanning 2021;2021: 9950131.
102. Buda, M et al. Accuracy of 3-dimensional computer-aided manufactured single-tooth implant definitive casts. J Prosthet Dent. 2018;120(6):913–918.
103. Papaspyridako, P et al. Digital workflow: In vitro accuracy of 3D printed casts generated from complete-arch digital implant scans. J Prosthet Dent. 2020;124(5):589–593.

8 Digital Implant Prosthodontics

Yu Pan, Edmond H. N. Pow, Katherine C. M. Leung, and Walter Y. H. Lam

Dental implants are increasingly favored for restoring edentulous patients due to their superior support, stability, and comfort compared to traditional complete dentures [1–3]. While screw-retained implants are preferred, achieving a passive fit between the suprastructure and supporting implants is often challenging. Misfits over 50 µm can lead to detrimental stress at the bone-implant interface, causing complications [4, 5] (**Figure 8.1**).

The conventional workflow for screw-retained implants is lengthy and technically demanding, with misfit corrections requiring sectioning and soldering [6, 7]. Complications like veneer chipping and screw fractures are common, with a 10-year complication rate of 67% and 21%, respectively [8]. A study found that greater misfits in complete-arch implants correlated with more screw-related issues [9].

To address these challenges, a digital workflow has emerged, gaining acceptance for its accuracy and efficiency [10]. This process involves three stages: data acquisition (using handheld intraoral scanners [IOS] or laboratory scans), computer-aided design (CAD) to create a virtual framework, and computer-aided manufacturing (CAM) for fabricating implant frameworks through CNC milling or 3D printing [11].

8.1 CLINICAL THRESHOLD

There is no consensus on acceptable distortion levels in implant-supported prostheses. Jemt et al. [4] reported mean 3D distortions of 111 ± 50 µm and 91 ± 51 µm between implants and frameworks in their one-year and five-year studies, respectively, deeming these clinically acceptable due to minimal marginal bone loss. Subsequent research set the upper limit of long-term distortion at 150 µm, supported by Jostad et al. [9], who assessed mean misfit in 30 patients with complete-arch prostheses over 19 years. This threshold has been adopted to define "implant success" by the US Department of Health and Human Services since 1979 [12].

Conversely, an in vitro study by Papaspyridakos et al. [5] proposed a lower threshold of 59 to 72 µm based on clinical fit and 3D distortions, though it was not correlated with clinical outcomes. Some studies noted unacceptable distortion levels of 192–366 µm [13] during data acquisition and 240–820 µm throughout the workflow [14]. While other research indicated good clinical fit and outcomes, quantitative measurements were lacking [10, 15, 16]. Most studies have short follow-up durations of one to four years, and techniques for assessing "clinical fit" varied, with tactile methods being inconsistent and radiographic methods likely underestimating misfits [17, 18].

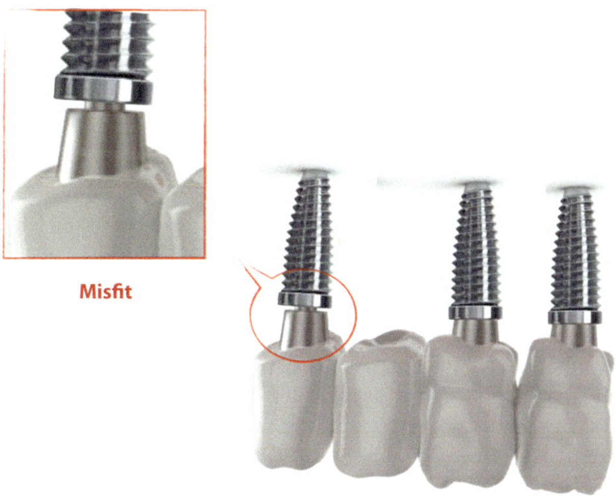

Figure 8.1 Misfit between the dental implant and the abutment.

DOI: 10.1201/9781003428541-8

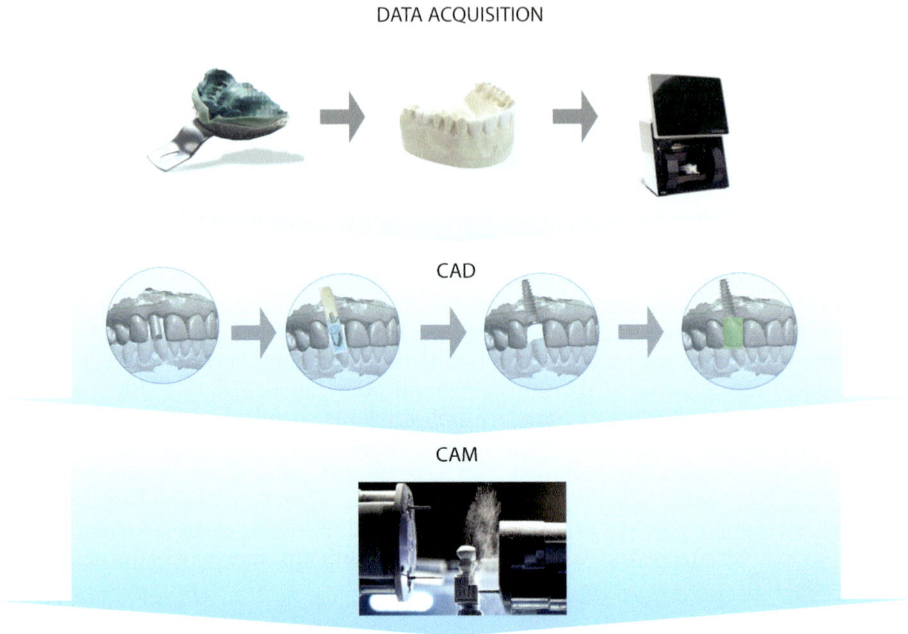

Figure 8.2 The analog-digital workflow.

8.2 DATA ACQUISITION STAGE

8.2.1 Analog-Digital Workflow

Analog-digital workflow involves digitizing the gypsum cast made from a conventional impression by high-precision laboratory scanners to obtain the digital model of the arch (**Figure 8.2**).

Laboratory scanners in dentistry, adapted from industrial optical scanners, often utilize structured light technology. This method employs structured light patterns to capture three-dimensional (3D) surface shape information from reflections [19]. The accuracy of these systems depends on the optical properties of the target surface and the quality of the sensor lens. Distortions or misinterpretations of light signals during reflection can affect scanning accuracy [20].

Studies indicate high trueness (5.3 ± 1.1 μm) and precision (1.6 ± 0.6 μm) for laboratory scanners with dentate models [21]. Trueness measures the agreement between test and reference measurements, while precision reflects test variability (ISO 5725-1) [22]. The International Organization for Standardization (ISO 12836) suggests using a geometric calibration block to evaluate scanner accuracy for indirect dental restorations [23] **(Figure 8.3)**.

The implant scenario differs from the dentate model in various ways, including the use of scan bodies for data acquisition and a focus on implant positioning rather than surface contour. These factors limit the applicability of tooth scanning accuracy studies to the implant context. A previous study [24] introduced a novel calibration object to assess laboratory scanner accuracy during implant scanning (**Figure 8.4**).

Results showed laboratory scanners were less accurate for implants than for dentate arches, experiencing distortion in tilted implant sites due to light access and turntable motion. In structured light 3D scanning, fringe patterns must reach the target surface unobstructed [25]. Tilted implants block light from undercuts [19], leading to low-intensity point clouds and reduced accuracy [26]. The turntable allows 360° rotation (–45° to 45°), needing to counteract gravity/vibrations for accurate positioning [25].

The trueness of laboratory scanners remains unaffected by inter-implant distance, with no significant differences between short and long spans. IOS may distort more with increased distance [27], as smaller wands limit visibility and require multiple stitched images, introducing errors [28, 29]. Laboratory scanners provide a wider view for direct 3D reconstruction, minimizing stitching errors [26].

Accuracy at the implant level is critical, as small deformations can amplify over distances (10 mm, height of scan body) [30]. Imaging near the implant is challenging due to reflections, undercuts, and

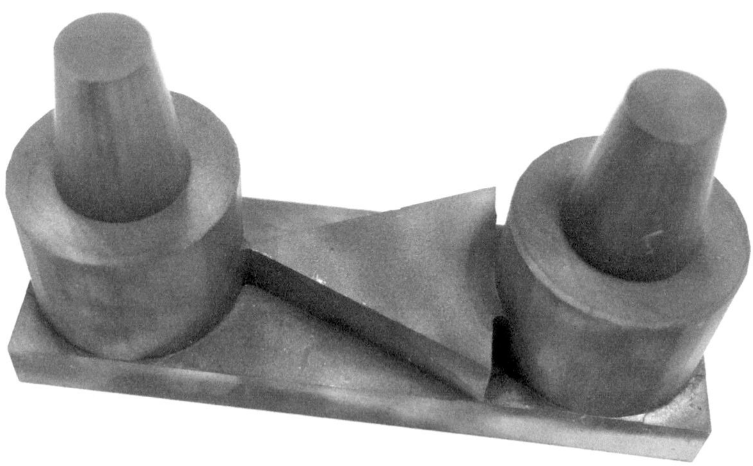

Figure 8.3 The calibration object proposed by ISO 12836 for indirect dental restorations.

gingival tissue [31]. The Zfx scanner offers vertical trueness of 2.6 µm for single implants, while horizontal accuracy in complete arch implants is vital. The IScan scanner shows lower horizontal distortion and better trueness at the implant level than the scan body. To enhance laboratory scanners, focus on mitigating unfavorable implant angulation in long spans and improving horizontal and vertical accuracy at the implant level.

8.2.1.1 Complete-Digital Workflow

Hand-held IOS are now available that can eliminate the need for a traditional impression, which is unpleasant for most patients (**Figure 8.5)** [32].

8.2.1.1.1 Mechanisms

Current IOS systems use optical mechanisms like confocal microscopy, optical triangulation, wavefront sampling, interferometry, stereophotogrammetry, structured light, laser, and video principles, with the first three primarily studied in one research area [33]. While IOS systems operate similarly to laboratory scanners, they are smaller for intraoral use. Light signals convert to point clouds in 3D images with depth and spatial data, but limited view frames capture only small areas per image (**Figure 8.6**). Therefore, complete arches are reconstructed by stitching multiple 3D images, introducing "stitching error," especially for long-span and complete-arch scanning [34].

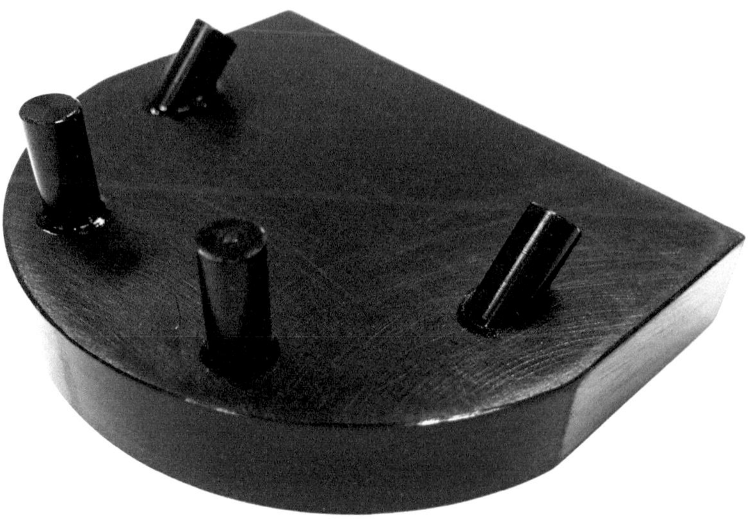

Figure 8.4 The custom-made calibration object is specifically designed for complete-arch implant situations.

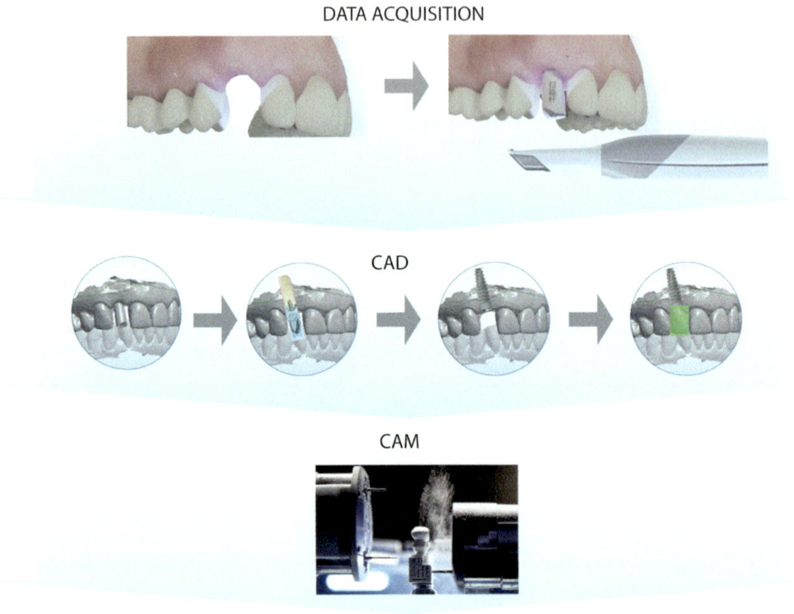

Figure 8.5 The complete digital workflow.

In triangulation devices, light signals reflect off surfaces and are captured by camera sensors, determining 3D point positions [35, 36]. These scanners report trueness and precision of about 70 μm and 60 μm, respectively [28, 37, 38]. Optical triangulation is more sensitive to environmental factors, requiring a clear view, making it hard to capture undercuts and affecting data quality [35].

Active wavefront sampling systems use a smaller wand and one camera for depth [34]. Recent software improved the 3M True Definition's trueness and precision to 10–30 μm and 30–40 μm [28, 37–40]. However, light powder dusting is still needed, making the process inconvenient [41].

8.2.1.1.2 Single and Short-Span Implant Scanning

Multiple studies indicate that IOS can achieve trueness of 6–45 μm, comparable to conventional polyether impressions for single and short-span implant-supported prostheses. Unlike natural

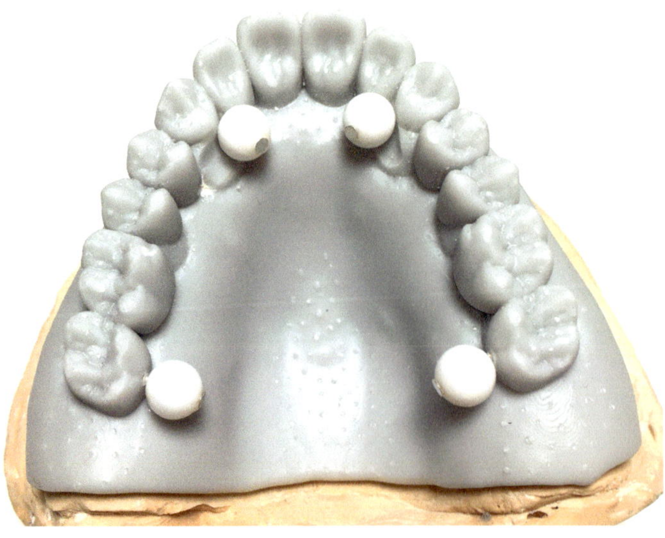

Figure 8.6 The calibration object proposed by ISO 20896 to assess the accuracy of hand-held IOS.

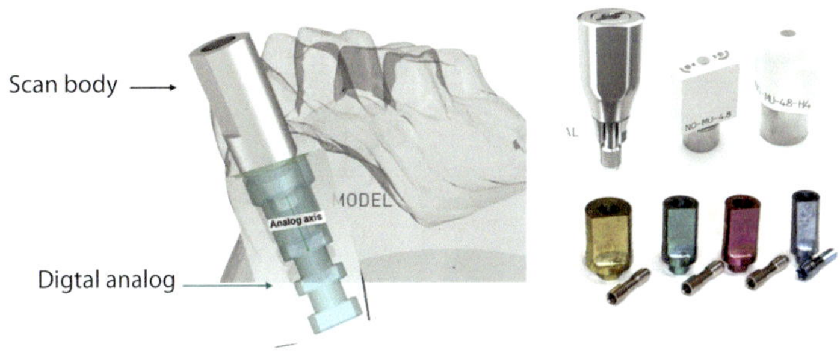

Figure 8.7 Implant scan body is connected to the dental implant to indicate its location and angulation.

teeth, dental implants are not directly scanned due to being submerged in alveolar bone; instead, they are scanned using a connector called a "scan body" (**Figure 8.7**).

Implant scan bodies are essential for transferring dental implant location and orientation from clinical to digital environments [42]. Accurate transfer relies on four assumptions: (1) The physical scan body matches its CAD library; (2) it connects precisely with the implant; (3) the virtual scan matches the physical scan body; and (4) the virtual scan aligns with the CAD library. Research is limited, but some studies indicate scan bodies can affect accuracy [43], and many commercially available options lack rigorous testing [31]. A perfect fit is crucial; gaps of 36 μm and 11 μm were noted by Stimmelmayr et al. [44]. Hand-tightened screws can cause displacements over 100 μm [45], leading to errors with multiple scan bodies.

Repositioning can create linear errors of 27.6 μm after reinsertion [46], while random repositioning may increase distortion by 10%. The connection fit between the scan body and implant is critical [47], with external implants tolerances of 12–44 μm and internal-hexagon implants of 58–86 μm [48]. Recent advancements have reduced tolerances to 4–7 μm [30], underscoring the need for tighter tolerances to minimize distortion.

8.2.1.1.3 Complete-Arch Scanning

Distortion increases significantly from < 20 μm in the first quadrant to > 100 μm in the second quadrant [49, 50, 51]. This distortion may account for two-thirds of the total clinical tolerance, highlighting the poor reliability of using IOS in cross-arch situations. Errors accumulate when stitching multiple small-view images together [26, 52]. Additionally, accurate stitching in edentulous regions can be compromised due to the absence of reference landmarks [53] (**Figure 8.8**).

Several techniques have been proposed to enhance accuracy in the second quadrant. One study found that fiducial dots, dental floss, and painting the palate did not improve scanning accuracy [43], whereas two other studies showed that extended scan bodies and auxiliary devices minimized stitching errors in cross-arch scans, reducing distortions for trueness from 125 to 64 μm and for

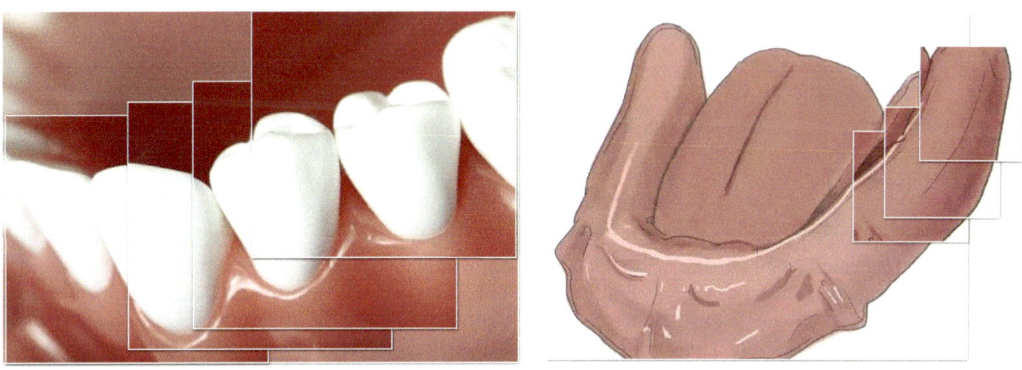

Figure 8.8 In dentate arches, multiple stitching of the scan images is more accurate with well-defined landmarks. Contrarily, such landmarks are lacking in the edentulous ridge, which makes recognition and registration of the matching images more difficult.

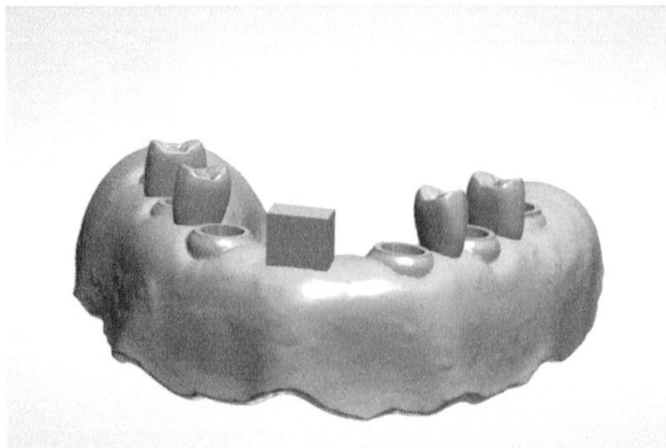

Figure 8.9 The auxiliary device is comprised of an opaque resin base and several well-defined landmarks.

precision from 84 to 63 μm [54, 55]. Another in vitro study introduced a novel auxiliary device that improved accuracy using well-defined landmarks and opaque surfaces (**Figure 8.9**) [56].

Several techniques aim to improve accuracy in the second quadrant. One study found fiducial dots, dental floss, and painting the palate ineffective [43]. In contrast, two studies showed that extended scan bodies and auxiliary devices reduced stitching errors in cross-arch scans, improving trueness from 125 to 64 μm and precision from 84 to 63 μm [54, 55]. A novel device utilizing defined landmarks decreased linear and angular distortion beyond clinical thresholds by 75% and 40%, respectively [56]. A resin base covering the mucosa could enhance IOS accuracy [53]. Scanning trueness declines with translucent substrates like enamel due to light distortion [57, 58], while glossy surfaces may also compromise performance [26], making opaque resin preferable.

IOS vary in tolerance to substrate differences; confocal microscopy scanners are less sensitive than active triangulation scanners 53]. Distinct landmarks can reduce inter-molar distortions by up to 60 μm, but Mizumoto et al. [43] found techniques like painting the palate ineffective, likely due to the limitations of spherical landmarks causing inaccuracies [59].

8.3 CAD STAGE

Tooth-supported CAD/CAM restorations are created based on scanned surface models, requiring conversion of scan bodies into CAD models that identify 3D implant positions [60] (**Figure 8.7**). The commonly used CAD software in dental laboratories is highly automated, with non-editable algorithms and parameters during processing [61]. The accuracy of this software is unclear, as manufacturers do not disclose it, and implant libraries provided by manufacturers or third parties often lack quality control, leaving their accuracies uncertain. As a result, the CAD stage is often viewed as a "closed black box" [11, 60].

Various factors can impact accuracy during the CAD processing stage. A recent study quantified deviations produced when scanned digital data matched implant library data [62]. Although these deviations appear clinically insignificant, they may propagate downstream in the digital workflow, contributing to errors in definitive prostheses.

8.3.1 Manufacturing Tolerance

Manufacturing tolerance is crucial for accuracy in CAD processing, as commercial scan body sizes (output) often differ from their CAD library counterparts (input). Most manufacturers do not specify precision, but a study indicated that tolerances of 2–25 μm could cause 50–130 μm deviations in virtual implant positions [63], underscoring its importance in transferring implant positions digitally.

8.3.2 Inaccurate Scanning

Inaccurate scanning can distort the final virtual model [28]. Scanning accuracy relies on quality point clouds from projected light signals [64], and the shape of the scan body plays a role; a dome-shaped body showed less deviation than a cuboidal one [62, 65]. Sharp edges can introduce noise complicating post-processing [66, 67], while surface contours are essential for virtual alignment, as high-curvature points aid recognition [35, 68]. The dome shape also prevents sliding during alignment [35].

8.3.3 Implant Library

To minimize virtual alignment errors, the CAD model design in the implant library is vital. The cuboidal scan body's four rectangular planes lack distinct angles, hindering matching accuracy [62]. In

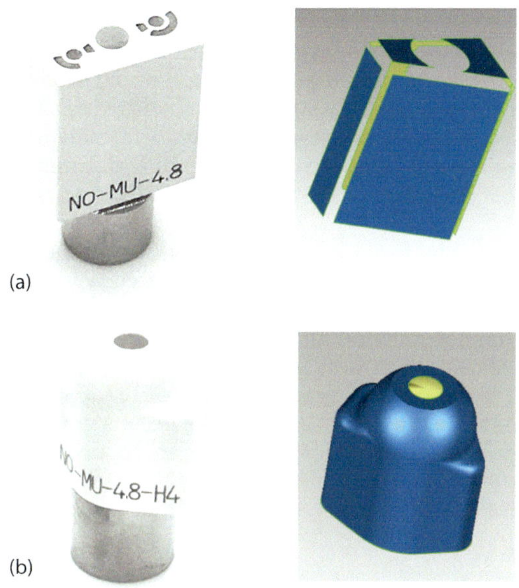

Figure 8.10 (a) The cuboidal scan body and the corresponding implant library and (b) the dome-shaped scan body and the corresponding implant library.

contrast, the dome-shaped scan body's CAD model is shorter than its physical counterpart, reducing distortion in border areas and ensuring reliable point clouds for matching [35] (**Figure 8.10**).

Therefore, implant scan bodies should be designed with rounded edges, high curvature, and smooth surfaces with asymmetrical features. Any sharp corners or edges should be avoided. The implant library should also be dimensionally identical to the physical scan body.

8.4 MANUFACTURING STAGE

After creating the CAD model, CAM software determines block and burs specifications, machining sequences, and process instructions [11]. CAM tasks are typically done in dental labs, allowing manual adjustments of machining parameters, unlike in-office systems with pre-set settings. Manufacturing may use subtractive or additive techniques.

8.4.1 CNC Milling

Milling is the most accurate method for fabricating implant frameworks [69, 70], with theoretical CNC tolerances around 25 µm and surface roughness of 1–6 µm [71]. Reported accuracy of milled frameworks is about 55 µm [69, 72–79], with mean marginal misfit of 100 µm [80–83], exceeding theoretical tolerances. Accuracy is influenced by milling device stability, drill bit design and wear, and cutting speed [11, 60, 71, 84, 85], while block material type does not significantly affect accuracy [84, 86, 87].

8.4.2 CNC Milling Followed by Post-Sintering

Pre-sintered zirconia and cobalt-chromium (Co-Cr) blocks are preferred to reduce drill bit wear [82]. Pre-sintered blocks must be milled larger due to 20–30% shrinkage post-sintering. Accuracies for complete-arch zirconia frameworks are comparable or slightly lower [78, 80, 83, 88–91], while significant distortions may occur in pre-sintered metal frameworks [82, 92]. Framework accuracy is affected by span and block volume contraction [86, 93].

8.4.3 AM Techniques

Four additive manufacturing (AM) techniques (SLA, DMLS, SLM, EBM) are commonly used, with SLA for interim polymer prostheses and others for definitive metal frameworks [75, 92, 94, 95]. AM, being newer in implant dentistry, is less accepted than CNC milling, with accuracy for complete-arch frameworks generally lower (3D implant position: 75 µm, marginal misfit: 139 µm), often exceeding the clinical threshold of 150 µm [75, 92, 96]. AM frameworks can distort due to internal stress [97] and may require supplementary CNC milling for smooth interfaces [74], with combined techniques enhancing accuracy [69].

8.5 ERROR PROPAGATION OF THE ENTIRE DIGITAL WORKFLOW

Digital workflow in implant dentistry is favored for accuracy, efficiency, cost-effectiveness, and patient acceptance [10]. Impressions are obtained via IOS or digitizing gypsum casts [98]. CAD/CAM technologies have replaced traditional methods, with CAD/CAM titanium frameworks (26 ± 10 μm) being more accurate than conventional gold frameworks (261 ± 141 μm) [99]. The clinical acceptability of digital complete-arch frameworks is debated, with proposed thresholds of 91 ± 51 μm [4] and a linear tolerance of 150 μm [28, 100–102]. Angular distortion is estimated at 0.459 degrees [103].

In vitro studies often mislead by focusing on single workflow stages [39, 104, 105]. Clinical scanning accuracy ranges from 192–366 μm [13], while in vitro accuracy ranges from 6–344 μm [28, 38, 39, 72, 105–109]. Fabrication accuracy varies from 2 to 102 μm [78, 83, 89, 90, 110], with distortions mainly occurring during data acquisition and CAM stages. While IOS is initially more accurate than lab-scanned casts, it shows lower accuracy later due to stitching errors [29, 34]. Distortions can arise from operational factors during scanning [111] and inaccuracies in the analogue-digital workflow [112]. Laboratory-scanned gypsum casts exhibit greater accuracy, suggesting conventional impressions may still be optimal. CAD distortion in the analogue-digital workflow is negligible, but complete-digital workflows show more distortion, especially in the second quadrant. Errors in IOS may lead to CAD model misalignment [28, 66], with more distorted scans increasing secondary distortions in CAD.

8.6 GENERAL CONCLUSIONS

Laboratory scanning and CAD processing produce minimal distortions in the digital workflow for implant prostheses. While intraoral scanning shows promise for single and short-span implants, it introduces larger errors in complete-arch cases, which can be mitigated by using well-defined landmarks. The implant scan body is critical for accurate analogue to digital transfer, relying on its geometry and fit. Data acquisition and manufacturing produce the most errors in controlled conditions; overall linear distortion is clinically acceptable, but angular distortion is not. Greater errors are expected in clinical settings, with distortions propagating and accumulating through each workflow stage.

REFERENCES

1. Feine, JS et al. The McGill consensus statement on overdentures mandibular two-implant overdentures as first choice standard of care for edentulous patients. Gerodontology. 2002;19(1):3–4.
2. Lam, WY et al. A 2-part facebow for CAD-CAM dentistry. J Prosthet Dent. 2016;116(6):843–847.
3. Lam, WYH et al. A clinical technique for virtual articulator mounting with natural head position by using calibrated stereophotogrammetry. J Prosthet Dent. 2018;119(6):902–908.
4. Jemt, T et al. Prosthesis misfit and marginal bone loss in edentulous implant patients. Int J Oral Maxillofac Implants. 1996;11(5):620–625.
5. Papaspyridakos, P et al. Accuracy of implant casts generated with splinted and non-splinted impression techniques for edentulous patients: an optical scanning study. Clin Oral Implants Res. 2012;23(6):676–681.
6. Pan, Y et al. Implant framework misfit: a systematic review on assessment methods and clinical complications. Clin Implant Dent Relat Res. 2021;23(2):244–258.
7. Katsoulis, J et al. Misfit of implant prostheses and its impact on clinical outcomes. Definition, assessment and a systematic review of the literature. Eur J Oral Implantol. 2017;10(Suppl 1):121–138.
8. Papaspyridakos, P et al. A systematic review of biologic and technical complications with fixed implant rehabilitations for edentulous patients. Int J Oral Maxillofac Implants. 2012;27(1):102–110.
9. Jokstad, A et al. New 3D technologies applied to assess the long-term clinical effects of misfit of the full jaw fixed prosthesis on dental implants. Clin Oral Implants Res. 2015;26(10):1129–1134.
10. Cappare, P et al. Conventional versus digital impressions for full arch screw-retained maxillary rehabilitations: a randomized clinical trial. Int J Environ Res Public Health. 2019;16(5):829.
11. Tapie, L et al. Understanding dental CAD/CAM for restorations–the digital workflow from a mechanical engineering viewpoint. Int J Comput Dent. 2015;18(1):21–44.
12. Schnitman, PA et al. Recommendations of the consensus development conference on dental implants. J Am Dent Assoc. 1979;98:373–377.
13. Stimmelmayr, M et al. Implant impression techniques for the edentulous jaw: a summary of three studies. J Prosthodont. 2016;25(2):146–150.
14. Mandelli, F et al. Solid index impression protocol: a hybrid workflow for high accuracy and passive fit of full-arch implant-supported restorations. Int J Comput Dent. 2020;23(2):161–181.
15. Roig, E et al. Fit of complete-arch implant-supported prostheses produced from an intraoral scan by using an auxiliary device and from an elastomeric impression: a pilot clinical trial. J Prosthet Dent. 2021;128(3):404–414.
16. Turkyilmaz, I et al. Four-year outcomes of full-arch fixed dental prostheses using CAD/CAM frameworks: a retrospective review of 15 cases. J Clin Exp Dent. 2018;10(10):e1045–e1048.
17. Abduo, J et al. Assessing the fit of implant fixed prostheses: a critical review. Int J Oral Maxillofac Implants. 2010; 25(3):506–515.

18. Winter, W et al. Bone adaptation induced by non-passively fitting implant superstructures: a finite element analysis based on in vivo strain measurements. Int J Oral Maxillofac Implants. 2011;26(6):1288–1295.
19. Geng, J. Structured-light 3D surface imaging: a tutorial. Adv Opt Photonics. 2011;3(2):128–160.
20. Pereira, JRM et al. Effects of different coating materials on three-dimensional optical scanning accuracy. Adv Mech Eng. 2019;11(4):168781401984241.
21. Ender, A et al. Accuracy of complete-arch dental impressions: a new method of measuring trueness and precision. J Prosthet Dent. 2013;109(2):121–128.
22. ISO 5725-1, Accuracy (trueness and precision) of measurement methods and results. Part 1: General principles and definitions. International Organization for Standardization. 1994; Geneva: http://www.iso.org/iso/home.html.
23. ISO 12836, Dentistry- Digitizing devices for CAD/CAM systems for indirect dental restorations-Test methods for assessing accuracy. International Organization for Standardization. 2015; Geneva: http://www.iso.org/iso/home.html.
24. Pan, Y et al. Evaluation of laboratory scanner accuracy by a novel calibration block for complete-arch implant rehabilitation. J Dent. 2020;102:103476.
25. Várady, T et al. Reverse engineering of geometric models—an introduction. Comput Aided Des. 1997;29(4):255–268.
26. Sadlo, F, T. Weyrich, R. Peikert and M. Gross. A practical structured light acquisition system for point-based geometry and texture. Proceedings Eurographics/IEEE VGTC Symposium Point-Based Graphics. 2005: pp. 89–145, Stony Brook, NY, USA, 2005, doi: 10.1109/PBG.2005.194069
27. Tan, MY et al. Comparison of three-dimensional accuracy of digital and conventional implant impressions: effect of interimplant distance in an edentulous arch. Int J Oral Maxillofac Implants. 2019;34(2):366–380.
28. Vandeweghe, S et al. Accuracy of digital impressions of multiple dental implants: an in vitro study. Clin Oral Implants Res. 2017;28(6):648–653.
29. Huang, R et al. Improved scanning accuracy with newly designed scan bodies: an in vitro study comparing digital versus conventional impression techniques for complete-arch implant rehabilitation. Clin Oral Implants Res. 2020; 31(7):625–633.
30. Chia, VA et al. In vitro three-dimensional accuracy of digital implant impressions: the effect of implant angulation. Int J Oral Maxillofac Implants. 2017;32(2):313–321.
31. Mizumoto, RM et al. Intraoral scan bodies in implant dentistry: a systematic review. J Prosthet Dent. 2018;120(3):343–352.
32. Lam, WYH et al. Mapping intraoral photographs on virtual teeth model. J Dent. 2018;79:107–110.
33. Çakmak, G, et al. The effect of scanner type and scan body position on the accuracy of complete-arch digital implant scans. Clin Implant Dent Relat Res. 2020;22(4):533–541.
34. Logozzo, S et al. Recent advances in dental optics – part I: 3D intraoral scanners for restorative dentistry. Opt Lasers Eng. 2014;54:203–221.
35. Bernardini, F, et al. The 3D model acquisition pipeline. Comput Graph Forum. 2002;21(2):149–172.
36. Rusinkiewicz, S et al. Real-time 3D model acquisition. ACM Trans Graphics. 2002;21(3):438–446.
37. Di Fiore, A et al. Full arch digital scanning systems performances for implant-supported fixed dental prostheses: a comparative study of 8 intraoral scanners. J Prosthodont Res. 2019;63(4):396–403.
38. Imburgia, M et al. Accuracy of four intraoral scanners in oral implantology: a comparative in vitro study. BMC Oral Health. 2017;17(1):92.
39. Amin, S et al. Digital vs. conventional full-arch implant impressions: a comparative study. Clin Oral Implants Res. 2017;28(11):1360–1367.
40. Gimenez-Gonzalez, B et al. An in vitro study of factors influencing the performance of digital intraoral impressions operating on active wavefront sampling technology with multiple implants in the Edentulous Maxilla. J Prosthodont. 2017;26(8):650–655.
41. Hategan, SI et al. Powder and powder-free intra-oral scanners: digital impression accuracy. Prim Dent J. 2018;7(2):40–43.
42. Rutkunas, V et al. Accuracy of digital implant impressions with intraoral scanners. A systematic review. Eur J Oral Implantol. 2017;10(Suppl 1):101–120.
43. Mizumoto, RM et al. Accuracy of different digital scanning techniques and scan bodies for complete-arch implant-supported prostheses. J Prosthet Dent. 2019;123(1):96–104.
44. Stimmelmayr, M et al. Digital evaluation of the reproducibility of implant scanbody fit–an in vitro study. Clin Oral Investig. 2012;16(3):851–856.
45. Kim, J et al. Displacement of scan body during screw tightening: a comparative in vitro study. J Adv Prosthodont. 2020;12(5):307–315.
46. Pan, Y et al. Reproducibility of laboratory scanning of multiple implants in complete edentulous arch: effect of scan bodies. J Dent. 2020;96:103329.
47. Molinero-Mourelle, P et al. Microleakage assessment of CAD-CAM cobalt-chrome and zirconia abutments on a conical connection dental implant: a comparative in vitro study. Clin Oral Implants Res. 2022;33(9):945–952.
48. Braian, M et al. Tolerance measurements on internal- and external-hexagon implants. Int J Oral Maxillofac Implants. 2014;29(4):846–852.
49. Gimenez, B et al. Accuracy of a digital impression system based on parallel confocal laser technology for implants with consideration of operator experience and implant angulation and depth. Int J Oral Maxillofac Implants. 2014;29(4):853–862.
50. Gimenez, B et al. Accuracy of a digital impression system based on active triangulation technology with blue light for implants: effect of clinically relevant parameters. Implant Dent. 2015;24(5):498–504.
51. Gimenez, B et al. Accuracy of a digital impression system based on active wavefront sampling technology for implants considering operator experience, implant angulation, and depth. Clin Implant Dent Relat Res. 2015;17(1):e54–e64.
52. Molinero-Mourelle, P et al. Photogrammetric and intraoral digital impression technique for the rehabilitation of multiple unfavorably positioned dental implants: a clinical report. J Oral Implantol. 2019;45(5):398–402.
53. Dutton, E et al. The effect different substrates have on the trueness and precision of eight different intraoral scanners. J Esthet Restor Dent. 2020;32(2):204–218.
54. Huang, RX et al. Improved scanning accuracy with newly designed scan bodies: an in vitro study comparing digital versus conventional impression techniques for complete-arch implant rehabilitation. Clin Oral Implants Res. 2020;31(7):625–633.

55. Iturrate, M et al. Accuracy analysis of complete-arch digital scans in edentulous arches when using an auxiliary geometric device. J Prosthet Dent. 2019;121(3):447–454.
56. Pan, Y et al. Improving intraoral implant scanning with a novel auxiliary device: an in-vitro study. Clin Oral Implants Res. 2021;30(12):1466–1473.
57. Bocklet, C et al. Effect of scan substrates on accuracy of 7 intraoral digital impression systems using human maxilla model. Orthod Craniofac Res. 2019;22(Suppl 1):168–174.
58. Bunsch, E, et al. Art documentation quality in function of 3D scanning resolution and precision. Springfield VA: IS&T; 2011.78690D-78690D-78611.
59. Maintz, JBA et al. A survey of medical image registration. Med Image Anal. 1998;2(1):1–36.
60. Tapie, L et al. Understanding dental CAD/CAM for restorations–accuracy from a mechanical engineering viewpoint. Int J Comput Dent. 2015;18(4):343–367.
61. Pan, Y et al. Comparison of the virtual techniques in registering single implant position with a universal-coordinate system: an in vitro study. J Dent. 2022;117:103925.
62. Pan, Y et al. Does the geometry of scan bodies affect the alignment accuracy of computer-aided design in implant digital workflow: an in vitro study? Clin Oral Implants Res. 2021;33(3):313–321.
63. Schmidt, A et al. Influence of the accuracy of intraoral scanbodies on implant position: differences in manufacturing tolerances. Int J Prosthodont. 2019;32(5):430–432.
64. Del Corso, M et al. Optical three-dimensional scanning acquisition of the position of osseointegrated implants: an in vitro study to determine method accuracy and operational feasibility. Clin Implant Dent Relat Res. 2009;11(3):214–221.
65. Gonzalez de Villaumbrosia, P et al. In vitro comparison of the accuracy (trueness and precision) of six extraoral dental scanners with different scanning technologies. J Prosthet Dent. 2016;116(4):543–550.e541.
66. Wang, J et al. Feature-Preserving surface reconstruction from unoriented, noisy point data. Computer Graphics Forum. 2013;32(1):164–176.
67. Rudolph, H et al. Matching point clouds: limits and possibilities. Int J Comput Dent. 2002;5(2–3):155–164.
68. Rodolà, E et al. A simple and effective relevance-based point sampling for 3D shapes. Pattern Recognition Letters. 2015;59:41–47.
69. Ciocca, L et al. Manufacturing of metal frameworks for full-arch dental restoration on implants: a comparison between milling and a novel hybrid technology. J Prosthodont. 2019;28(5):556–563.
70. Molinero-Mourelle, P, et al. Effect of fabrication technique on the microgap of CAD/CAM cobalt-chrome and zirconia abutments on a conical connection implant: an in vitro study. Materials (Basel). 2021;14(9).
71. Lebon, N et al. Understanding dental CAD/CAM for restorations - dental milling machines from a mechanical engineering viewpoint. Part a: chairside milling machines. Int J Comput Dent. 2016;19(1):45–62.
72. Knechtle, N et al. Accuracy of digital complete-arch, multi-implant scans made in the edentulous jaw with gingival movement simulation: an in vitro study. J Prosthet Dent. 2021;128(3):468–478.
73. Paniz, G et al. The precision of fit of cast and milled full-arch implant-supported restorations. Int J Oral Maxillofac Implants. 2013;28(3):687–693.
74. Revilla-Leon, M et al. Discrepancy of complete-arch titanium frameworks manufactured using selective laser melting and electron beam melting additive manufacturing technologies. J Prosthet Dent. 2018;120(6):942–947.
75. Revilla-Leon, M et al. implant-prosthodontic discrepancy of complete-arch cobalt-chromium implant frameworks manufactured through selective laser melting additive manufacturing technology using a coordinate measuring machine. Int J Oral Maxillofac Implants. 2019;34(3):698–707.
76. Sierraalta, M, et al. Precision of fit of titanium and cast implant frameworks using a new matching formula. Int J Dent. 2012;2012:374315.
77. Svanborg, P et al. Additively manufactured titanium and cobalt-chromium implant frameworks: fit and effect of ceramic veneering. Int J Oral Maxillofac Implants. 2018;33(3):590–596.
78. Svanborg, P et al. Fit of 3Y-TZP complete-arch implant-supported fixed dental prostheses before and after porcelain veneering. J Prosthet Dent. 2019;122(2):137–141.
79. Svanborg, P et al. Fit of cobalt-chromium implant frameworks before and after ceramic veneering in comparison with CNC-milled titanium frameworks. Clin Exp Dent Res. 2015;1(2):49–56.
80. Tiossi, R et al. Effect of cyclic loading on the vertical microgap of long-span zirconia frameworks supported by 4 or 6 implants. J Prosthet Dent. 2014;112(4):828–833.
81. Uribarri, A et al. Marginal and internal fit of CAD/CAM frameworks in multiple implant-supported restorations: scanning and milling error analysis. Clin Implant Dent Relat Res. 2019;21(5):1062–1072.
82. Woo, HW et al. Precision of the milled full-arch framework fabricated using pre-sintered soft alloy: a pilot study. J Adv Prosthodont. 2018;10(2):128–131.
83. Yilmaz, B et al. Marginal discrepancy of CAD-CAM complete-arch fixed implant-supported frameworks. J Prosthet Dent. 2018;120(1):65–70.
84. Lebon, N et al. Understanding dental CAD/CAM for restorations–dental milling machines from a mechanical engineering viewpoint. Part B: labside milling machines. Int J Comput Dent. 2016;19(2):115–134.
85. Lebon, N et al. Influence of CAD/CAM tool and material on tool wear and roughness of dental prostheses after milling. J Prosthet Dent. 2015;114(2):236–247.
86. Abduo, J et al. Fits of implant zirconia custom abutments and frameworks: a systematic review and meta-analyses. Int J Oral Maxillofac Implants. 2019;34(1):99–114.
87. Astakhov, VP. Surface integrity – definition and importance in functional performance. In: Davim, J, eds. Surface Integrity in Machining. Springer; 2010: 1–35.
88. Al-Meraikhi, H et al. In vitro fit of CAD-CAM complete arch screw-retained titanium and zirconia implant prostheses fabricated on 4 implants. J Prosthet Dent. 2018;119(3):409–416.
89. Barbin, T et al. Biomechanical behavior of CAD/CAM cobalt-chromium and zirconia full-arch fixed prostheses. J Adv Prosthodont. 2020;12(6):329–337.
90. Katsoulis, J et al. Precision of fit of implant-supported screw-retained 10-unit computer-aided-designed and computer-aided-manufactured frameworks made from zirconium dioxide and titanium: an in vitro study. Clin Oral Implants Res. 2014;25(2):165–174.

91. Katsoulis, J et al. In vitro precision of fit of computer-aided design and computer-aided manufacturing titanium and zirconium dioxide bars. Dent Mater Off Publ Acad Dent Mater. 2013;29(9):945–953.
92. Tasin, S et al. Evaluation of strain distribution on an edentulous mandible generated by cobalt-chromium metal alloy fixed complete dentures fabricated with different techniques: an in vitro study. J Prosthet Dent. 2019;122(1):47–53.
93. Mai, HN et al. Comparative study of the fit accuracy of full-arch bar frameworks fabricated with different presintered cobalt-chromium alloys. Biomed Res Int. 2018;2018:1962514.
94. Barbin, T et al. 3D metal printing in dentistry: an in vitro biomechanical comparative study of two additive manufacturing technologies for full-arch implant-supported prostheses. J Mech Behav Biomed Mater. 2020;108:103821.
95. Kim, J, et al. Influence of the postcuring process on dimensional accuracy and seating of 3D-printed polymeric fixed prostheses. Biomed Res Int. 2020;2020:2150182.
96. Revilla-Leon, M et al. Influence of scan body design and digital implant analogs on implant replica position in additively manufactured casts. J Prosthet Dent. 2020;124(2):202–210.
97. Alharbi, N et al. Additive manufacturing techniques in prosthodontics: where do we currently stand? A critical review. Int J Prosthodont. 2017;30(5):474–484.
98. Ahlholm, P et al. Digital versus conventional impressions in fixed prosthodontics: a review. J Prosthodont. 2018;27(1):35–41.
99. Paniz, G et al. The precision of fit of cast and milled full-arch implant-supported restorations. Int J Oral Maxillofac Implants. 2013;28(3):687–693.
100. Papaspyridakos, P et al. Digital workflow: in vitro accuracy of 3D printed casts generated from complete-arch digital implant scans. J Prosthet Dent. 2020;124(5):589–593.
101. Papaspyridakos, P et al. Digital workflow for implant rehabilitation with double full-arch monolithic zirconia prostheses. J Prosthodont. 2020;29(6):460–465.
102. Wulfman, C et al. Digital scanning for complete-arch implant-supported restorations: a systematic review. J Prosthet Dent. 2020;124(2):161–167.
103. Andriessen, FS et al. Applicability and accuracy of an intraoral scanner for scanning multiple implants in edentulous mandibles: a pilot study. J Prosthet Dent. 2014;111(3):186–194.
104. Abdel-Azim, T et al. The influence of digital fabrication options on the accuracy of dental implant-based single units and complete-arch frameworks. Int J Oral Maxillofac Implants. 2014;29(6):1281–1288.
105. Ciocca, L et al. In vitro assessment of the accuracy of digital impressions prepared using a single system for full-arch restorations on implants. Int J Comput Assist Radiol Surg. 2018;13(7):1097–1108.
106. Mutwalli, H et al. Trueness and precision of three-dimensional digitizing intraoral devices. Int J Dent. 2018;2018:5189761.
107. Bilmenoglu, C et al. In vitro comparison of trueness of 10 intraoral scanners for implant-supported complete-arch fixed dental prostheses. J Prosthet Dent. 2020;124(6):755–760.
108. Mangano, FG et al. Trueness and precision of four intraoral scanners in Oral implantology: a comparative in vitro study. PLoS One. 2016;11(9):e0163107.
109. Braian, M et al. Trueness and precision of 5 intraoral scanners for scanning edentulous and dentate complete-arch mandibular casts: a comparative in vitro study. J Prosthet Dent. 2019;122(2):129–136.e122.
110. Revilla-Leon, M et al. Discrepancy at the implant abutment-prosthesis interface of complete-arch cobalt-chromium implant frameworks fabricated by additive and subtractive technologies before and after ceramic veneering. J Prosthet Dent. 2020;125(5):795–803.
111. Reich, S et al. Do "cut out-rescan" procedures have an impact on the accuracy of intraoral digital scans? J Prosthet Dent. 2020;125(1):89–94.
112. Papaspyridakos, P et al. Accuracy of implant impressions for partially and completely edentulous patients: a systematic review. Int J Oral Maxillofac Implants. 2014;29(4):836–840.

9 Guided Endodontics

Digital Flow Applied to Endodontics

Leonardo dos Santos Barroso, Kusai Baroudi, Gustavo Moreira de Almeida, and Adriana Marques Nunes

9.1 INTRODUCTION

Endodontics, the branch of dentistry concerned with the treatment of dental pulp and tissues surrounding the roots of teeth, has witnessed significant advancements in recent years. One of the most notable developments is the integration of guided techniques, which have transformed the way that endodontic procedures are performed. Guided endodontics is a precise and minimally invasive approach that relies on advanced imaging, computer technology, and three-dimensional (3D) printing to enhance treatment planning, execution, and outcomes and also is a recent resource for dealing with clinical challenges in a safer and more precise way. It is defined as a computer-assisted therapy approach, which was primarily developed to localize calcified root canals in a minimally invasive way [1, 2].

From a historical perspective point of view, the concept of guided endodontics can be traced back to the early use of radiographic templates and stents to aid in endodontic access and canal navigation. However, it was the advent of cone beam computed tomography (CBCT) and the subsequent integration of computer-aided design and computer-aided manufacturing (CAD/CAM) that truly propelled guided endodontics into the modern era. These technological advances have enabled clinicians to visualize and plan endodontic procedures with unprecedented accuracy.

The idea came from the concepts of implantology and guided surgeries. Zehnder et al. [2] investigated a technique in which a CBCT file was overlayed with an intraoral scanned file in an implantology planning software to create an endodontic intervention planning for calcified root canals. The authors described the technique and showed an excellent result in dealing with calcified canals. In a laboratory study, 60 single rooted teeth were mounted on six maxillary jaw models. Each tooth was submitted to a CBCT and to intraoral digital scanning, and the files were matched in a planning CoDiagnostix™ software. Access cavities, sleeves, and templates for guiding the procedure were planned virtually. Then templates were printed in a 3D printer. Each tooth had its own specific template, and access surgeries were accomplished by two operators. The objective was to assess the accuracy of technique and to observe if a different operator could interfere with the result. The results showed that all canals were accessed and negotiated after cavity preparation with a low deviation angle (mean of 1.81°), and there was no influence of the different operator.

The conclusions of this study reinforced the use of this technique, which was first described in a clinical situation in which an upper central incisor was involved [1]. A 15-year-old female patient presented with acute apical periodontitis, and a radiographic exam showed an obliteration from the pulp chamber to the middle third of the root. The position of the canal and the situation were judged as too risky to be accomplished with traditional resources such as an operating microscope. Thus, a computed guided approach was developed using the technique described above. The patient was submitted to a CBCT and an intraoral scan where digital imaging and communications in medicine (DICOM) files and stereolithography (STL) files were overlaid in a planning software. The bur type and its trajectory were planned on computer and a template with a sleeve was 3D-printed. The template was positioned, and the canal was found 9 mm away from the apex. Root canal preparation was carried out with rotary instruments, and after chemo-mechanical debridement, intracanal dressing was used to help with controlling microbial infections and symptoms. After four weeks, the canal was filled with epoxy filling material, and the access cavity was restored with resin composite. Control follow-up after 15 months showed excellent results with absence of signs and symptoms in addition to the existence of radiographic normality of periapical structures.

From this point, the technique was spread all over the world, and several studies were performed with the aim of investigating it and to propose improvements. Several case reports have been published showing successful outcomes.

Pulp canal obliteration (PCO) associated with traumatic injury in anterior teeth results from accelerated deposition of dentin within the root canal space [3]. This reparative process develops as a pulpal response to severed neurovascular supply during trauma [4, 5]. An observational study from Jacobsen and Kerekes [5] showed that 78 out of 122 teeth injured by trauma and followed up for 10 years developed total obliteration of pulp canal space in addition to 44 partial obliterations.

 DOI: 10.1201/9781003428541-9

Oginni et al. [6] also found similar results, and as a consequence of this, calcific metamorphosis pulp necrosis occurs and, therefore, root canal treatment must be accomplished to control infection and its harm to periapical tissues. The authors reported a 27% risk of pulp necrosis in such teeth.

The most frequent sign of PCO is tooth discoloration and this is present in 70–80% of teeth [7]. Internal bleaching is an inexpensive, stable, and conservative aesthetic treatment, and thus root canal treatment is also indicated for such condition [8].

The aim of the guided technique is to allow safe, conservative, and less time-consuming access to the challenging anatomy of such teeth and help to treat or prevent apical periodontitis. In these cases, preparing an adequate access cavity and identifying the canal orifice can be challenging and may create a massive loss of tooth structure that is associated with a higher risk of fracture [9] and a high failure rate [10]. Magnifying glasses, operative microscopes, and CBCT exams can be used for better guidance. Nevertheless, it may be difficult for the operator, especially a novice, to interpret the CBCT images and create a mental guide while performing the treatment manually. Guided endodontics emerged to solve these problems, reducing the risk of perforations and other iatrogenic problems by creating a specific pathway for root canal access and instrumentation [11, 12].

Guided endodontics represents a significant paradigm shift in the practice of endodontics, offering the potential to improve treatment outcomes while minimizing invasiveness. With ongoing advancements in technology and increased adoption by clinicians, guided endodontics is poised to play an increasingly integral role in the future of endodontic care, ultimately benefiting both practitioners and patients alike.

9.2 CLINICAL APPLICATION

Because of its precision and possibilities, guided endodontics is currently recommended for all situations that somehow impair pulp canal space localization and negotiation, such as calcified canals, post-traumatic pulp canal obliteration, and dentin dysplasia [13].

a. *Complex Anatomy*: Guided techniques are particularly valuable when dealing with teeth that have complex root canal systems, such as partial or total pulp canal obliterations and molars with multiple canals or curved roots.
b. *Re-Treatment Cases*: In cases of failed root canal treatments, guided endodontics can aid in the safe and efficient removal of post materials such as fiber posts and the negotiation of previously inaccessible canals.
c. *Minimally Invasive Access*: Guided access openings allow for minimal removal of tooth structure while ensuring precise entry into the pulp chamber.
d. *Dental Trauma*: Traumatically injured teeth with fractured roots can benefit from guided endodontics to locate and negotiate fragmented root segments.
e. *Apical Surgeries*: Guided endodontics can assist in assessing the proximity of vital structures when planning for incision, osteotomy, apicectomy, and retropreparation as well [1, 12, 14].

9.3 BENEFITS OF GUIDED ENDODONTICS

9.3.1 Precision and Accuracy

The precise planning and execution facilitated by guided endodontics lead to accurate root canal treatment, minimizing the risk of procedural errors and improving long-term success rates.

9.3.2 Enhanced Efficiency

By providing a clear roadmap for the entire treatment process, guided endodontics increases efficiency, reduces chair time, enhances patient comfort, and improves overall workflow in dental practice.

9.3.3 Minimized Radiation Exposure

The integration of CBCT scans for treatment planning minimizes the need for additional radiographic exposure during the procedure, promoting patient safety and reducing radiation risks.

9.3.4 Improved Predictability

Guided procedures result in more predictable treatment outcomes, contributing to higher success rates.

It is important to make clear that there are two distinct types of computer-assisted techniques: static and dynamic. Both use DICOM files from CBCT and STL files from intraoral scanning. Static guided endodontics aims to allow a straight-line access to pulp canal space and is recommended for straight-rooted teeth. Dynamic guided endodontics is a real-time technique and requires deep mastery from the operator (Kulinkovych-Levchuk et al., 2022). Both will be discussed later in this chapter.

9.4 STATIC GUIDED ENDODONTICS DIGITAL FLOW

9.4.1 Cone Beam Computed Tomography (CBCT)

CBCT is a 3D imaging technology that employs a cone-shaped X-ray beam to capture detailed cross-sectional images of a patient's anatomy, particularly the oral and maxillofacial regions. Unlike conventional two-dimensional (2D) X-rays, CBCT provides high-resolution, 3D images that are vital for endodontic procedures.

Guided endodontics relies heavily on high-resolution 3D imaging techniques such as CBCT, which provide detailed information about tooth anatomy and surrounding structures. This technology allows for precise preoperative assessments, virtual treatment planning, and the creation of digital guides for guiding instruments during the procedure.

The role of CBCT in guided endodontics:

- *Enhanced Diagnosis*: CBCT offers a comprehensive view of both the tooth and surrounding structures, allowing endodontists to diagnose and evaluate complex cases more accurately. It aids in the detection of hidden canals, calcified canals, and anomalies that may be missed in traditional radiographs.
- *Treatment Planning*: Guided endodontics relies heavily on meticulous treatment planning. CBCT images provide precise measurements of tooth length, curvature, and the number of canals, enabling the endodontist to plan the procedure with utmost accuracy. This reduces the risk of complications during treatment.
- *Minimally Invasive Approach*: The 3D images obtained from CBCT scans enable endodontists to create customized guides for root canal access and instrumentation. These guides facilitate minimally invasive procedures, reducing the removal of healthy tooth structure and ensuring that treatment is focused only on the affected area.
- *Predictable Outcomes*: With CBCT-guided endodontics, endodontists can visualize the entire root canal system and its complexities before starting treatment. This leads to more predictable outcomes, a higher success rate, and a reduced likelihood of complications, such as instrument fractures or missed canals.
- *Improved Patient Experience*: Patients benefit from CBCT-guided endodontics as well. The precise planning and execution of root canal procedures reduce chair time and discomfort. Patients can often complete treatment in a single visit, resulting in a more positive overall experience.
- *Research and Education*: CBCT technology has also revolutionized endodontic research and education. Dentists and endodontists can use CBCT scans to teach and train future practitioners effectively. It has become an invaluable tool in dental education.
- *Risk Mitigation*: CBCT helps in identifying any potential complications in advance, such as proximity to critical anatomical structures like nerves or adjacent teeth. This allows for careful treatment planning and risk mitigation strategies.
- *Follow-up and Assessment*: After treatment, CBCT scans can be used to assess the success of the procedure and ensure that no residual infection or issues remain, further enhancing patient care and outcomes.

CBCT stands out for its ability to produce high-resolution 3D images of anatomical structures. Unlike conventional 2D radiography, CBCT captures volumetric data, providing clinicians with a comprehensive view of complex structures. This 3D capability is particularly advantageous in fields such as maxillofacial surgery, orthopedics, and radiation therapy planning, where precise spatial information is vital. CBCT devices offer a flexible field of view (FOV) that can be tailored to the specific clinical requirements. This customization allows healthcare professionals to focus on the region of interest while limiting unnecessary radiation exposure to adjacent tissues. For instance, in dental CBCT, the FOV can be adjusted to capture a single tooth or encompass the entire maxillofacial region [15].

It employs a cone-shaped X-ray beam and 2D detector to capture multiple 2D images during a single rotation around the patient's head. These 2D images are then reconstructed into a high-resolution 3D volume dataset. The result is a detailed representation of the patient's dental anatomy, offering axial, sagittal, and coronal views with isotropic voxels, which facilitate precise measurements and evaluation of root canal morphology and periapical lesions. This high level of detail is crucial for identifying subtle abnormalities, evaluating bone density, and planning intricate surgical procedures. In dental applications, CBCT can discern minuscule dental structures, facilitating precise treatment planning [16].

One of the salient features of CBCT is its capacity to deliver relatively low radiation doses to patients while maintaining image quality. This is achieved through specialized hardware and software optimizations, including cone-shaped X-ray beams, pulsed X-ray delivery, and adaptive dose management. Consequently, CBCT minimizes patient exposure, making it a safer alternative to conventional CT scans. Its systems are renowned for their rapid image acquisition, typically completing a scan in a matter of seconds. This speed is advantageous in clinical settings, reducing patient discomfort and minimizing motion artifacts. It is especially valuable in emergency cases and for patients who may have difficulty remaining still during imaging [17].

DICOM is universally recognized for storing, transmitting, and managing medical imaging data. In the context of guided endodontics, DICOM files play a crucial role in acquiring, processing, and utilizing 3D image data for precise diagnosis and treatment planning. DICOM files are the standard output format for most modern imaging devices used in dentistry, including CBCT scanners and intraoral radiography systems. These files contain detailed information about the patient, imaging parameters, and the actual image data. DICOM's universal compatibility ensures that images obtained from various devices can be seamlessly integrated into the endodontic workflow [18].

Endodontists can use specialized software to manipulate and enhance DICOM images for a more detailed examination of root canal anatomy and surrounding structures. This capability is invaluable for identifying complex canal configurations and optimizing treatment plans [16]. DICOM files serve as the foundation for virtual guided endodontic procedures. Using specialized software, endodontists can overlay the DICOM data onto real-time images during treatment, providing a dynamic and precise guide for instrument placement, irrigation, and obturation. Moreover, this image file can be overlayed with STL to allow planning and 3D printing of a static template to guide the endodontic access. This technology enhances procedural accuracy and reduces the risk of iatrogenic errors [18].

In the realm of modern endodontics, CBCT has emerged as a game changer. Its ability to provide detailed, 3D images and facilitate precise treatment planning and execution has significantly improved the success rates and patient experiences in guided endodontics. This technology has become an indispensable tool for endodontists, ensuring that root canal treatments are performed with the highest level of precision and predictability, ultimately leading to improved patient outcomes.

9.4.2 Digital Scanning

Intraoral scanning technology has ushered in a new era of precision and efficiency in various dental disciplines, including endodontics. This section aims to delve into the specifics of intraoral scanning and its profound relationship with guided endodontics, highlighting the ways in which this technology has revolutionized the field.

Intraoral scanning involves the use of specialized digital scanners to capture high resolution, 3D images of the intraoral environment, including the teeth, soft tissues, and surrounding structures. These scanners employ a variety of technologies to create a detailed virtual model of the patient's oral anatomy. The resulting digital impressions serve as a foundation for precise treatment planning by providing clinicians with a detailed, 3D representation of the tooth and its surrounding structures. This digital model allows for the assessment of canal morphology, the identification of anomalies, and the planning of access cavities with a high degree of accuracy [19–23].

Advantages of Intraoral Scanning in Guided Endodontics

- *Enhanced Precision*: Intraoral scanning provides highly accurate digital impressions, reducing the margin for error in guided endodontic procedures.
- *Minimized Patient Discomfort*: The noninvasive nature of intraoral scanning improves patient comfort, making it an attractive option for those with dental anxiety.
- *Efficient Workflow*: The digital workflow streamlines the entire guided endodontic process, reducing chairside time and enhancing the overall patient experience.
- *Improved Communication*: Intraoral scans facilitate clear communication between the endodontist and other dental specialists involved in interdisciplinary cases.

STL files serve as the foundation for generating accurate 3D models of dental anatomy, including teeth, roots, and surrounding tissues. These files are created through specialized intraoral scanning systems, CBCT, or digital impressions. The STL format efficiently stores the geometric data of these structures, enabling their visualization and manipulation in 3D space [24].

One of the primary advantages of STL files in guided endodontics is their utility in virtual treatment planning. Clinicians can import STL files into specialized software, allowing for detailed analysis of root canal morphology, assessment of anomalies, and precise planning of access cavities. This digital approach enhances treatment accuracy by providing a comprehensive view of the tooth's internal structure [25].

STL files are instrumental in guiding endodontic procedures. They enable the creation of 3D-printed surgical guides, which assist clinicians in navigating the root canal system accurately. These guides provide real-time feedback during the procedure, ensuring precise instrument placement, irrigation, and obturation. This technology minimizes the risk of iatrogenic errors and improves treatment outcomes [26].

Recent advancements in STL technology have further improved its utility in guided endodontics. Enhanced scanners and software allow for more detailed and accurate STL file generation. Additionally, innovations in 3D printing technology enable the production of biocompatible and patient-specific endodontic instruments and guides, tailored to the unique anatomy of each patient [27].

Intraoral scanning technology has become an indispensable tool in the arsenal of modern endodontics. Its seamless integration with guided endodontic techniques empowers clinicians to deliver precise, predictable, and patient-centered care. As technology continues to advance, the relationship between intraoral scanning and guided endodontics is expected to evolve, further enhancing the field's capacity to provide optimal outcomes for patients. Dental professionals should embrace this synergy to ensure the highest standards of care in endodontics.

9.4.3 Computer-Aided Planning (CAP)

Computer software plays a crucial role in guided endodontics. Specialized software enables the clinician to manipulate 3D images, identify canal morphology, plan access openings, and simulate instrumentation procedures. These virtual plans can then be used to create surgical guides, ensuring that the treatment is carried out exactly as planned. Digital planning software plays a significant role in guided endodontics and has revolutionized the way that endodontists plan and execute their procedures, leading to better outcomes and improved patient experiences [22, 28, 29].

Some features of this software is described below:

- *Image Acquisition and Analysis*: Digital planning software starts with the acquisition of high-resolution 2D and 3D images of the patient's teeth and surrounding structures. These images can be obtained through CBCT scans, intraoral scanners, or digital radiography. The software then analyzes these images to provide detailed information about the tooth's anatomy, including the number of canals, their morphology, and any potential challenges [15, 16].
- *Treatment Planning*: Endodontists can use digital planning software to create a comprehensive treatment plan. This involves identifying the precise location of the infected or damaged pulp, determining the length of the root canal, and selecting the appropriate instruments and materials for the procedure. The software aids in visualizing the root canal system in 3D, making it easier to plan for complex cases [25, 30].
- *Virtual Navigation*: One of the key advantages of digital planning software in guided endodontics is the ability to navigate the root canal system virtually. The software provides a clear view of the canal's shape, curvature, and any obstructions. This information helps the endodontist to choose the correct path for instrumentation and reduces the risk of perforations or missed canals [31, 32].
- *Customized Guides*: Some advanced digital planning software can generate customized guides for endodontic procedures. These guides can be 3D-printed or milled to assist the dentist during the actual treatment. They help to ensure that the instruments are guided precisely along the planned path, improving the accuracy of the procedure and reducing the risk of complications [33].
- *Real-time Feedback*: During the endodontic procedure, digital planning software can provide real-time feedback to the endodontist. This can include information about the depth of instrumentation, the location of files within the canal, and alerts if the treatment deviates from the planned path. This feedback allows for immediate adjustments and corrections, enhancing the overall quality of treatment [34, 35].

- *Record Keeping and Documentation*: Digital planning software also serves as a valuable tool for record keeping and documentation. It allows endodontists to store detailed records of each procedure, including images, treatment plans, and real-time data. This documentation is essential for monitoring patient progress and for future reference [36, 37].
- *Patient Communication*: Digital planning software can facilitate communication with patients by providing visual representations of their dental condition and the planned treatment. This helps patients to better understand the procedure, its importance, and the expected outcomes, leading to increased patient satisfaction and trust [16, 38].

One of the pivotal aspects of computer-aided planning (CAP) in guided endodontics is precise treatment planning. The software allows endodontists to create a comprehensive virtual treatment plan by identifying precisely the location of infected or damaged pulp, determining the root canal length, and selecting appropriate instruments and materials. CAP technology provides 3D visualization of the root canal system, facilitating the planning of complex cases [39].

Advanced CAP technology can generate customized guides and templates for endodontic procedures. These guides provide precise guidance for instrument placement during the actual treatment. 3D-printed or milled guides ensure accuracy and facilitate the pre-planned path for instrumentation, resulting in enhanced procedural precision [29].

In conclusion, digital planning software has become an indispensable tool in guided endodontics. It enables endodontists to plan and execute root canal treatments with a level of precision and confidence that was previously unattainable. This technology not only improves the success rates of these procedures but also enhances the overall patient experience by reducing discomfort and the need for repeat treatments. As technology continues to advance rapidly, digital planning software will likely play an even more prominent role in the field of endodontics.

There are several software programs and applications designed to aid in guided endodontics planning. However, please note that the field of software applications is constantly evolving, and new tools may emerge. Here are some examples of guided endodontics planning software:

- *Simplant by Dentsply Sirona*: Simplant is a widely used software for guided implant placement, but it also offers tools for endodontic planning, including root canal treatment planning.
- *Planmeca Romexis Endodontic Imaging Software*: Planmeca Romexis offers a specific endodontic imaging software that helps with visualization and planning of endodontic procedures.
- *3D Diagnostix*: 3D Diagnostix provides software solutions for guided implant surgery planning, but it also offers tools for endodontic planning and visualization.
- *Materialise ProPlan CMF*: While primarily known for craniofacial surgical planning, Materialise ProPlan CMF can also be utilized for endodontic treatment planning involving complex cases.
- *Kodak 3D Imaging Software*: Kodak offers software for dental imaging and treatment planning, which can be utilized for endodontic planning, including root canal treatments.
- *Dentiq Guide by Dentiq Dental Solutions*: Dentiq Guide is a comprehensive dental implant planning and surgical guide design software that can also be used for endodontic treatment planning.
- *XNav Technologies X-Guide*: X-Guide is primarily designed for guided implant surgery, but it can also assist in endodontic procedures by providing 3D guidance during root canal treatments.

Please verify the latest updates and features of these software programs to ensure they meet your specific needs for guided endodontics planning. Always consult with dental professionals and conduct thorough research to choose the most suitable software for your practice.

9.4.4 Templates

Guided endodontics often involves the use of templates or surgical guides, which are designed based on the digital impressions obtained through intraoral scanning. These guides facilitate precise access cavity preparation by directing the drill to the exact location and depth needed to reach the root canal system. This minimizes unnecessary removal of tooth structure and reduces the risk of iatrogenic damage.

The utilization of templates or surgical guides in guided endodontics has garnered substantial attention. Templates play a fundamental role in achieving precise access cavity preparation, minimizing the removal of healthy tooth structure, and reducing the risk of procedural complications.

9.4.4.1 Role of Templates in Guided Endodontics

The models can be printed in 3D using a subtractive CAD/CAM system or additive printers and must contain an extension over the area of tooth to be opened (sleeve). There must be a hole in this location with the exact diameter of the drill to be used for the procedure. In general, when planning the template, a metal washer is placed on the sleeve with the exact diameter compatible with the drill to be used. However, there is the possibility of planning and printing the template with the sleeve without using the metal washer. We recently had a case using a template without a metal washer with good results. We noticed in other cases that the use of a metal washer generates more friction on the drill during drilling, and the resulting heat could enable drill fracture. We noticed much less friction and consequent heat with a sleeve without the metal washer.

One of the most significant advances in guided endodontics has been the development and use of templates generated through digital impressions and CAD/CAM technology. These templates offer unparalleled precision in guiding the endodontic drill to the exact location and depth required within the tooth's anatomy. This level of accuracy is fundamental in minimizing the risk of iatrogenic damage, such as root perforations, ledge formation, or excessive dentin removal. Laboratory investigations have shown minimal deviation angles as low as 1.59° when using guided templates, underscoring their high degree of predictability and control during access preparation [40].

The precision afforded by these templates also directly contributes to the minimization of invasive procedures. Since the drill path is carefully preplanned and executed with fidelity, vital tooth structure is preserved. This conservation is critical for maintaining the long-term biomechanical integrity of the tooth and reducing the necessity for subsequent restorative interventions. Moreover, the use of templates in guided endodontics contributes significantly to clinical efficiency. By optimizing the trajectory and depth of drilling, the overall chairside time is reduced, which not only improves clinical workflow but also enhances patient comfort and satisfaction with the procedure.

Clinical studies have provided robust evidence supporting the benefits of template-guided endodontics. Buchgreitz et al. and Zehnder et al. demonstrated in laboratory settings that guided approaches significantly improve procedural success rates while reducing the incidence of common technical complications when compared to conventional access techniques [2, 41].

These findings confirm that templates represent a pivotal innovation in contemporary endodontic practice, allowing clinicians to deliver highly accurate, efficient, and patient-centered treatments. As guided endodontics becomes more accessible, these tools are likely to become routine in complex clinical cases, bolstering practitioner confidence and improving clinical outcomes.

Technologically, the creation of templates for endodontic access involves either subtractive CAD/CAM systems or additive 3D printing processes. Regardless of the manufacturing method, the template must include a sleeve over the area of the tooth to be accessed. This sleeve typically includes a precisely sized hole that matches the diameter of the drill intended for use. In most cases, a metallic washer is inserted into the sleeve to provide this precision fit. However, it is also possible to fabricate the template entirely in resin without a metal washer.

In recent clinical experience, templates without metal washers were used with favorable results. It was observed that metal washers, while providing structural reinforcement, also increased friction during the drilling process. This additional friction may generate heat and contribute to premature drill wear or even fracture. Conversely, the use of a sleeve made entirely of printed resin was associated with less friction and reduced thermal generation during osteotomy, enhancing safety and control.

In summary, the integration of templates into guided endodontic protocols represents a major step forward in minimally invasive dentistry. Backed by scientific evidence and practical validation, these resources provide an effective strategy for overcoming anatomical challenges, reducing iatrogenic risks, and delivering more predictable outcomes for patients.

9.4.5 Template Adjustment and Placement

Although the scanning process is very accurate, in our personal experience, some templates may present areas that hinder template placement. Therefore, before starting the procedure itself, the template must be adapted and tested on patients. This care is necessary to check its adaptation and stability. During the treatment, it is essential that the template remains properly locked and static, so that the drill follows its trajectory accurately.

One way we have found to precisely identify such retention points in templates is to use a copy pencil. The template is installed in the patient's mouth and where a point is identified that prevents full adaptation, the template is removed and the tooth/region that presents the interference is marked with a copy pencil. The template is placed again and when removed, the interference point is marked so that grinding can be carried out with a milling cutter. The procedure is repeated until the template is fully fitted and adapted to its position, properly stable and locked.

9.4.6 Clinical Procedure

This section now aims to provide a summary description of the flow of procedures for performing guided endodontics.

As discussed earlier in this chapter, when an obstruction in the root canal system is identified and endodontic treatment is planned, the following steps should be followed:

1. Request CBCT with the smallest possible FOV of the region of the involved tooth. A smaller FOV will provide higher definition images of the intervention area.
2. For the best results in 3D planning, also request an 8 × 8 FOV, full-arch computed tomography with lip, cheek, and tongue retraction.
3. Request intraoral scanning, which must include the bottom of the vestibule and hard palate.
4. Overlay the DICOM and STL files in the digital planning software, defining the diameter and trajectory according to the tooth anatomy. The target point is the apical region on a straight-line path. Plan and design the template with a sleeve of at least 6 mm above the drilling point. This margin is important to ensure enough drill position stabilization. Remember that drill must be kept in position with no lateral variation during the drilling process. Another important observation is that the template must have an opening in teeth to ease and guide its installation. There are companies where such files can be sent by email and the planning and 3D printing of the templates are properly carried out. Search for possibilities in your region.
5. Once the template has been 3D-printed, it is important to test and adjust it. Install the template on the patient and check its adaptation and stability. If points that prevent its full adaptation exist, wear these points successively until the appropriate position is found and the template is locked.
6. Once the template check adaptation is complete, anesthetize and proceed with rubber dam installation. Then, install the template and mark with a pencil the drilling point in the tooth surface. Remove the template and with a diamond round bur make an opening in the pencil-marked area by breaking enamel layer.
7. As the drill approaches the apical third of the root, it is recommended to interrupt the mechanical instrumentation and proceed with a manual #10 file to verify the presence and patency of the canal. Despite the high accuracy of digital planning, anatomical variations may still occur. In a documented case by Krastl et al., the canal lumen was identified 4 mm before the depth anticipated by the virtual planning, reinforcing the importance of intraoperative verification [1].
8. Once the predetermined depth is achieved, use a prepended #08 or #10 K-file to locate the canal lumen and accomplish endodontic treatment. During this localization procedure, EDTA solutions, ultrasonically activated, might be used to clean the area and remove mineralized crystals that may block the canal entrance.

See **Figures 9.1 and 9.2**.

9.4.7 Technique Limitations

The clinical viability and implementation of guided endodontics have been extensively documented in numerous case reports over recent years. These reports have demonstrated the technique's effectiveness in managing challenging anatomical situations and in improving the predictability of access cavity preparations [11, 14, 41–53].

In clinical research, Buchgreitz et al. [41] confirmed the feasibility of guided endodontic access in a series of 50 cases, where root canals were successfully located and negotiated in all instances. This evidence supports the assertion that guided access cavity preparation can be performed with a high degree of safety and effectiveness. The technique is particularly well-suited for teeth with straight roots or for the straight portions of curved canals, especially in anterior regions, where there is typically sufficient space for template installation and precise drill positioning. Although its primary application has been reported in anterior teeth, there is growing literature demonstrating its successful use in posterior teeth as well, provided spatial and anatomical considerations are properly addressed [14].

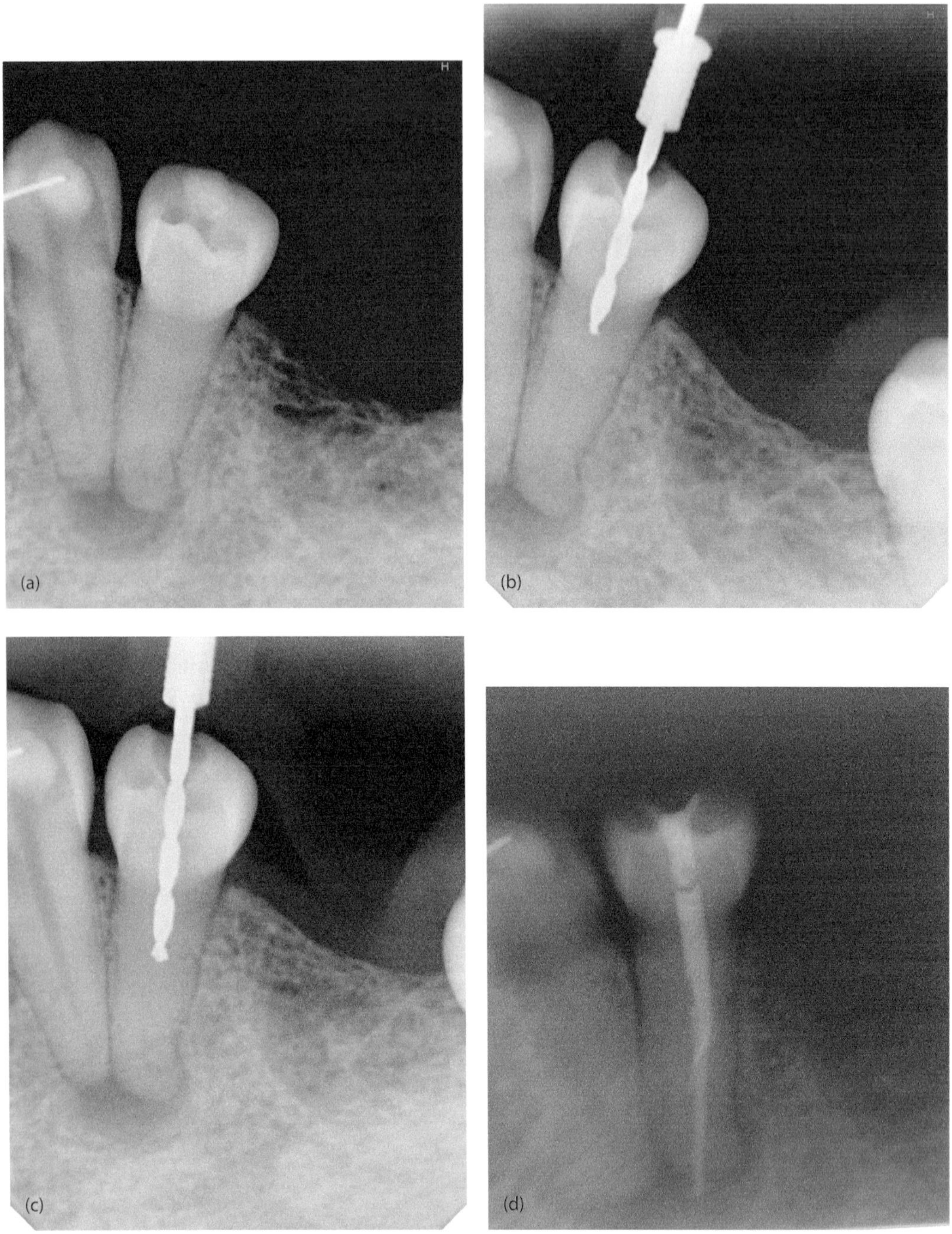

Figure 9.1 A radiographic clinical sequence of the guided endodontics approach: (a) Initial radiograph of a lower premolar with an apical radiolucency and pulp space obliteration (patient was asymptomatic and had a trauma luxation history). (b) First control of drill depth. (c) Final drilling control. (d) Final radiograph with endodontic filling along the root canal.

Nevertheless, despite its advantages, guided endodontics is not without limitations. The technique requires considerable time for planning, including digital analysis, software manipulation, and 3D printing of the customized template. Moreover, it necessitates the acquisition of high-resolution CBCT images, which contribute to an increased radiation dose for the patient. Additionally, the overall cost of treatment may be elevated due to the combination of CBCT, intraoral scanning, and

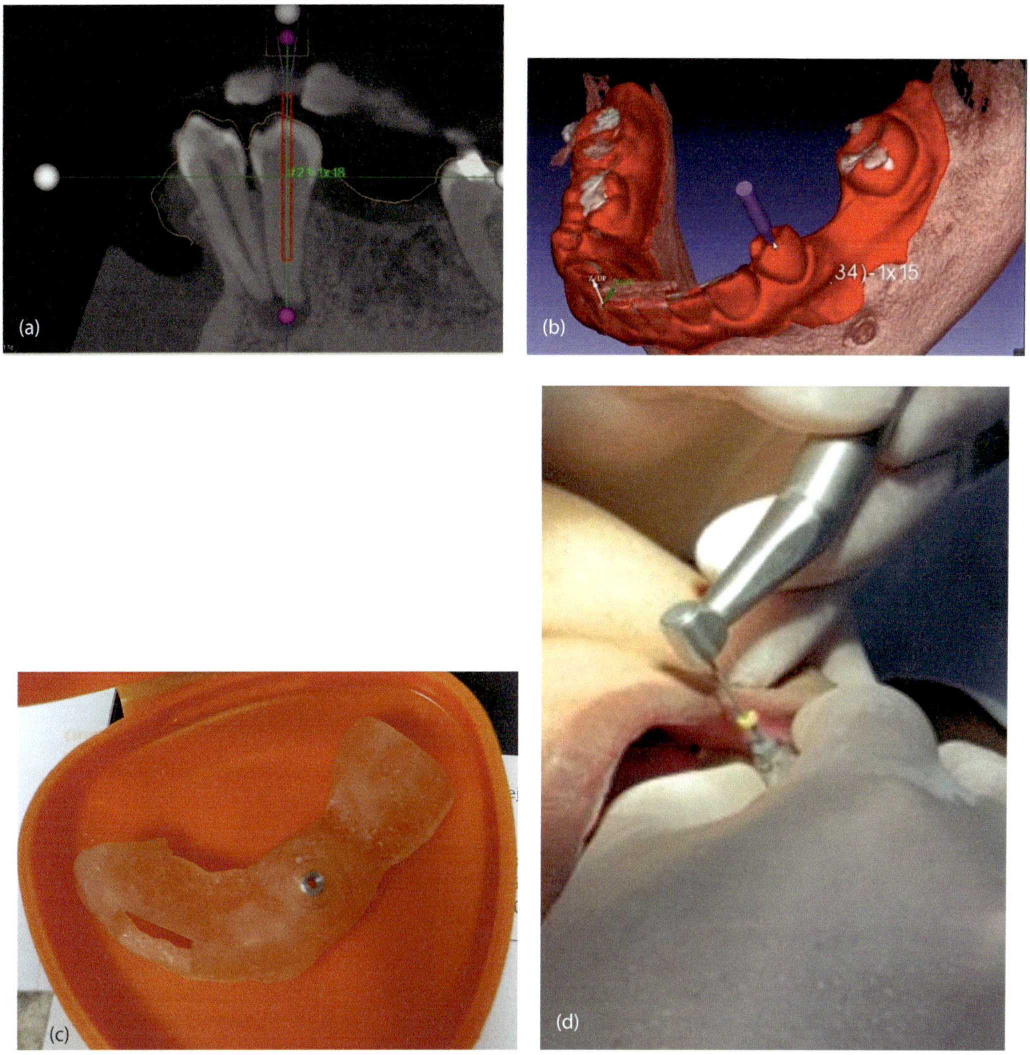

Figure 9.2 The digital flow sequence of the endodontic guide approach: (a) Initial planning of drilling direction in the DICOM file (Computed-aided planning). (b) Template design and planning. (c) 3D-printed template in the CAD/CAM system. (d) Guided access being performed.

template fabrication processes. These factors can pose challenges to the widespread implementation of guided endodontics, particularly in resource-limited settings.

9.4.8 Failure of Technique

Fonseca-Tavares et al. [54] published a clinical case report describing a failure in the execution of guided endodontic technique and the subsequent implementation of a surgical solution. The report highlighted the critical importance of achieving proper bone fixation to ensure adequate stabilization of the template during the drilling procedure. According to the authors, inaccuracies arising from manual mesh merging during the digital planning phase contributed to an unfavorable deviation of the drill path, resulting in root perforation. The misplacement of the guide led the bur to deviate from the planned trajectory and communicate with the lateral periodontal ligament. To manage this complication, a surgical approach was adopted: The perforation site was sealed, and an apicoectomy was performed to address the periapical infection. The adopted surgical strategy yielded satisfactory clinical and radiographic outcomes. This case underscores that despite the precision typically associated with guided endodontics, complications may arise, and when they do, surgical intervention can serve as a viable and effective solution.

9.5 DYNAMIC GUIDED ENDODONTICS

Although static navigation in guided endodontics relies on a prefabricated template to guide the drilling procedure – thereby minimizing dependency on the operator's manual skills – dynamic navigation introduces a different paradigm. It operates as a real-time progress-monitoring system in which the clinician's expertise plays a significant role in achieving precise outcomes. Similar to static systems, dynamic navigation depends on the fusion of DICOM images obtained from CBCT and STL files generated from intraoral scanning. These datasets are overlaid within specialized planning software to create a highly accurate digital replica of the tooth and its surrounding structures. Once integrated with dynamic navigation systems, this synergy enables clinicians to visualize and track endodontic instruments in real time, ensuring safe canal navigation and reducing the risk of procedural errors.

In this workflow, the merged datasets are loaded into a dynamic navigation platform, which includes a stereo camera and a real-time tracking system. The system projects the virtual plan onto a monitor, allowing the operator to follow the exact position and orientation of the drill within axial, sagittal, and coronal planes. This visual guidance, although highly effective, demands advanced motor coordination and visual-spatial awareness, since the operator must focus on the monitor rather than the patient's mouth while performing the procedure. Notably, the origin of dynamic navigation systems can be traced back to developments in implantology, where they have been widely utilized for precision placement of dental implants [55].

In earlier versions of this technique, physical reference markers had to be attached to the patient's dentition prior to CBCT acquisition to enable accurate spatial tracking. However, more recent technological advances now allow these reference points to be planned digitally and fabricated via 3D printing, streamlining the process. During the access cavity preparation, the position and motion of the drill are continuously displayed in real time on the system monitor, offering immediate visual feedback and improved procedural control [56].

A significant advantage of dynamic over static navigation lies in its flexibility and speed. Because dynamic systems do not require the fabrication of physical templates, they are particularly advantageous in emergency scenarios, allowing immediate treatment of patients experiencing acute dental pain without waiting for a guide to be produced [57].

9.5.1 Technique Accuracy

The accuracy and efficacy of dynamic navigation in guided endodontics have been evaluated in several in vitro studies, demonstrating promising results when compared to traditional freehand approaches. Chong et al. [58], in an experimental study on extracted teeth, reported that dynamic navigation systems were able to detect root canals in 26 out of 29 cases. In two of the remaining teeth – both maxillary molars – only one canal could be located due to tracking difficulties, while in the third case, also a maxillary molar, the preparation deviated from the planned trajectory.

Zubizarreta-Macho et al. [59] conducted a comparative analysis between static navigation, dynamic navigation, and freehand access preparation. Their results indicated that both navigation techniques were significantly more accurate than the freehand method. However, the angular deviation observed in static navigation reached an average of 10°, which is notably higher than values reported in other studies, where deviations as low as 1.3° have been documented.

Using a model of 138 3D-printed teeth with simulated PCO, Jain et al. [60] demonstrated that dynamic navigation could accurately detect root canals, with an average angular deviation of 1.7°, a result comparable to those achieved through static navigation.

In another study, Dianat et al. [61] evaluated 60 extracted teeth with PCO and found that dynamic navigation resulted in access cavities that were not only more accurate in terms of linear and angular deviation, but also more conservative. Moreover, the navigated procedures required less time to visualize the root canal systems when compared to the freehand group.

Similarly, Torres et al. [62] assessed the precision of dynamic navigation in accessing heavily calcified canals using 3D-printed models and concluded that the system offers high accuracy. However, the authors emphasized the importance of operator training and recognized a learning curve associated with this technique.

Connert et al. [57] also tested a miniaturized dynamic navigation system and showed that even inexperienced operators could prepare minimally invasive access cavities with outcomes similar to experienced clinicians when using the navigated approach. In contrast, freehand procedures showed significant discrepancies, including greater loss of dental structure.

A systematic review and meta-analysis conducted by Mekhdieva et al. [63] reinforced these findings, highlighting that dynamic navigation contributes to reduced operating time, improved accuracy, minimal substance loss, and lower rates of iatrogenic complications. Nevertheless, the authors acknowledged that clinical trials remain scarce, limiting the strength of evidence supporting dynamic navigation's widespread use.

Despite its benefits, dynamic navigation systems also present notable limitations. One of the primary concerns is the high cost of acquisition and maintenance. Additionally, unlike static navigation – which relies on physical guides – dynamic systems demand constant operator interaction and advanced visual-motor coordination, as the clinician must focus on a monitor rather than directly on the operative field. This shift in focus requires adaptation and can be a barrier to some practitioners. Furthermore, some currently available systems are large and bulky, which may hinder their integration into smaller clinical settings or reduce maneuverability during procedures.

9.6 FUTURE DIRECTIONS

The field of guided endodontics continues to evolve rapidly, with ongoing research focused on enhancing software accuracy, expanding the range of clinical indications, and reducing costs associated with the technology. One of the most promising areas of advancement lies in the integration of artificial intelligence and robotics, which holds potential to further increase precision, automation, and efficiency in both static and dynamic navigation procedures.

Although guidance through templates and sleeves already constitutes a sophisticated technique, clinical demands suggest the need for a broader variety of commercially available drills with different diameters and lengths. This is especially important for a more patient-centered approach, particularly when accessing teeth in posterior regions where spatial constraints limit the use of standard guides.

Among the most innovative perspectives for the future is the incorporation of magnetic resonance imaging (MRI) into dental diagnostics and guided procedures. MRI presents the notable advantage of eliminating ionizing radiation, which is particularly desirable in pediatric dentistry due to children's increased sensitivity to radiation exposure [64]. In a proof-of-principle study, Leontiev et al. [65] demonstrated that MRI-based planning could enable the preparation of precise access cavities in a laboratory environment. Using a splint filled with a hydrous gel to aid in visualization, the MRI data was successfully superimposed with surface scans, allowing for accurate assessment of root canal location. The root canal system was visualized in 91 out of 100 test cases, with a mean angular deviation of 1.82°. Despite the promising results, clinical application of this method remains pending, as MRI equipment is not yet accessible to dental professionals. However, continued technological development may pave the way for its future implementation.

Furthermore, the demand for prospective clinical trials remains a priority to strengthen the scientific basis and validate the long-term efficacy and safety of guided endodontics in real-world practice. High-quality in vivo studies are essential to address limitations of current in vitro investigations and to establish reliable clinical protocols.

Looking ahead, Connert et al. [56] suggest that reducing the size of navigation systems would greatly improve operability and ergonomics during patient care. Moreover, they emphasize that systems should be able to digitally plan and integrate reference markers, eliminating the need for a second CBCT scan if one has already been acquired. Ideally, these systems would no longer depend on physical markers and would instead rely on the patient's own anatomical structures for orientation.

Another prospective advancement in guided endodontics is the application of augmented reality (AR) in dynamic navigation. AR technology allows for the overlay of navigation paths and radiographic imagery directly onto the operator's view of the operative field via head-up displays or integrated microscopes. This integration facilitates simultaneous visualization of both real and virtual environments, potentially improving operator control and focus. While AR has shown feasibility in neurosurgical applications [66], its use in endodontics remains at a conceptual stage. Song et al. [67] proposed its implementation in endodontic practice, but clinical application has yet to be realized.

REFERENCES

1. Krastl, G, Zehnder, MS, Connert, T, Weiger, R, Kühl, S. Guided endodontics: a novel treatment approach for teeth with pulp canal calcification and apical pathology. Dent Traumatol. 2016;32(3):240–246.
2. Zehnder, MS, Connert, T, Weiger, R, Krastl, G, Kühl, S. Guided endodontics: accuracy of a novel method for guided access cavity preparation and root canal location. Int Endod J. 2016;49(10):966–972.
3. Ricucci, D, Loghin, S, Lin, LM, Spångberg, LS, Tay, FR. Is hard tissue formation in the dental pulp after the death of the primary odontoblasts a regenerative or a reparative process? J Dent. 2014;42(9):1156–1170.
4. Andreasen, FM, Zhijie, Y, Thomsen, BL, Andersen, PK. Occurrence of pulp canal obliteration after luxation injuries in the permanent dentition. Endod Dent Traumatol. 1987;3(3):103–15.

5. Jacobsen, I, Kerekes, K. Long-term prognosis of traumatized permanent anterior teeth showing calcifying processes in the pulp cavity. Scand J Dent Res. 1977;85(7):588–98.
6. Oginni, AO, Adekoya-Sofowora, CA, Kolawole, KA. Evaluation of radiographs, clinical signs and symptoms associated with pulp canal obliteration: an aid to treatment decision. Dent Traumatol. 2009;25(6):620–625.
7. Robertson, A, Andreasen, FM, Bergenholtz, G, Andreasen, JO, Norén, JG. Incidence of pulp necrosis subsequent to pulp canal obliteration from trauma of permanent incisors. J Endod. 1996;22(10):557–560.
8. Martin-Biedma, B, Gonzalez-Gonzalez, T, Lopes, M, Lopes, L, Vilar, R, Bahillo, J et al. Colorimeter and scanning electron microscopy analysis of teeth submitted to internal bleaching. J Endod. 2010;36(2):334–337.
9. Lang, H, Korkmaz, Y, Schneider, K, Raab, WH. Impact of endodontic treatments on the rigidity of the root. J Dent Res. 2006;85:364–368.
10. Cvek, M, Granath, L, Lundberg, M. Failures and healing in endodontically treated non-vital anterior teeth with post-traumatically reduced pulpal lumen. Acta Odontol Scand. 1982;40:223–228.
11. Loureiro, MAZ, Silva, JA, Chaves, GS, Capeletti, LR, Estrela, C, Decurcio, DA. Guided endodontics: the impact of new technologies on complex case solution. Aust Endod J. 2021;47(3):664–671.
12. McCabe, PS, Dummer, PM. Pulp canal obliteration: an endodontic diagnosis and treatment challenge. Int Endod J. 2012;45:177–197.
13. Decurcio, DA, Bueno, MR, Silva, JA, Loureiro, MAZ, Damião Sousa-Neto, M, Estrela, C. Digital planning on guided endodontics technology. Braz Dent J. 2021;32(5):23–33.
14. Lara-Mendes, STO, Barbosa, CFM, Santa-Rosa, CC, Machado, VC. Guided endodontic access in maxillary molars using cone-beam computed tomography and computer-aided design/computer-aided manufacturing system: a case report. J Endod. 2018;44:875–879.
15. Scarfe, WC, Farman, AG, Sukovic, P. Clinical applications of cone-beam computed tomography in dental practice. J Can Dent Assoc. 2009;75(10):705–707.
16. Patel, S, Durack, C, Abella, F et al. Cone beam computed tomography in endodontics - a review. Int Endod J. 2012; 45(1):3–15.
17. Ludlow, JB, Ivanovic, M. Comparative dosimetry of dental CBCT devices and 64-slice CT for oral and maxillofacial radiology. Oral Surg Oral Med Oral Pathol Oral Radiol Endod. 2008;106(1):106–114.
18. Leal, F, Campos, PSF, Carrasco, L et al. Digital dentistry: the use of DICOM files for 3D printing in endodontics. Braz Dent J. 2019;30(4):354–360.
19. Nedelcu, R, Olsson, P, Nyström, I et al. Finish line distinctness and accuracy in 7 intraoral scanners versus conventional impression: an in vitro descriptive comparison. BMC Oral Health. 2013;13(1):12.
20. Patzelt, SB, Emmanouilidi, A, Stampf, S et al. Accuracy of full-arch scans using intraoral scanners. Clin Oral Investig. 2016;20(7):1487–1494.
21. Tang, L, Sun, Y, Chen, Z et al. Application of intraoral scanning technology in computer-aided design of dental occlusal splint. J Healthcare Eng. 2018;2018:2643512.
22. Vasudavan, S, Hicks, ML, Abughazaleh, K et al. Digital workflow for guided endodontics: a case report. Case Rep Dent. 2019;2019:4587401.
23. Vasudavan, S, Hicks, ML, Abughazaleh, K et al. Integration of intraoral scanning and 3D printing for guided endodontic surgery: a novel approach. Case Rep Dent. 2020;2020:8871309.
24. Tanimoto, Y, Higuchi, D, Hatuno, K et al. In vitro evaluation of a digital system for guided endodontic surgery. PLoS One. 2019;14(8):e0221480.
25. Abella, F, Teixidó, LM, Patel, S et al. Cone-beam computed tomography analysis of the root canal morphology of maxillary first and second premolars in a Spanish population. J Endod. 2011;37(10):1396–1401.
26. Sun, Y, Wang, W, Chuang, KC et al. A novel guided endodontic access cavity design and its effect on root canal length determination accuracy: a cone-beam computed tomographic study. J Endod. 2020;46(7):982–989.
27. Li, H, Li, X, Ge, W et al. Application of 3D printing technology in guiding root canal therapy of complex root morphology. J Healthcare Eng. 2021;2021:5529536.
28. Welk, A, Splieth, C, Wiedemeier, D et al. Accuracy of intraoral and extraoral digital data acquisition for dental restorations. J Appl Oral Sci. 2017;25(6):548–554.
29. Zheng, D, Benderli, Y, Meyer, CA et al. Accuracy of 3D-printed endodontic surgical guides created from CBCT. J Endod. 2019;45(4):437–442.
30. Tchorz, JP, Wrbas, KT, Hellwig, E et al. 3D versus 2D imaging in root canal diagnosis. J Dent. 2013;41(5):382–386.
31. Durack, C, Patel, S. Cone beam computed tomography in endodontics. Braz Dent J. 2012;23(3):179–191.
32. Wang, Y, He, W, Zhu, M et al. Evaluation of root canal morphology of maxillary molars in a Chinese population using cone-beam computed tomography. BMC Oral Health. 2021;21(1):293.
33. Vázquez de la Torre, CJ, Sánchez-Turrión Andreu, J, Figueiredo, R et al. Evaluation of digital guided endodontic access cavities: a pilot clinical study. J Clin Exp Dent. 2019;11(4):e327–e333.
34. Rödig, T, Kupis, J, Konietschke, F et al. Accuracy of endodontic working length determination using cone beam computed tomography. Int Endod J. 2017;43(9):1523–1527.
35. Vasconcelos, KF, Nejaim, Y, Haiter-Neto, F et al. Detection of simulated periapical lesions with two cone-beam computed tomography units and digital periapical radiography. Int Endod J. 2012;45(9):817–826.
36. Kruse, C, Spin-Neto, R, Maret, D et al. Assessment of root canal treatment outcomes: an evaluation of different assessment criteria in panoramic radiographs, intraoral periapical radiographs, and cone-beam computed tomography scans. J Endod. 2016;42(6):910–916.
37. Moiseiwitsch, JR. Clinical uses of digital imaging in endodontics. Dent Clin North Am. 2002;46(2):249–267.
38. Nascimento, EHL, Gaia, BF, Pozza, DH et al. Can cone-beam computed tomography detect changes in dentin after root canal dressing with antibiotic paste? A randomized clinical trial. J Endod. 2020;46(10):1377–1385.
39. González-Martín, O, Li, X, Vera, J et al. Evaluation of root canal anatomy in human permanent teeth in a Chinese subpopulation using cone-beam computed tomography. BMC Oral Health. 2017;17(1):161.
40. Connert, T, Zehnder, MS, Weiger, R, Kühl, S, Krastl, G. Microguided endodontics: accuracy of a miniaturized technique for apically extended access cavity preparation in anterior teeth. J Endod. 2017;43:787–790.

41. Buchgreitz, J, Buchgreitz, M, Bjørndal, L. Guided endodontics modified for treating molars by using an intracoronal guide technique. J Endod. 2019;45:818–823.
42. Casadei, BA, Lara-Mendes, STO, Barbosa, CFM, Araújo, CV, Freitas, CA, Machado, VC et al. Access to original canal trajectory after deviation and perforation with guided endodontic assistance. Aust Endod J. 2020;46:101–116.
43. Fonseca Tavares, WL, Diniz Viana, AC, de Carvalho, MV, Feitosa Henriques, LC, Ribeiro Sobrinho, AP. Guided endodontic access of calcified anterior teeth. J Endod. 2018;44:1195–1199.
44. Hegde, SG, Tawani, G, Warhadpande, M, Raut, A, Dakshindas, D, Wankhade, S. Guided endodontic therapy: management of pulp canal obliteration in the maxillary Central incisor. J Conserv Dent. 2019;22:607–611.
45. Ishak, G, Habib, M, Tohme, H, Patel, S, Bordone, A, Perez, C et al. Guided endodontic treatment of calcified lower incisors: a case report. Dent J. 2020;8:74.
46. Kamburoğlu, K, Koç, C, Sönmez, G, Çapçı, A. 3D printing in endodontics: report of three clinical cases with innovative approaches. Int J Comput Dent. 2021;24:317–328.
47. Krug, R, Volland, J, Reich, S, Soliman, S, Connert, T, Krastl, G. Guided endodontic treatment of multiple teeth with dentin dysplasia: a case report. Head Face Med. 2020;16:27.
48. Lara-Mendes, STO, Barbosa, CFM, Machado, VC, Santa-Rosa, CC. A new approach for minimally invasive access to severely calcified anterior teeth using the guided endodontics technique. J Endod. 2018;44:1578–1582.
49. Llaquet Pujol, M, Vidal, C, Mercadé, M, Muñoz, M, Ortolani-Seltenerich, S. Guided endodontics for managing severely calcified canals. J Endod. 2021;47:315–321.
50. Maia, LM, de Carvalho, MV, da Silva, N, Brito Júnior, M, da Silveira, RR, Moreira Júnior, G et al. Case reports in maxillary posterior teeth by guided endodontic access. J Endod. 2019;45:214–218.
51. Tavares, WLF, Ferreira, MVL, de Carvalho, MV, Braga, T, Amaral, RR, Cohen, S. Antimicrobial photodynamic therapy and guided endodontics: a case report. Photodiagnosis Photodyn Ther. 2020;31:101935.
52. Todd, R, Resnick, S, Zicarelli, T, Linenberg, C, Donelson, J, Boyd, C. Template-guided endodontic access. J Am Dent Assoc. 2021;152:65–70.
53. Torres, A, Shaheen, E, Lambrechts, P, Politis, C, Jacobs, R. Microguided endodontics: a case report of a maxillary lateral incisor with pulp canal obliteration and apical periodontitis. Int Endod J. 2019;52:540–549.
54. Fonseca-Tavares, WL, de Oliveira Murta Pedrosa, N, Moreira, RA, Braga, T, de Carvalho Machado, V, Ribeiro Sobrinho, AP et al. Limitations and management of static-guided endodontics failure. J Endod. 2022;48(2):273–279.
55. Marquardt, P, Witkowski, S, Strub, J. Three-dimensional navigation in implant dentistry. Eur J Esthet Dent. 2007;2:80–98.
56. Connert, T, Weiger, R, Krastl, G. Present status and future directions – guided endodontics. Int Endod J. 2022;55(Suppl. 4): 995–1002.
57. Connert, T, Leontiev, W, Dagassan-Berndt, D, Kühl, S, ElAyouti, A, Krug, R et al. Real-time guided endodontics with a miniaturized dynamic navigation system versus conventional freehand endodontic access cavity preparation: substance loss and procedure time. J Endod. 2021;47:1651–1656.
58. Chong, BS, Dhesi, M, Makdissi, J. Computer-aided dynamic navigation: a novel method for guided endodontics. Quintessence Int. 2019;50:196–202.
59. Zubizarreta-Macho, A, Munoz, AP, Deglow, ER, AgustinPanadero, R, Alvarez, JM. Accuracy of computer aided dynamic navigation compared to computer-aided static procedure for endodontic access cavities: an in vitro study. J Clin Med. 2020;9:129.
60. Jain, SD, Carrico, CK, Bermanis, I. 3-dimensional accuracy of dynamic navigation technology in locating calcified canals. J Endod. 2020;46:839–845.
61. Dianat, O, Nosrat, A, Tordik, PA, Aldahmash, SA, Romberg, E, Price, JB et al. Accuracy and efficiency of a dynamic navigation system for locating calcified canals. J Endod. 2020;46:1719–1725.
62. Torres, A, Boelen, GJ, Lambrechts, P, Pedano, MS, Jacobs, R. Dynamic navigation: a laboratory study on the accuracy and potential use of guided root canal treatment. Int Endod J. 2021;54:1659–1667.
63. Mekhdieva, E, Del Fabbro, M, Alovisi, M, Scotti, N, Comba, A, Berutti, E, Pasqualini, D. Dynamic navigation system vs. free-hand approach in microsurgical and non-surgical endodontics: a systematic review and meta-analysis of experimental studies. J Clin Med. 2023;12:5845.
64. Dula, K, Bornstein, MM, Buser, D, Dagassan-Berndt, D, Ettlin, DA, Filippi, A et al. SADMFR guidelines for the use of cone-beam computed tomography/digital volume tomography. Swiss Dent J. 2014;124:1169–1183.
65. Leontiev, W, Bieri, O, Madörin, P, Dagassan-Berndt, D, Kühl, S, Krastl, G et al. Suitability of magnetic resonance imaging for guided endodontics: proof of principle. J Endod. 2021;47:954–960.
66. Contreras Lopez, WO, Navarro, PA, Crispin, S. Intraoperative clinical application of augmented reality in neurosurgery: a systematic review. Clin Neurol Neurosurg. 2019;177:6–11.
67. Song, T, Yang, C, Dianat, O, Azimi, E. Endodontic guided treatment using augmented reality on a head-mounted display system. Healthcare Technol Lett. 2018;5:201–207.

10 Advances of Digital Technology in Oral Tissue Engineering

Mahdieh Alipour and Juan Manual Taboas

10.1 INTRODUCTION

Digital dentistry, the application of computers in imaging, treatment planning, and implant design, has made significant advances in dental medicine [1]. In recent years, its application in oral tissue engineering has gained momentum due to its potential to revolutionize dental treatments and therapies. By harnessing the capabilities of digital tools and techniques, researchers and clinicians can design and fabricate complex structures with precise specifications, creating patient-specific solutions for improved oral tissue regeneration and restoration [2, 3].

One area where digital technology has had a profound impact is in the design and fabrication of scaffolds for tissue engineering. Computer-aided design (CAD), computer-aided manufacturing (CAM), and solid free-form fabrication (aka 3D printing) provide the ability to create patient-specific scaffolds with optimal structural and mechanical properties [4–6]. Precise fabrication of scaffolds using CAD, CAM, and 3D printing techniques has allowed for the creation of complex three-dimensional structures with tailored physical properties, promoting improved tissue growth and regeneration [7–10]. Additionally, digital imaging techniques such as computed tomography (CT) and magnetic resonance imaging (MRI) have played a crucial role in providing detailed anatomical data and facilitating accurate diagnosis, treatment planning, and postoperative assessment in dental procedures [11, 12]. In addition, digital workflows enable clinicians to assess the biocompatibility of dental materials and select suitable materials for scaffold fabrication [13, 14]. The integration of advanced imaging techniques and digital technologies allows for in vivo evaluation of tissue growth and regeneration, providing valuable insights into the effectiveness and long-term stability of tissue-engineered constructs [15].

Digital dentistry has facilitated interdisciplinary collaboration in oral tissue engineering. Dentists, engineers, and scientists can collectively work on treatment planning and design processes, leveraging their respective expertise to optimize treatment outcomes [16, 17]. This collaboration enhances the effectiveness of oral tissue engineering strategies and encourages innovation in the field.

Despite the promising advancements, challenges and limitations exist in the implementation of digital technology in oral tissue engineering. These include the need for standardized protocols, the cost of equipment and materials, and the requirement for further research to establish the long-term clinical outcomes of digital techniques [18, 19]. However, with ongoing research and development, the future of digital technology in oral tissue engineering is promising. The integration of digital tools and techniques has opened new possibilities for personalized and patient-specific solutions, enhancing the outcomes of oral tissue regeneration and restoration. While challenges remain, ongoing advancements in digital technology are expected to further improve the field of oral tissue engineering.

The objective of this chapter is to provide a comprehensive overview of the recent advances in digital dentistry and its applications in oral tissue engineering. Additionally, we discuss the challenges and limitations associated with the implementation of digital dentistry in tissue engineering, as well as the future perspectives and potential for further advancements.

10.2 DIGITAL IMAGING TECHNIQUES

Digital imaging techniques play a critical role in the field of oral tissue engineering, providing valuable information for accurate diagnosis, treatment planning, and the design of patient-specific solutions [20]. These advanced imaging modalities have revolutionized the way clinicians assess oral structures and guide the fabrication of scaffolds for tissue regeneration [21]. In this section, the key digital imaging techniques used in oral tissue engineering and their applications will be explored.

10.2.1 Intraoral Scanners

Intraoral scanners are digital imaging devices used to capture detailed images of the intraoral structures, including teeth and soft tissues [22]. These scanners utilize optical or laser-based technologies to create digital impressions of the oral cavity, replacing traditional dental impressions, e.g., Cadent's iTero Digital Impression System and 3M ESPS's Lava Chairside Oral Scanner. Intraoral scans provide accurate and highly detailed images that can be used for CAD of restorations, prostheses, and patient-specific scaffolds for tissue engineering [23, 24]. The use of intraoral scanners reduced the need for physical impressions, reduced patient discomfort, and streamlined the digital workflow, eliminating the need for digital scanning of oral impressions [25].

DOI: 10.1201/9781003428541-10

10.2.2 Computed Tomography (CT), Cone Beam Computed Tomography (CBCT), and MicroCT (Micro-Computed Tomography) Imaging

CT imaging utilizes multiple X-ray images from different angles to reconstruct a 3D volume representation of the patient's anatomy. CT scans provide high-resolution images of mineralized tissues such as bone and teeth, making them valuable for various dental applications. In the craniofacial region, CT imaging aids in the identification of pathologies, such as tumors or cysts, facilitating treatment planning and guiding the design of patient-specific scaffolds [26, 27]. Cone beam computed tomography (CBCT) is popular in dental medicine because it is faster and employs a lower radiation dose than conventional CT [28, 29] CBCT employs a cone-shaped X-ray beam as opposed to the fan-shaped beam of conventional CT. CBCT is particularly valuable for implant planning, orthodontics, and evaluating dental structures.

Micro-computed tomography (microCT) is also a powerful imaging technique that has become instrumental in oral tissue engineering research. This high-resolution imaging modality allows for the non-destructive analysis of small samples with exceptional detail but precludes live imaging in human patients due to radiation doses, long scanning times, and sample size limitations. MicroCT provides valuable insights into the microarchitecture and internal structures of oral tissues, such as bone and dental structures, enabling researchers to analyze intricate features at a micro level [30, 31]. With the ability to generate 3D reconstructions, microCT facilitates accurate measurements of parameters such as porosity, surface area, and volume, which are essential for evaluating the quality and properties of tissue-engineered constructs [32, 33]. Moreover, microCT allows for the longitudinal assessment of tissue regeneration and remodeling over time in small animal models such as rodents, providing valuable information on the efficacy and stability of oral tissue engineering approaches [34, 35]. Overall, the application of microCT in oral tissue engineering research has significantly advanced our understanding of tissue formation and integration, helping to optimize scaffold design and fabrication processes [36, 37].

Ho et al. assessed the adequacy of dental cone-beam computed tomography (CBCT) and micro-computed tomography (micro-CT) for measuring trabecular bone structural parameters, including bone volume fraction (BV/TV), specific bone surface (BS/BV), trabecular thickness (Tb.Th.), and trabecular separation (Tb.Sp.), using cellular synthetic bone phantoms across four density groups (0.12–0.32 g/cm^3). While strong correlations were observed between the two techniques (Spearman ρ ranging from 0.81 to 0.96, all $p < 0.001$), CBCT measurements yielded systematically higher BV/TV and Tb.Th. values, lower BS/BV, and variable Tb.Sp. (smaller in low-density groups but slightly larger in high-density ones) compared to micro-CT, resulting in significant absolute differences that warrant further validation for targeted clinical applications (**Figure 10.1**) [32].

10.2.3 Magnetic Resonance Imaging (MRI)

MRI is another valuable digital imaging technique utilized in oral tissue engineering. MRI utilizes magnetic fields and radio waves to generate the volumetric representation of soft tissue [38, 39]. This non-invasive imaging modality allows for the evaluation of soft tissue structures, such as muscles, ligaments, and blood vessels, which are crucial considerations in the design of scaffolds for tissue

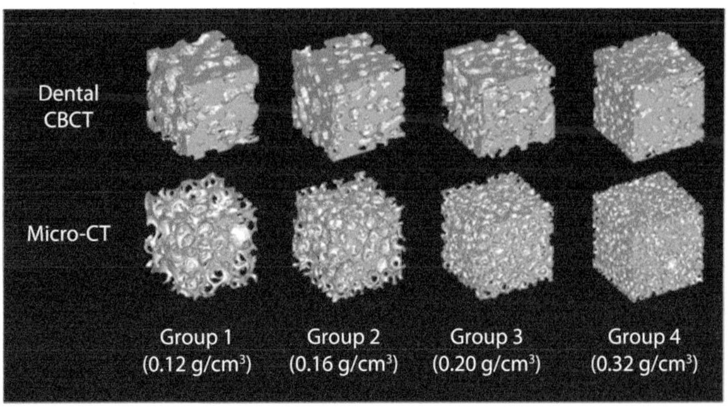

Figure 10.1 The 3D models of the synthetic cellular bone, using dental CBCT and microCT. (Copyright 2013, by the authors. Licensee Springer Nature. Open-access article distributed under the terms of the Creative Commons Attribution License.)

Table 10.1: Advantages and Disadvantages of the MRI Technique

Advantages	Disadvantages
1. Non-invasive.	1. Claustrophobia.
2. No detrimental effect as it uses non-ionizing radiation.	2. Expensive and very noisy.
3. Helps to differentiate soft tissue from one another due to contrast resolution.	3. Contraindicated in patients with cardiac pacemakers, implantable defibrillators, etc.
4. Multiplanar image (sagittal, coronal, oblique) can be obtained.	4. Bone marrow gives a signal but bone doesn't.
5. Safe for pregnant women and children.	5. Distinction between malignant and benign tumors is difficult.
6. Artifacts with dental fillings are not seen.	
7. Manipulation of the image can be done.	

Source: Copyright 2016, by the authors. Open-access article distributed under the terms of the Creative Commons Attribution License. See Ref. [42].

engineering [40, 41]. Better prognosis can be achieved by utilizing MRI in diagnosis and treatment planning, such as jaw lesions and temporomandibular joint disorders (TMDs) [42]. The most common application of MRI in the craniofacial region is in the diagnosis of various lesions, inflammatory conditions affecting the facial skeleton, and examination of the salivary glands, maxillary sinuses, and masseter muscles [42, 43]. The advantage and disadvantages of this technique are summarized by Niraj et al. in **Table 10.1** [42].

10.3 COMPUTER-AIDED DESIGN (CAD) AND COMPUTER-AIDED MANUFACTURING (CAM)

CAD and CAM technologies have revolutionized various industries, including dental medicine. CAD involves the use of specialized software to create digital models and designs of objects or structures. In the context of digital dentistry, CAD software enables the precise design and customization of dental prostheses, implants, scaffolds, and other components used in reconstructive procedures [44]. Once the digital design is complete, the data is transferred to the CAM system, which utilizes computer-controlled machinery to manufacture the physical objects based on the CAD model. CAM technology allows for the automated production of highly accurate and intricately designed oral tissue engineering constructs. It encompasses various manufacturing techniques, such as milling, 3D printing, and laser cutting, depending on the specific requirements of the application [45, 46]. Conventional CAM involves the selective removal of material to fabricate the designed part (subtractive or indirect fabrication), while 3D printing involves the selective deposition of material to build the part (additive or direct fabrication). In general, conventional CAM (e.g., mills, laser cutters, and CNC routers) provides faster fabrication of solid objects, while 3D printing simultaneous fabrication of different parts with enhanced control over their internal architecture [47]. In addition to their design and manufacturing capabilities, CAD and CAM technologies facilitate interdisciplinary collaboration in oral tissue engineering. They allow for seamless data exchange between clinicians, researchers, and engineers, promoting efficient communication and integration of expertise from various fields [48].

Furthermore, CAM with 3D printing has made inroads into dental practice. The ability to fabricate multiple patient-specific parts without retooling machinery has been a critical advantage driving the inroad of 3D printing in dental applications of orthodontics, surgical modeling, and implant guides [47]. On the other hand, the CAD models allow for the customization and optimization of designs, considering factors such as shape, size, and mechanical properties [49]. The CAD software facilitates the virtual planning of oral reconstructive procedures, aiding in surgical guidance, implant placement, and prosthetic restoration design [50–52]. This approach facilitates optimal functional and esthetic outcomes, improving the success rates and longevity of dental implants. The lower cost and technical burdens of 3D printing have turned it into a promising tool in dental practices with the in-house fabrication of highly accurate and customized trial dentures, aligners, guards and splints, bleaching and bonding trays, and some types of crowns [53].

In summary, the integration of CAD and CAM technologies has revolutionized oral tissue engineering by providing advanced tools for the design, customization, and fabrication of tissue-engineered constructs. These technologies enhance the precision, efficiency, and reproducibility of oral tissue engineering processes, ultimately leading to improved treatment outcomes and patient satisfaction.

10.4 TYPES OF SOLID FREE FORM (SFF) FABRICATION IN ORAL TISSUE ENGINEERING

Several solid free form (SFF) techniques exist, and many have been applied for the needs of modern dental medicine (**Figure 10.2**). Some of these have been used in oral tissue engineering using various materials [54].

Stereolithography (STL) is the earliest developed SFF technique. It involves the use of a laser to selectively cure a liquid photopolymer resin layer by layer, resulting in the creation of complex 3D structures. This method requires material waste in the fabrication of support structures that are later removed. These support building parts where not all pieces are interconnected within a single layer, holding them in place until interconnected in subsequent layers. These must be removed post-lithography. STL has been utilized in the fabrication of dental models, surgical guides, and prostheses [55].

Digital light processing (DLP) is a competitive technology for STL. DLP utilizes a digital micromirror device (DMD) to project an entire image onto the liquid photopolymer resin at one time, resulting in faster build times than STL. However, DLP also requires the use of support structures. This technique offers high printing speed and excellent resolution, making it suitable for fabricating dental models, prostheses, and surgical guides [56].

Laminated object manufacturing (LOM) involves the layer-by-layer cutting and bonding of thin sheets of materials such as paper, plastic, or metal. LOM is generally used in lower-resolution builds and consumes much material akin to unused ink on a typewriter ribbon. LOM allows for the creation of 3D objects with good mechanical strength, making it suitable for the production of anatomical models, dental splints, and temporary prostheses [57].

Fused deposition modeling (FDM) is another commonly employed SFF technique in dental medicine. FDM utilizes a thermoplastic filament that is extruded through a heated nozzle and deposited layer by layer to build the desired object. Similar to STL and DLP, FDM requires support structures. This technique offers versatility in material selection and has been utilized in the fabrication of dental models, orthodontic appliances, and surgical guides [58].

Selective laser sintering (SLS) is an SFF technique that utilizes a high-powered laser to selectively fuse powdered materials together to form a solid object. SLS can work with a wide range of biocompatible materials, including polymers and metals. In this technique, the metal powder

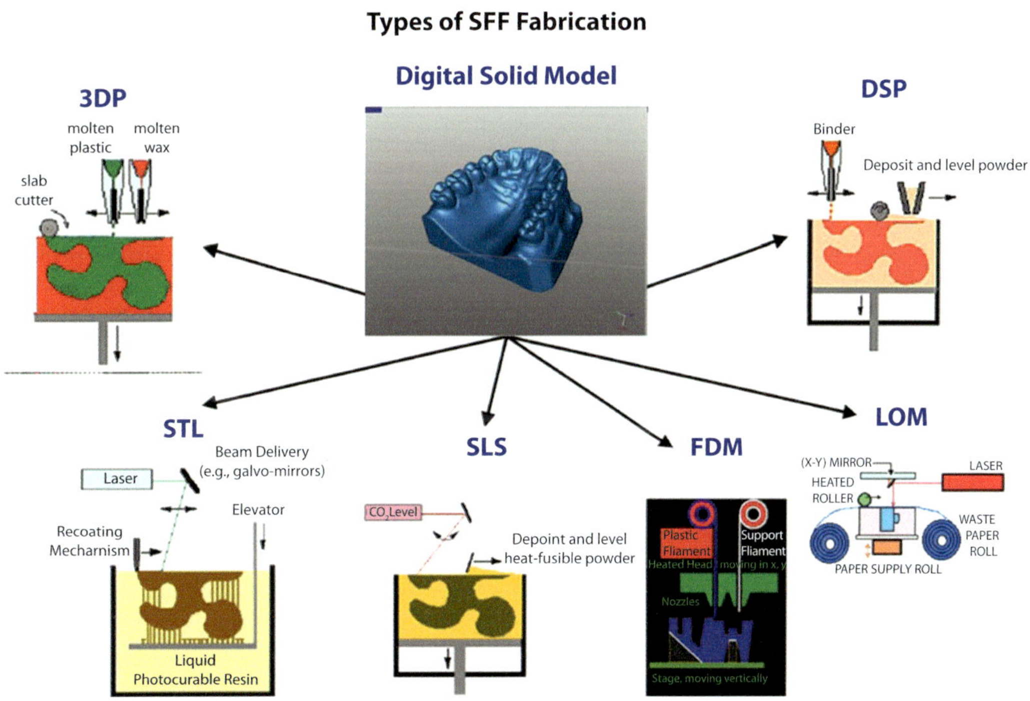

Figure 10.2 Different types of solid form fabrication (SFF). *Abbreviations*: 3DP, three-dimensional printing; DLP, digital light projection; DSP, direct shell production; FDM, fused deposition modeling; LOM, laminated object manufacturing; SLS, selective laser sintering; STL, stereolithography.

bed serves as the support for building structure and thus is an efficient use of material. This technique has been used for the production of dental frameworks, implants, and customized surgical tools [59].

Three-dimensional printing (3DP) is a versatile SFF technique that utilizes various printing technologies, including binder jetting and material jetting. In binder jetting, the material powder bed serves as the support structure, akin to SLS. With material jetting, multiple nozzles are used to print the build and support materials. These techniques enable the creation of complex oral constructs using a range of materials such as ceramics, polymers, and metals.

Furthermore, 3DP has applications in the fabrication of dental implants, bone graft substitutes, and drug delivery systems [60]. However, precise control over scaffold porosity and internal pore architecture parameters, including pore geometry, size, interconnectivity, orientation, and branching, is essential for optimizing nutrient diffusion, interstitial fluid, blood flow, cell growth and function, tissue differentiation, scaffold's mechanical function, and the mechanical properties of the regenerated tissue [61, 62]. For example, biphasic or multiphasic scaffolds offer a solution for guiding the growth of different tissues while meeting distinct mechanical and biological requirements. These scaffolds can be designed with discrete regions optimized for selective tissue growth by utilizing different material types, material properties, internal architectures (e.g., porosity, pore interconnectivity), and cells and biological factors. This approach allows tailored support for each tissue type and facilitates their respective growth and development within the scaffold, enhancing the overall regenerative process [62–65].

In a study by Rasperini et al., the authors applied a 3D-printed bioresorbable scaffold and signaling growth factor to treat a large periodontal osseous defect, marking the first reported case of its kind in humans [66].

For endodontic applications, a 3D printed scaffold containing polycaprolactone (PCL) and mineral tioxide aggregate (MTA) was fabricated, and their bioactivity was tested on human dental pulp stem cells. These scaffolds demonstrated the high regenerative potential of these scaffolds for regenerative endodontics (RET) [66]. In another study, the 3D-printed scaffold containing biodentine and PCL promoted the differentiation ability of human dental pulp cells (hDPCs) [67]. Overall, it has been shown that 3D-printed scaffolds provided a better structure for the attachment, proliferation, and regeneration of hDPSCs [67].

For TMJ applications, Wei et al. used 3D CT reconstruction and 3D printing of the mandible in a goat model; they used this approach of utilizing 3D reconstruction of CT and 3D printers to provide a promising method for TMJ regeneration, offering potential advancements in the field (**Figure 10.3**) [68].

10.5 CHALLENGES AND FUTURE PERSPECTIVES

While significant progress has been made in the field of digital technology in dental regenerative medicine, there are several challenges and limitations that need to be addressed for its broader implementation in clinical settings. One of the key challenges is the ability to fabricate complex oral tissue structures with precise tissue architecture and functionality. Ensuring the proper organization and integration of different cell types and extracellular matrix components within the printed constructs remains a significant hurdle [69]. Another challenge lies in the development of suitable bioink materials that can support cell viability, proliferation, and differentiation during the printing process. Bioinks should possess appropriate mechanical properties, biocompatibility, and biodegradability while promoting the desired cell behavior and tissue regeneration, a challenging feat [70]. Vascularization is another critical aspect that needs to be addressed in the printing of oral tissues. The successful integration of a functional vascular network within the printed constructs is essential for providing oxygen and nutrients to the cells, as well as supporting their long-term survival and tissue integration [71]. Moreover, scaling up the bioprinting process for larger defects presents logistical challenges. Ensuring a consistent and reliable deposition of cells and biomaterials over a larger printing area while maintaining the desired structural integrity and functionality of the printed constructs is a complex task [72]. Furthermore, the translation of digital models into clinically applicable printed constructs requires advancements in imaging techniques, data processing, and software algorithms. Accurate and detailed patient-specific models are necessary to achieve optimal outcomes in oral tissue engineering [73]. Lastly, there are regulatory and ethical considerations that need to be addressed in the implementation of digital technology in oral tissue engineering. Ensuring the safety, efficacy, and long-term performance of printed constructs, as well as addressing concerns regarding intellectual property and patient privacy, are critical aspects that require attention. Despite these challenges, ongoing research and collaboration between scientists, engineers, and clinicians continue to drive advancements in the field. With further developments in

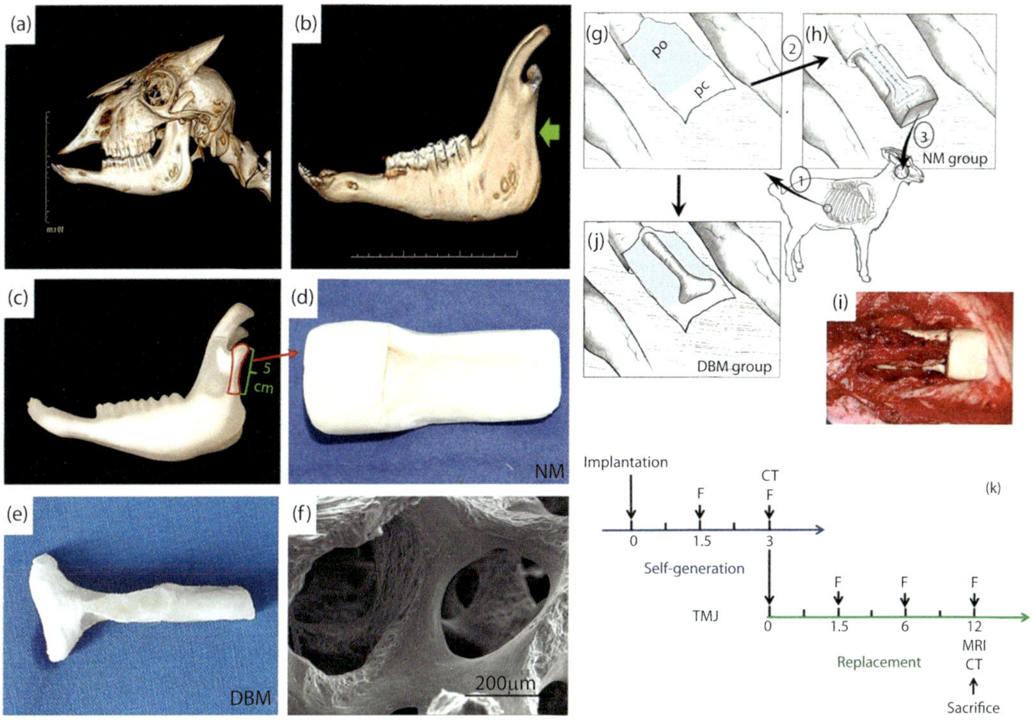

Figure 10.3 Preparation of the temporomandibular joint negative mold (NM) for the guided self-generation procedure in a goat model. (a) Based on cranial 3D CT, (b) the mandible was reconstructed and (c) printed in 3D. (d) A hydroxylapatite NM of the TMJ and mandibular ramus, 5cm in length, was obtained. (e) After removal of a segment of the 3rd or 4th rib and costicartilage counting from caudally (#1), the regenerative unit was prepared from the costal perichondrium and periosteum (#2). (f) Schematic illustration and (g) intraoperative view of the NM-guided tissue self-generation chamber, including the previously prepared periosteum/perichondrium piece in combination with the NM. Finally, the self-generated tissue was used for autologous replacement in the temporomandibular joint (#3). (h) In the control group, the TMJ/mandibular ramus DBM scaffold was wrapped with the previously prepared periosteum/perichondrium. In both groups, the perichondrium covered the designated articular surface, and the periosteum enclosed the osseous part. (i) An allogenic DBM scaffold of the same size served as a positive control, which was examined for (j) microstructure and porosity by scanning electron microscopy. (k) The study timeline consisted of two stages, construct self-generation and replacement, during which fluorescent labeling of osteogenesis and radiologic, histologic, and immunohistochemical analyses were performed. *Abbreviations*: DBM, demineralized bone matrix; F, fluorescent labeling; NM, negative mold; pc, perichondrium; po, periosteum. Copyright 2016, by the authors, Nature publication. Open-access article distributed under the terms of the Creative Commons Attribution License.

bioink formulations, printing techniques, and tissue maturation strategies, the potential for digital technology to revolutionize oral tissue engineering is promising.

REFERENCES

1. Oberoi, G et al. 3D printing—encompassing the facets of dentistry. Front Bioeng Biotechnol. 2018;6:172.
2. Eldeeb, AE et al. Biomaterials for tissue engineering applications and current updates in the field: a comprehensive review. AAPS PharmSciTech. 2022;23(7):267.
3. Arifin, N et al. A comprehensive review of biopolymer fabrication in additive manufacturing processing for 3D-tissue-engineering scaffolds. Polymers. 2022;14(10):2119.
4. Cui, M et al. Exploration and preparation of patient-specific ciprofloxacin implants drug delivery system via 3D printing technologies. J Pharmaceut Sci. 2021;110(11):3678–3689.
5. Saito, E et al. Experimental and computational characterization of designed and fabricated 50: 50 PLGA porous scaffolds for human trabecular bone applications. J Mater Sci Mater Med. 2010;21:2371–2383.
6. Yang, PJ, Temenoff, JS. Engineering orthopedic tissue interfaces. Tissue Eng Part B Rev. 2009;15(2):127–141.
7. Yan, Y et al. Layered manufacturing of tissue engineering scaffolds via multi-nozzle deposition. Mater Lett. 2003;57(18):2623–2628.
8. Eshraghi, S, Das, S. Micromechanical finite-element modeling and experimental characterization of the compressive mechanical properties of polycaprolactone – hydroxyapatite composite scaffolds prepared by selective laser sintering for bone tissue engineering. Acta Biomater. 2012;8(8):3138–3143.

9. Denry, I, Kuhn, LT. Design and characterization of calcium phosphate ceramic scaffolds for bone tissue engineering. Dent Mater. 2016;32(1):43–53.
10. Diaz-Gomez, L et al. Three-dimensional printing of tissue engineering scaffolds with horizontal pore and composition gradients. Tissue Eng Part C Methods. 2019;25(7):411–420.
11. Li, Q et al. Review of spectral imaging technology in biomedical engineering: achievements and challenges. J Biomed Optics. 2013;18(10):100901.
12. Moharamzadeh, K et al. Tissue-engineered oral mucosa. J Dent Res. 2012;91(7):642–650.
13. Ashammakhi, N et al. Biodegradable implantable sensors: materials design, fabrication, and applications. Adv Funct Mater. 2021;31(49):2104149.
14. Barrere, F et al. Advanced biomaterials for skeletal tissue regeneration: instructive and smart functions. Mater Sci Eng R: Rep. 2008;59(1–6):38–71.
15. Emara, A, Shah, R. Recent update on craniofacial tissue engineering. J Tissue Eng. 2021;12:20417314211003735.
16. Etajuri, EA, Suliman, E, Mahmood, WAA, Ibrahim, N, Buzayan, M, Mohd, NR. Deviation of dental implants placed using a novel 3D-printed surgical guide: an in vitro study. Dent Med Probl. 2020;57(4):359–362.
17. Yeung, M et al. Accuracy and precision of 3D-printed implant surgical guides with different implant systems: an in vitro study. J Prosthet Dent. 2020;123(6):821–828.
18. Mironov, V et al. Biofabrication: a 21st century manufacturing paradigm. Biofabrication. 2009;1(2):022001.
19. Alipour, M, Aghazadeh, M. Cell microencapsulation. In: Sefat F et al., eds. Principles of Biomaterials Encapsulation, vol. 1. Woodhead Publishing; 2023:459–482.
20. Guzzi, EA, Tibbitt, MW. Additive manufacturing of precision biomaterials. Adv Mater. 2020;32(13):1901994.
21. Nyberg, EL et al. 3D-printing technologies for craniofacial rehabilitation, reconstruction, and regeneration. Ann Biomed Eng. 2017;45:45–57.
22. Mangano, C et al. Combining intraoral scans, cone beam computed tomography and face scans: the virtual patient. J Craniofac Surg. 2018;29(8):2241–2246.
23. Hou, X et al. An overview of three-dimensional imaging devices in dentistry. J Esthet Restorat Dent. 2022;34(8):1179–1196.
24. Zandparsa, R. Digital imaging and fabrication. Dent Clin. 2014;58(1):135–158.
25. AlRumaih, HS. Clinical applications of intraoral scanning in removable prosthodontics: a literature review. J Prosthodont. 2021;30(9):747–762.
26. Nejatian, T et al. Digital dentistry. In: Advanced Dental Biomaterials. Elsevier; 2019:507–540.
27. Hong, CJ et al. Clinical applications of three-dimensional printing in otolaryngology–head and neck surgery: a systematic review. Laryngoscope. 2019;129(9):2045–2052.
28. Pauwels, E et al. An exploratory study of contrast agents for soft tissue visualization by means of high resolution X-ray computed tomography imaging. J Microscop. 2013;250(1):21–31.
29. White, SC, Pharoah, MJ. The evolution and application of dental maxillofacial imaging modalities. Dent Clin N Am. 2008;52(4):689–705.
30. Vásárhelyi, L et al. Microcomputed tomography–based characterization of advanced materials: a review. Mater Today Adv. 2020;8:100084.
31. Chaurand, P et al. Multi-scale X-ray computed tomography to detect and localize metal-based nanomaterials in lung tissues of in vivo exposed mice. Sci Rep. 2018;8(1):1–11.
32. Ho, JT, et al. Trabecular bone structural parameters evaluated using dental cone-beam computed tomography: cellular synthetic bones. Biomed Eng. 2013;12(1):115.
33. van Lenthe, GH et al. Nondestructive micro-computed tomography for biological imaging and quantification of scaffold–bone interaction in vivo. Biomaterials. 2007;28(15):2479–2490.
34. Lienemann, PS et al. Longitudinal in vivo evaluation of bone regeneration by combined measurement of multi-pinhole SPECT and micro-CT for tissue engineering. Sci Rep. 2015;5(1):10238.
35. Zuncheddu, D et al. Quality control methods in musculoskeletal tissue engineering: from imaging to biosensors. Bone Res. 2021;9(1):46.
36. Costa, PF et al. Advanced tissue engineering scaffold design for regeneration of the complex hierarchical periodontal structure. J Clin Periodontol. 2014;41(3):283–294.
37. Hollister, S et al., eds. Image based design and manufacture of scaffolds for bone reconstruction. IUTAM Symposium on Synthesis in Bio Solid Mechanics: Proceedings of the IUTAM Symposium held in Copenhagen, Denmark, 24–27 May 1998; 2002: Springer.
38. Ventura, SR et al. Application of MRI and biomedical engineering in speech production study. Comput Methods Biomech Biomed. Eng. 2009;12(6):671–681.
39. Gray, CF et al. Advanced imaging: magnetic resonance imaging in implant dentistry: a review. Clin Oral Implants Res. 2003;14(1):18–27.
40. Klontzas, ME, Protonotarios, A. High-resolution imaging for the analysis and reconstruction of 3D microenvironments for regenerative medicine: an application-focused review. Bioengineering. 2021;8(11):182.
41. Xu, H et al. Monitoring tissue engineering using magnetic resonance imaging. J Biosci Bioeng. 2008;106(6):515–527.
42. Niraj, LK et al. MRI in dentistry – a future towards radiation free imaging – systematic review. J Clin Diagnostic Res. 2016;10(10):ZE14.
43. Tanasiewicz, M. Magnetic resonance imaging in human teeth internal space visualization for requirements of dental prosthetics. J Clin Exp Dent. 2010;2(1):e6–11.
44. Burke, S, Sinclair, R. Computer-aided design (CAD) and computer-aided manufacturing (CAM) of apparel and other textile products. In: Textiles and Fashion. Elsevier; 2015:671–703.
45. Taneva, E et al. 3D scanning, imaging, and printing in orthodontics. Issues Contemporary Orthodont. 2015;148(5): 862–867.
46. Haghnegahdar, L et al. From IoT-based cloud manufacturing approach to intelligent additive manufacturing: industrial internet of things – an overview. Int J Adv Manufacturing Technol. 2022:1–18.
47. Tayebi, L et al. 3D printing methods applicable in oral and maxillofacial surgery. In: 3D Printing in Oral & Maxillofacial Surgery. Springer International Publishing; 2021:11–60.
48. Amini, AR et al. Bone tissue engineering: recent advances and challenges. Crit Rev Biomed Eng. 2012;40(5).

49. Honigmann, P et al. Patient-specific surgical implants made of 3D printed PEEK: material, technology, and scope of surgical application. BioMed Res Int. 2018;2018(1):4520636.
50. Abdulla, MA et al. CAD-CAM technology: a literature review. Al-Rafidain Dent J. 2020;20(1):95–113.
51. D'souza, KM, Aras, MA. Applications of computer-aided design/computer-assisted manufacturing technology in dental implant planning. J Dent Implants. 2012;2(1):37.
52. Anderson, J et al. Endodontic applications of 3D printing. Int Endodont J. 2018;51(9):1005–1018.
53. Van Noort, R. The future of dental devices is digital. Dent Mater. 2012;28(1):3–12.
54. Kumar, M, Sharma, V. Additive manufacturing techniques for the fabrication of tissue engineering scaffolds: a review. Rapid Prototyping J. 2021;27(6):1230–1272.
55. Melchels, FP et al. A review on stereolithography and its applications in biomedical engineering. Biomaterials. 2010; 31(24):6121–6130.
56. Chaudhary, R et al. Additive manufacturing by digital light processing: a review. Prog Addit Manuf. 2023;8(2):331–351.
57. Dhavalikar, P et al. Biomedical applications of additive manufacturing. In: Biomaterials Science. Elsevier; 2020:623–639.
58. Chakraborty, D et al. Extruder path generation for curved layer fused deposition modeling. Comput Aided Des. 2008;40(2):235–243.
59. Mazzoli, A. Selective laser sintering in biomedical engineering. Med Biol Eng Computing. 2013;51:245–256.
60. Sears, NA et al. A review of three-dimensional printing in tissue engineering. Tissue Eng Part B Rev. 2016;22(4):298–310.
61. Taboas, J et al. Indirect solid free form fabrication of local and global porous, biomimetic and composite 3D polymer-ceramic scaffolds. Biomaterials. 2003;24(1):181–194.
62. Schek, RM et al. Engineered osteochondral grafts using biphasic composite solid free-form fabricated scaffolds. Tissue Eng. 2004;10(9–10):1376–1385.
63. Lee, CH et al. Three-dimensional printed multiphase scaffolds for regeneration of periodontium complex. Tissue Eng Part A. 2014;20(7–8):1342–1351.
64. Chen, J et al. Hydrogel to guide chondrogenesis versus osteogenesis of mesenchymal stem cells for fabrication of cartilaginous tissues. Biomed Mater. 2020;15(4):045006.
65. Gehlen, J et al. Tomographic volumetric bioprinting of heterocellular bone-like tissues in seconds. Acta Biomater. 2023;156:49–60.
66. Rasperini, G et al. 3D-printed bioresorbable scaffold for periodontal repair. J Dent Res. 2015;94(9_suppl):153S–157S.
67. Ho, CC et al. The effects of biodentine/polycaprolactone three-dimensional-scaffold with odontogenesis properties on human dental pulp cells. Int Endodont J. 2018;51:e291–e300.
68. Wei, J et al. Autologous temporomandibular joint reconstruction independent of exogenous additives: a proof-of-concept study for guided self-generation. Scientific Rep. 2016;6(1):1–9.
69. Chen, F-M, Liu, X. Advancing biomaterials of human origin for tissue engineering. Progress Polymer Sci. 2016;53:86–168.
70. Mobaraki, M et al. Bioinks and bioprinting: a focused review. Bioprinting. 2020;18:e00080.
71. Hann, SY et al. Recent advances in 3D printing: vascular network for tissue and organ regeneration. Translat Res. 2019;211:46–63.
72. Ngo, TD et al. Additive manufacturing (3D printing): a review of materials, methods, applications and challenges. Compos B Eng. 2018;143:172–196.
73. Jin, Z et al. 3D printing of physical organ models: recent developments and challenges. Adv Sci. 2021;8(17):2101394.

11 Technical and Biological Basis in Tooth Preparation for Chairside Digital Flow

Marina Amaral, Ana Maria Estivalete Marchionatti, Laís Regiane Silva-Concílio, and Vinícius Felipe Wandscher

11.1 INTRODUCTION

Chairside digital workflow in fixed prosthodontics integrates digital technologies, such as intraoral scanners and computer-aided design/computer-aided manufacturing (CAD/CAM) systems in the dental office to enhance efficiency and effectiveness for the placement of fixed dental restorations. Some technical and biological aspects of teeth abutments/preparations may be considered when aiming to optimize the digital workflow in fixed prosthodontics, since specific features may influence the whole process from treatment planning to restoration placement.

Deep margin elevation (DME), immediate dentin sealing (IDS), and finishing preparation techniques may affect clinical and laboratory processes in the digital workflow. DME is a clinical approach used to manage subgingival margins in crown preparations. It improves the accessibility and visibility of the margin, facilitating better impression accuracy and cementation of the final restoration. IDS consists of applying the adhesive system to dentin directly after tooth preparation, before impression, resulting in improvement of bond strength and bonding stability of CAD/CAM restorations, but it may affect the trueness and precision of scanning. The different tooth preparation finishing procedures may also affect scanning accuracy.

This chapter discusses such points in the preparation of teeth that will receive an indirect restoration through digital workflow, presenting their advantages, disadvantages, and proposals to avoid or reduce inaccuracy of scanning and improve the process.

11.2 THE CERVICAL MARGIN ELEVATION AND THE DIGITAL WORKFLOW

Indirect restorations often have margins located subgingivally, which may cause biological and operative difficulties [1]. Subgingival margins can be challenging to access and to control moisture and contamination, leading to inadequate marginal integrity and ultimately compromising the longevity and aesthetics of the restoration. Deep margin elevation (DME), also referred to as proximal box elevation, cervical margin relocation or coronal margin relocation, represents a conservative clinical strategy for managing subgingival margins in indirect restorations. This approach consists of placing a direct restorative material to relocate a cervical margin originally positioned below the gingival level to a supragingival location, thereby facilitating subsequent restorative procedures [2, 3]. Materials commonly used for DME include conventional composite resins, flowable composites, bulk-fill composite resins, and self-adhesive resin-based luting materials [2]. Composite resin seems to be the most favorable material for this purpose [2, 4].

Replacing the cervical margin coronally presents various benefits, including facilitating rubber dam isolation, impression taking, bonding, and removing cement excess of indirect restorations, as well as avoidance of unnecessary tissue sacrifice. DME is a less invasive approach in comparison with other alternatives to manage subgingival defects, such as surgical crown lengthening, orthodontic eruption, and surgical extrusion. Frequently, such approaches may lead to further attachment loss, root and furcation exposures, dentinal hypersensitivity, unfavorable aesthetics, and unfavorable crown/root proportion [1, 5].

DME exhibits a high level of clinical sensitivity, particularly when conducted on deep subgingival margins [6]. DME is technically more complex when enamel is absent at the margin and dentin and/or cementum are exposed [1]. To perform DME procedure, complete isolation of the operative field and ability to effectively position a matrix properly, isolating margins and ensuring a perfect seal, are needed [7]. For DME, a matrix is positioned in order to seal the subgingival margin, ensuring that no gingival tissue or rubber dam is entrapped in between. It is preferable to use a curved matrix to achieve an adequate emergence profile and contour for margins located in the region of the CEJ [1, 8]. For deep lesions, the "matrix-in-a-matrix" technique can be used by sliding a sectioned fragment of metal matrix between the margin and the existing matrix [5, 8]. Immediate dentin sealing is recommended, followed by the application of a composite resin base to elevate the margin by approximately 2 mm. Polishing strips and flexible disks are used for the finishing process. To eliminate any composite resin flashes, a no. 12 blade or a sickle scaler can be used, and interdental flossing is also performed to ensure that there are no overhangs. A bitewing radiograph is necessary to check the

 DOI: 10.1201/9781003428541-11

presence of overhangs or gaps. Careful follow-up is essential to monitor soft tissue health [6, 8] and to assess the potential need for surgical intervention [8]. When endodontic therapy is needed, it is recommended whenever possible to perform DME first to enable proper absolute isolation for the root canal treatment [1, 8].

Technically and biologically, DME indication relies on the possibility of placing a rubber dam in the gingival sulcus and on the respect to the biological width [1, 5, 8]. Long-term clinical studies focused on the periodontal health of teeth restored with margin elevation are still needed, but current evidence shows that well-defined subgingival composite restorations are compatible with gingival health when biological width is preserved [6, 9]. Some authors suggest that a healthy and noninflammatory periodontium can be achieved under certain conditions even when there is biological width invasion [10, 11]. One study suggests that DME can be clinically successful when there is violation of the biological width to a limited extent under the precondition of patient's strict oral regular hygiene with individually adapted interproximal brushes [10]. Another study states that in cases in which subgingival proximal caries lead to deep cavities where there is already a destruction of the gingival attachment, there is no regeneration of a normal periodontal attachment apparatus on the restorative material if DME can be performed with proper isolation and bonding; instead, a situation with another kind of biologic width (mainly composed by a longer junctional epithelium along the composite resin and a smaller connective attachment on the dentin below the material), seems healthy and well-tolerated by the periodontium [11].

The main advantage of combining deep margin elevation and digital workflow is saving time. Unlike other surgical and orthodontic approaches to manage subgingival defects, DME can be performed in one session [2]. Therefore, the combination of DME and chairside digital workflow provides the opportunity for same-day indirect restorations. However, when DME is performed as the initial step, how does it affect the subsequent clinical procedures and the overall performance of indirect restorations obtained by chairside digital workflow?

Obtaining mechanical and biologically adequate indirect restorations is often hindered or even considered impossible when deep subgingival proximal defects are present because the proper execution of the clinical steps needed (cavity preparation, impression taking, and moisture-free adhesive cementation) is impaired [3, 8]. In this sense, the presence of an elevated cervical margin facilitates or even enables the execution of all subsequent clinical procedures required prior to the completion of the indirect restoration. **Table 11.1** explains the advantages of DME in each step.

Table 11.1: Clinical Steps and Respective Advantages of Performing Deep Margin Elevation

Clinical Step	Advantages of DME
1. Preparation	Considering the preparation phase, removal of overcuts and a slight cavity convergence (with tapered or at least parallel cavity walls) for the insertion of a restoration are required [12]. When DME is performed, it is possible to apply a flowable composite resin (ideally a highly filled composite) to seal sharp margins, fill undercuts, flatten the cavity floor, and optimize the cavity geometry, which allows a more conservative preparation with no removal of healthy dental tissue to suppress undercuts and to obtain a satisfactory path of insertion for the proximal boxes [8, 12]. In addition, DME will generate an appropriate contour and emergence profile if a curved matrix is used [8].
2. Digital impression	With respect to the impression-taking step, achieving an accurate and precise image during digital impression is a prerequisite to obtain a good-quality indirect restoration [3]. However, cavity margins extending subgingivally in severely damaged teeth may difficult scanning [12], especially in the molar region due to the limited space and limitations imposed by the scanning depths of the digital system. After DME, digital scanning becomes simpler, accelerates, and provides a more accurate image than with a deep cavity [3].
3. Restoration design	Deep cervical margins have difficulty creating an appropriate emergence profile and a favorable contact point for the restoration [1]. Margin elevation reestablishes anatomical conditions so that an indirect restoration with a gingival emergence profile and a suitable contact point can be designed and manufactured.
4. Rubber dam isolation	After cervical margin is raised, isolation of the operatory field with a rubber dam becomes technically easier, ensuring safe delivery of the definitive restoration under a contamination-free adhesive cementation [8].
5. Cementation	The presence of saliva and blood is difficult to control in subgingival margins and may hamper adhesive bonding, leading to possible restauration failure [3]. After cervical margin relocation, rubber dam isolation of the working field for reliable luting procedures becomes feasible [13]. Also, light-curing through an indirect restoration may be improved when proximal margins have a reduced depth and the removal of resin cement excesses in the sulcus may be better controlled if the margin is repositioned supragingivally [13].

Besides facilitating the clinical procedures, DME seems to be beneficial for the overall performance of indirect restorations. When the restoration adhesion is considered, the proximal composite may reduce polymerization shrinkage stresses [13]. The presence of an elevated margin has a positive impact on the bond strength of composite inlays using self-adhesive resin cement or does not affect bond strength for a total-etch resin cement.

Regarding the mechanical behavior, the shorter proximal extensions provided by DME positively impacts the strength of indirect restorations: Complete seating to the preparation margin resulting in improved marginal adaptation reduces stresses during functional loading and may prevent long-term tooth fracture from loading [13, 14]. Many studies showed that DME performed on 2 mm below the cemento-enamel junction cavities has no detrimental effect on the fracture strength of lithium disilicate inlays and onlays [14], resin nanoceramic onlays [15], feldspathic ceramic and resin-nanoceramic onlays [13], and monolithic zirconia crowns [16]. Another study suggested that bulk-fill composite is preferred for margin elevation in relation to conventional composite resin in terms of fracture strength of teeth restored with lithium-disilicate endocrowns [17]. Also, DME does not impair fatigue failure load of for leucite-reinforced glass–ceramics and indirect resin composite inlays [18]. In addition, fracture pattern is not different for teeth with DME in comparison to teeth without margin elevation [13–16].

The marginal integrity is also a crucial factor to avoid leakage and restoration failure. Achieving an adequate adhesion and proper sealing to deep cervical dentin can be challenging, especially below the cemento-enamel junction. When we consider marginal quality of indirect restorations cemented on elevated margins, we have three interfaces: (1) between the indirect restoration and the luting cement; (2) between the luting cement and the composite, and (3) between the composite and dentin. The luting cement/composite and the indirect restoration/luting cement interfaces should not be considered troublesome: The optimal precision of the CAD/CAM digital workflow provides a very good marginal adaptation of the indirect restoration to the preparation margins, resulting in adequate marginal seal. However, the main source of concern is the composite-dentin interface [19]. Various studies demonstrate that composite restorations used for cervical margin elevation do not affect margin quality [15, 20–22]. Other studies showed lower seal in the composite-dentin interface than when restorations are cemented directly on dentin [17, 19, 23]. However, it must be taken into consideration that the perfect scenario would be bonding indirect restorations directly to dentin, but such situation is not always feasible under concrete clinical conditions. For such cases, DME has been proven to be promising enough to encourage the technique use [23].

Thus, DME stands as a viable treatment option to optimize chairside digital workflow. Even though randomized clinical trials are necessary to evaluate longevity, the existing literature so far indicates that cervical margin relocation can be used successfully prior to indirect restorations as an alternative with a low level of complications over a relatively long time [24].

11.3 CLINICAL CASE 1 (FIGURES 11.1–11.16)

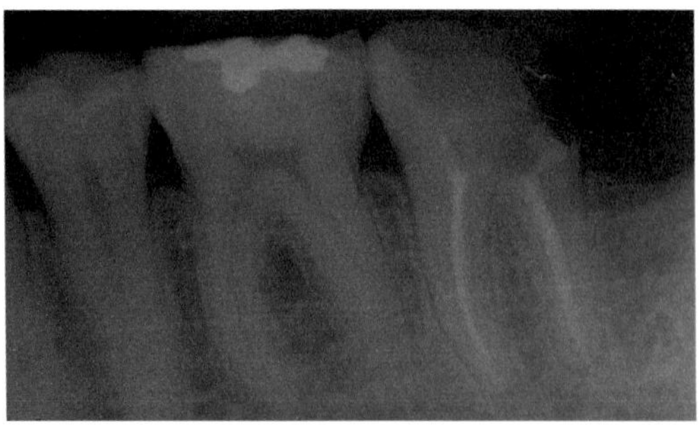

Figure 11.1 Radiographic image of tooth 47. Dentin margin at gingival level.

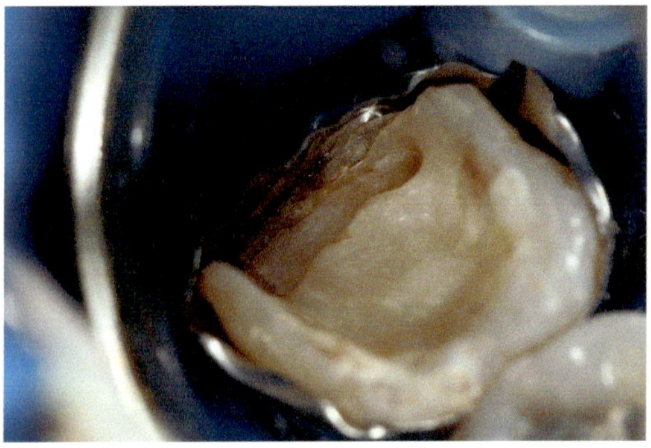

Figure 11.2 Absolute isolation using the rubber dam, clamp n° 200 with dental separation ring and metallic matrix.

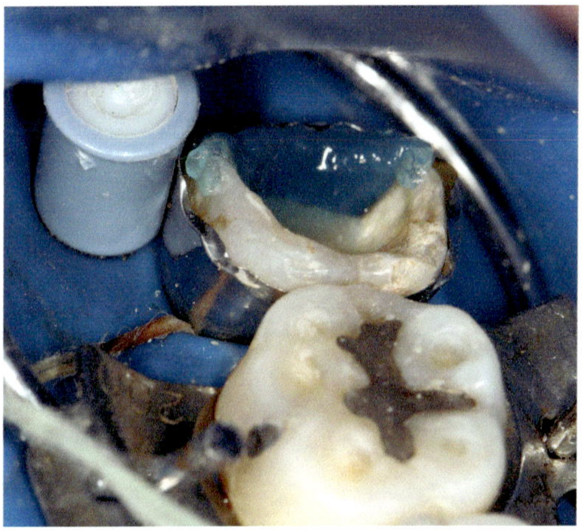

Figure 11.3 Acid etching.

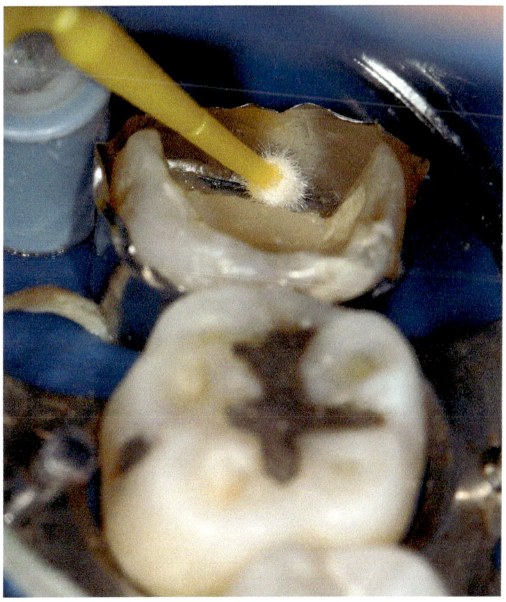

Figure 11.4 System adhesive application.

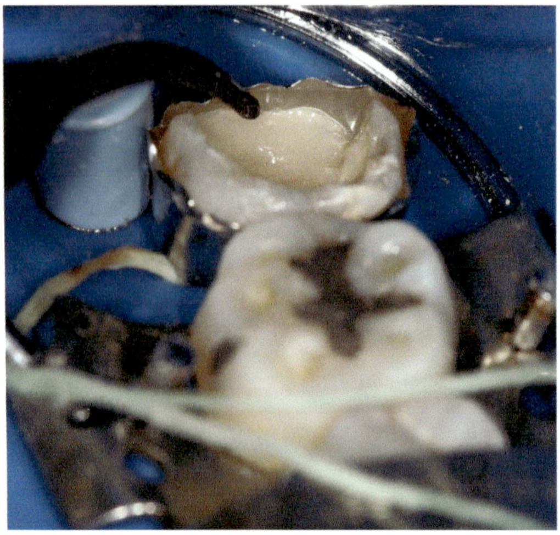

Figure 11.5 Composite resin flow application.

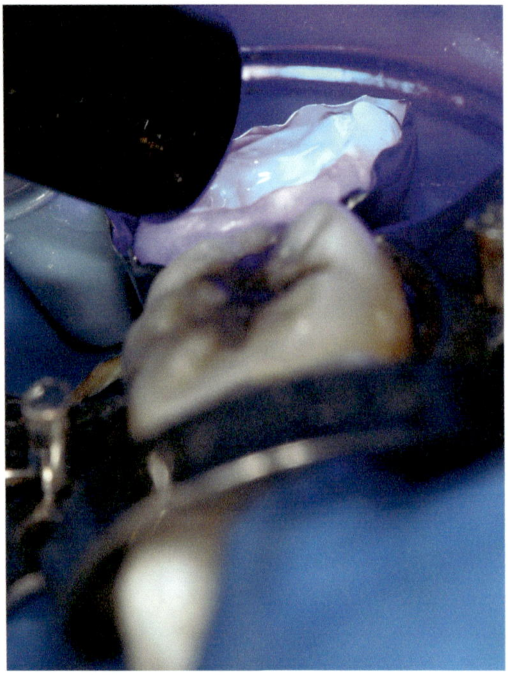

Figure 11.6 Photoactivation.

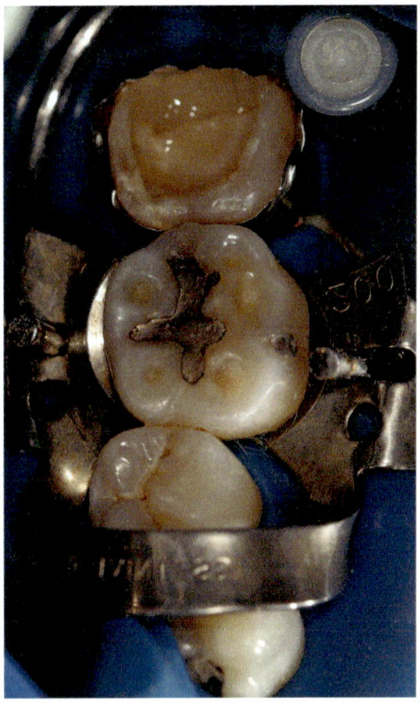

Figure 11.7 Margin elevation finished.

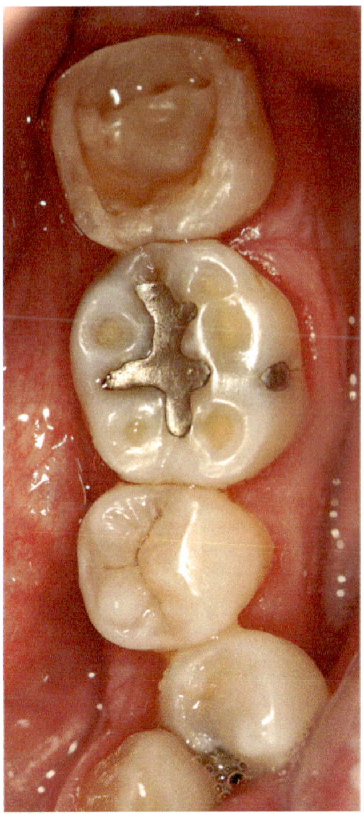

Figure 11.8 Absolute isolation removed.

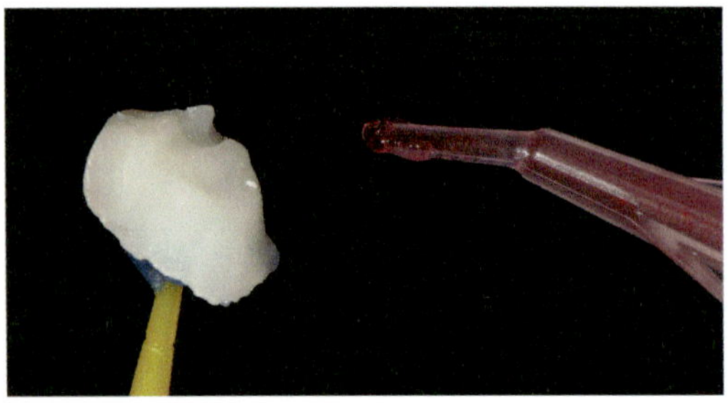

Figure 11.9 Lithium disilicate inlay acid fluoridric etching.

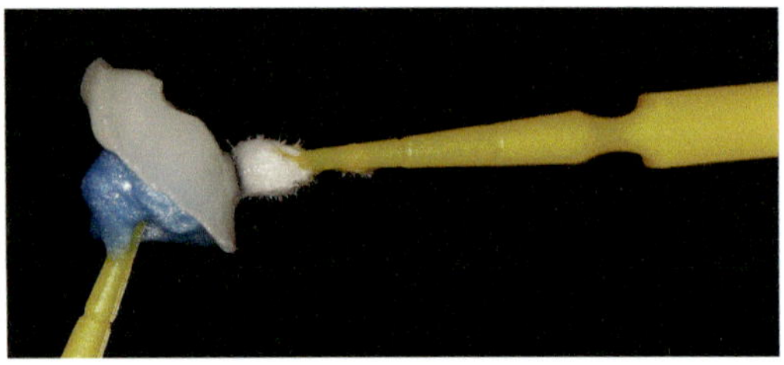

Figure 11.10 Silane application.

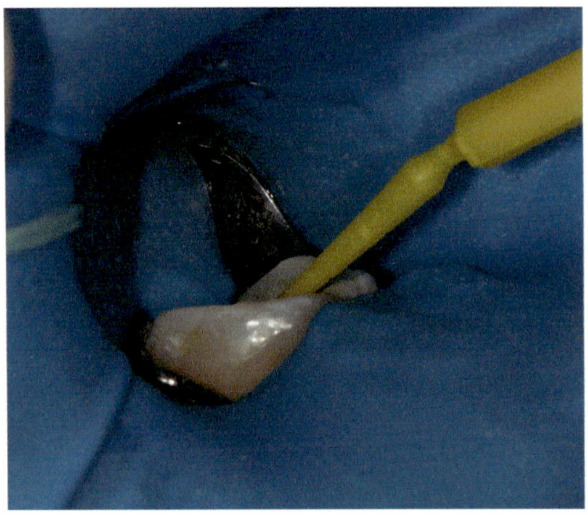

Figure 11.11 Universal adhesive application on tooth.

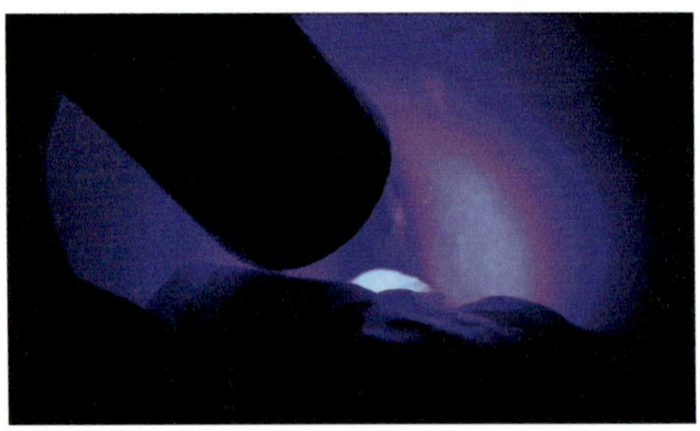

Figure 11.12 Photoactivation.

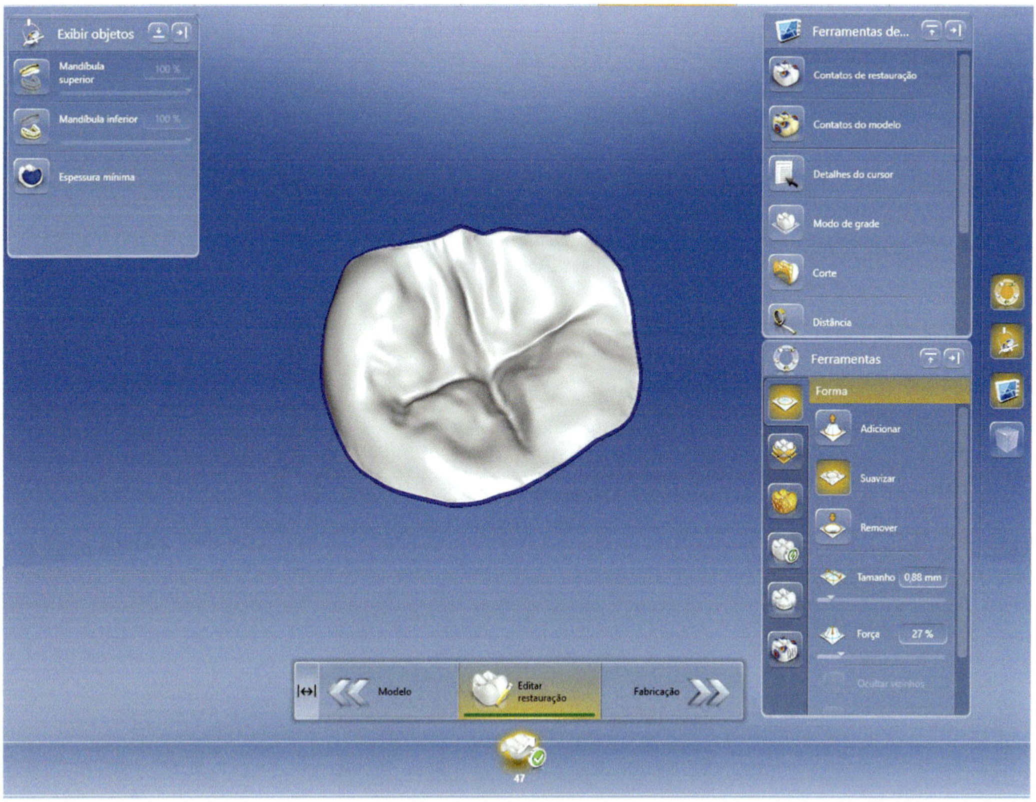

Figure 11.13 Virtual lithium disilicate inlay project.

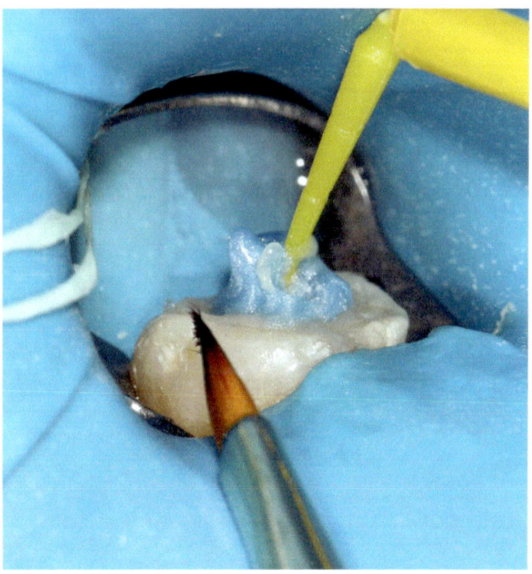

Figure 11.14 Inlay cementation.

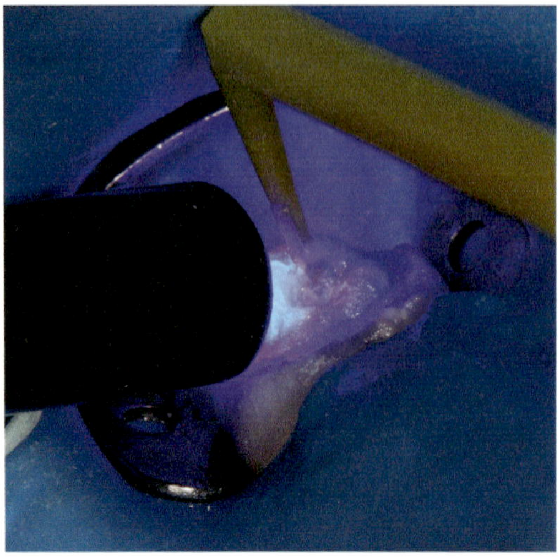

Figure 11.15 Resin cement activation.

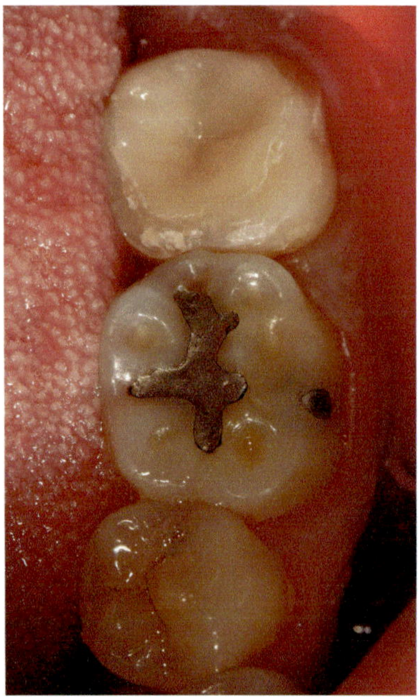

Figure 11.16 Restoration finished.

11.4 CLINICAL CASE 2 (FIGURES 11.17–11.22)

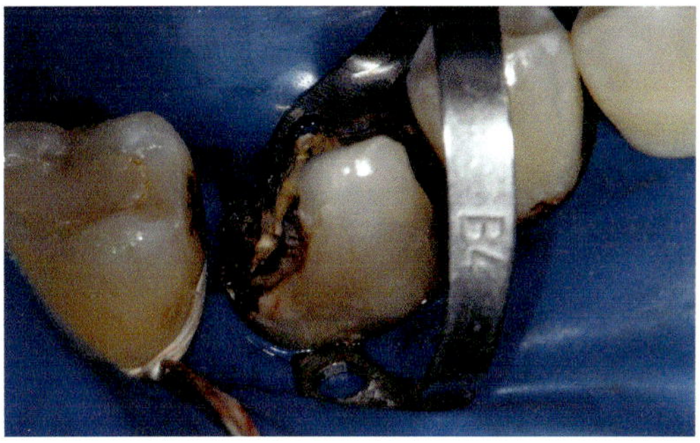

Figure 11.17 Tooth 36 with OMD amalgam restoration removed.

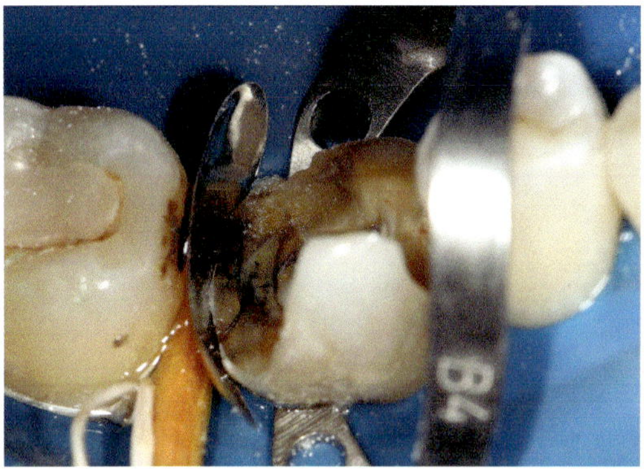

Figure 11.18 Secondary caries remotion and metallic matrix adaptation with wood edge.

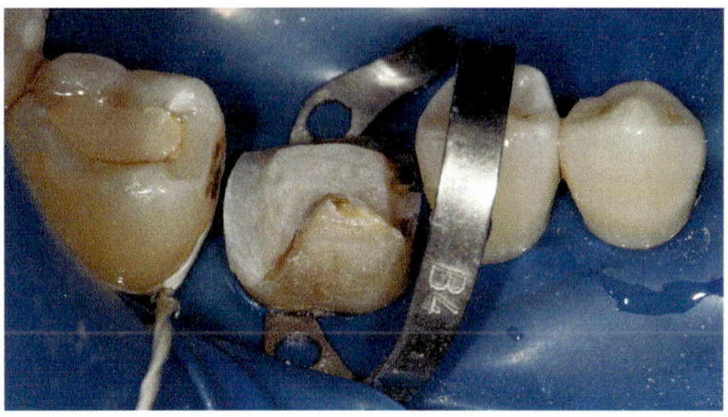

Figure 11.19 Margin elevation with composite resin and immediate dentin sealing (Optibond FL – Kerr and Beautifull Flow Plus 00 – Shofu) followed by preparation.

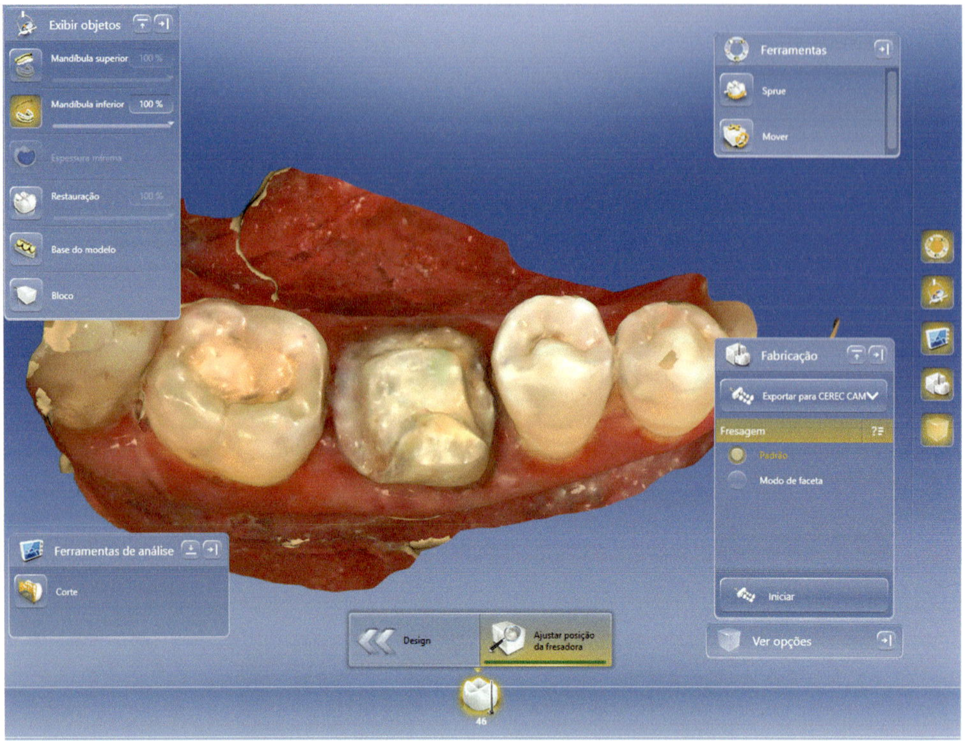

Figure 11.20 Intraoral scanning of tooth 36.

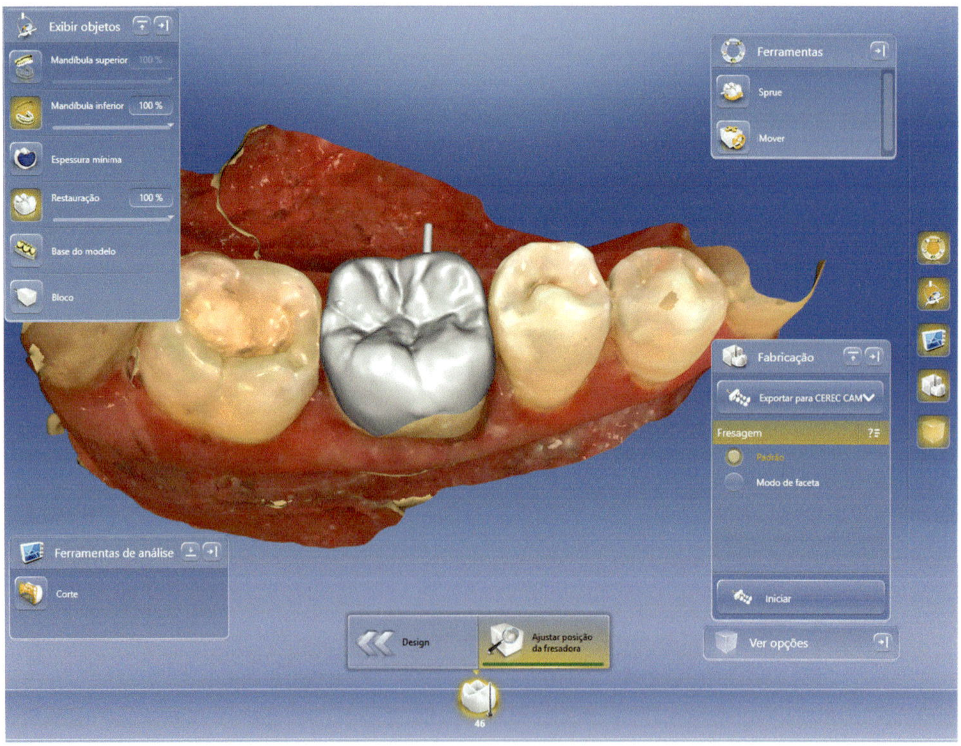

Figure 11.21 Virtual project overlay restoration.

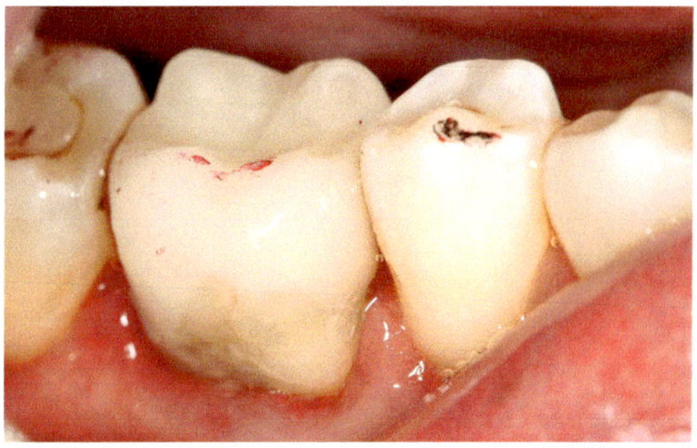

Figure 11.22 Cerec blocks overlay adhesively cemented.

11.5 CLINICAL CASE 3 (FIGURES 11.23–11.31)

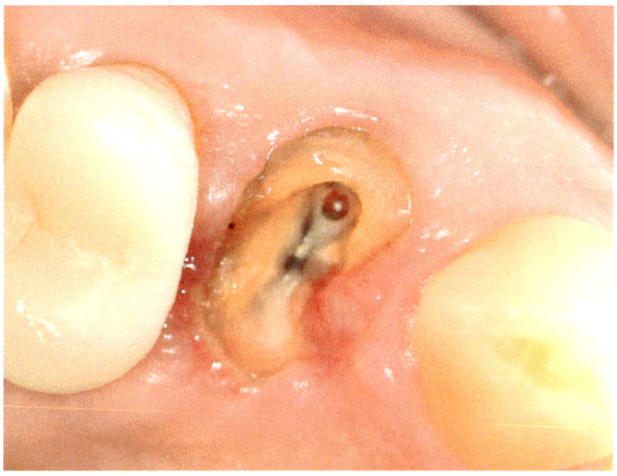

Figure 11.23 Initial situation.

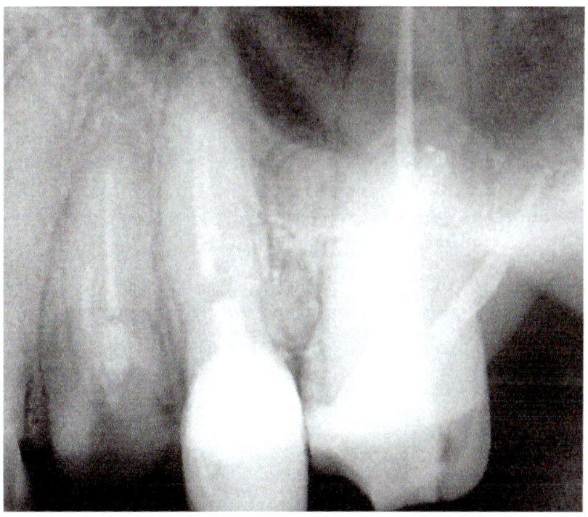

Figure 11.24 Initial radiography.

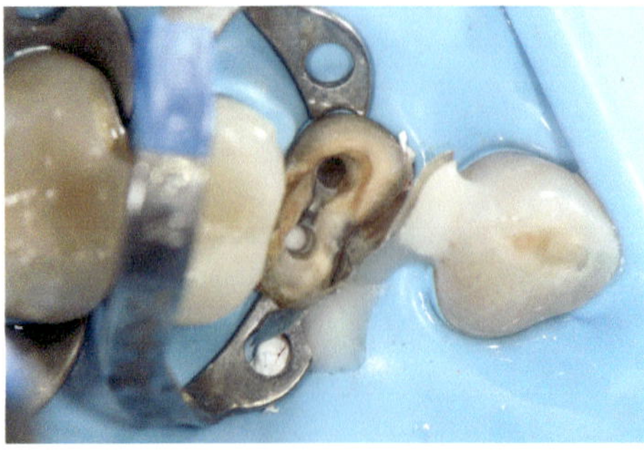

Figure 11.25 Rubber dam isolation, metallic matrix adapted with polytetrafluoroethylene tape and resin flow. This procedure facilitates tooth isolation to endodontic treatment.

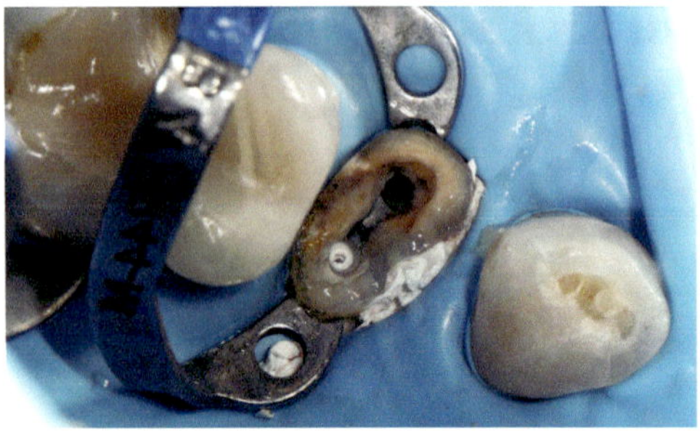

Figure 11.26 Metallic matrix removed. The polytetrafluoroethylene tape promotes the metallic matrix cervical adaptation.

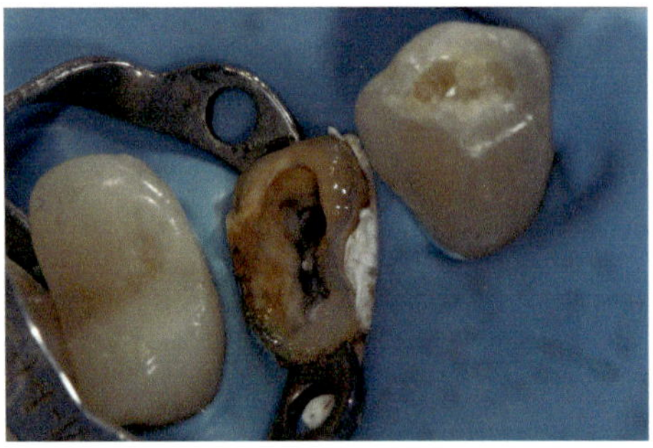

Figure 11.27 Observe the cervical margin reconstructed with the gingival retraction. The margin was adhesively reconstructed (Optibond FL – Kerr and Beautifull Flow Plus 00 – Shofu).

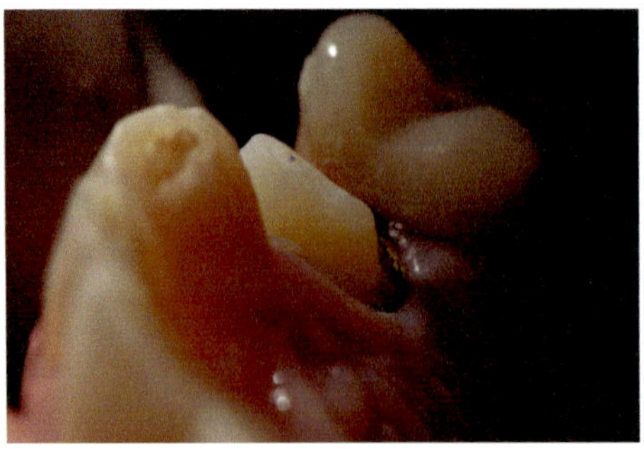

Figure 11.28 Tooth 14 reconstructed with fiber post (Hi Rem Post – Overfibers) and composite core (AllCem Core – FGM). Abutment ready for intraoral scanning with double wire gingival retraction.

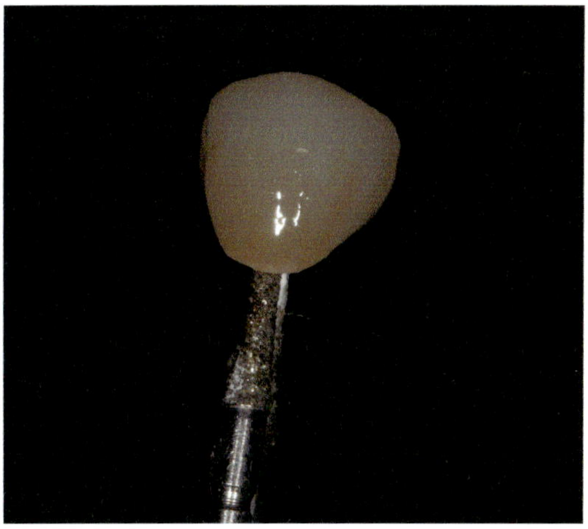

Figure 11.29 Polymer infiltrated ceramic network crown (Brava blocks – FGM).

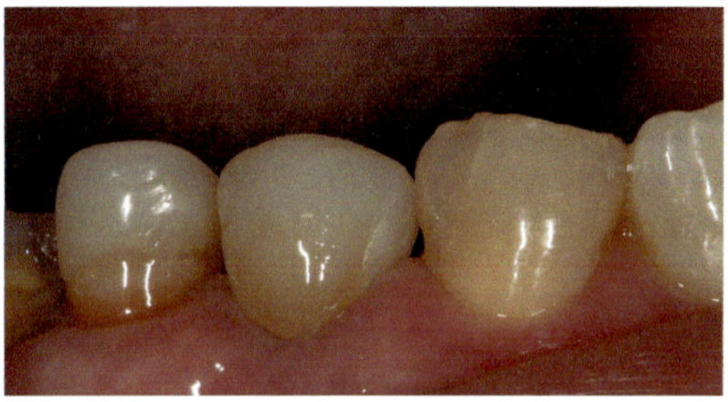

Figure 11.30 Composite hybrid crown adhesively cemented with universal adhesive (Gluma Bond Universal – Kulzer) and dual resin cement (NX3 – Kerr).

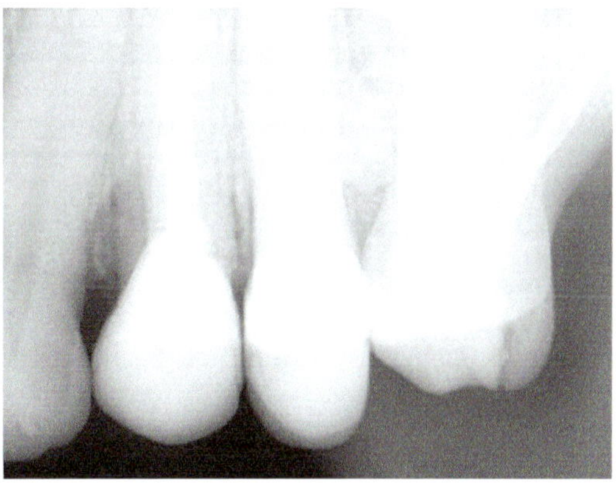

Figure 11.31 Final radiography.

11.6 THE PREPARATION MARGIN IN THE DIGITAL WORKFLOW

In oral rehabilitation that uses indirect restorations, the biological, mechanical, and aesthetic principles must be followed to obtain a dental preparation that reaches functional and aesthetic demands. In this context, the gingival margin is an important region that promotes an adequate cervical delimitation, with enough space for a resistant cervical portion of the restoration, without overcontour, that enables the maintenance of periodontal health. An excessive marginal discrepancy in fixed dental prostheses may favor the onset of periodontal pathology, promote the development of secondary caries, and contribute to prosthesis fracture, ultimately increasing the risk of premature prosthetic failure [25, 26].

Compared with traditional procedures, a workflow using intraoral digital scanning (IOS) offers several advantages. Despite significant advances in digital impression technologies, the configuration of the preparation finish line continues to be a critical factor influencing the clinical performance of the abutment tooth [27, 28]. An adequate tooth preparation and a well-defined finish line contribute to the result of IOS accuracy, favoring the manufacturing of fixed dental prostheses with adequate contour and adaptation, and consequent long-term clinical success [29].

Accuracy is measured in terms of trueness and precision. Trueness is the deviation between the scanned object with IOS from its true geometry. On the other hand, precision is the deviation between the repeated scans of the identical object executed with the identical IOS and with similar parameters [30]. The accuracy of intraoral scanners is influenced by multiple variables, including variations in scanning strategies, the optical properties of the scanned substrate—such as reflectivity and translucency—the complexity of the tooth preparation and finish line geometry, the scanning distance, and the dimensions of the scanner head [31].

It remains necessary to determine whether conventional finish line configurations used for indirect restorations are equally suitable for digital workflows or whether modifications are needed to optimize intraoral scanning procedures. The current challenge lies in reassessing established preparation parameters to define designs that enable accurate IOS acquisition and reliable STL processing, ultimately allowing the fabrication of clinically acceptable restorations while preserving tooth structure and taking advantage of contemporary restorative materials and adhesive luting protocols [32].

The selection of the geometry of tooth preparation and finish line design also has a direct correlation with a satisfactory IOS obtained and well-adapted prostheses with integral margins. There was a significant effect of the finish line design on the accuracy of IOS [30, 32].

Regarding the geometry, less complex preparation promotes more accurate IOS. Partial preparation (i.e., inlay, onlay, overlay, and endocrown) requires a design with more angles, edges, and walls involved, when compared to full-crown preparations. This finding may be associated with preparations presenting a greater number of intracoronal axial walls, which increase surface complexity and make digital reconstruction more challenging, thereby raising susceptibility to errors caused by camera misalignment. The observed improvement may be explained by error patterns related to acute angles, which are influenced by both optical constraints and software processing limitations. When the tilt angle of the scanning camera surpasses the preparation's divergence angle, visual obstruction or interference can occur, compromising data acquisition [33, 34].

Ashraf et al. [35] evaluated four preparation configurations, including two intracoronal designs with divergence angles of 6° and 12°, and two extracoronal designs featuring convergence angles of 6° and 12°. The study demonstrated that greater convergence or divergence between opposing walls was associated with improved trueness, possibly because increased axial wall inclination enlarges the surface area available for scanning, thereby enhancing acquisition accuracy. Additionally, extracoronal preparations yielded superior results compared with intracoronal designs. A further explanation may be that intracoronal walls tend to generate shadowed areas during scanning, which can promote light scattering and lead to artifacts in the final digital image [29].

With regard to finish line designs, five types and their subtypes are typically used: chamfer (wide and narrow), deep chamfer, shoulder, rounded shoulder, and tangential [30, 32]. While certain studies have reported significant differences regarding the influence of finish line design on marginal adaptation when assessed through intraoral scanning workflows [36], other investigations have failed to observe similar effects [37]. Such discrepancies may be attributed to variations in methodologies employed for marginal fit assessment, as well as differences in restorative techniques and materials used in the fabrication of the restorations.

Finish lines well-defined with edges wide, rounded, and polished facilitate the IOS process and promote better indirect restorations. Overall, independent of the intraoral scanner system employed, chamfer finish lines tend to demonstrate superior trueness, whereas vertical preparation designs have been associated with greater precision [30, 32]. According to Shah et al. [38], shoulder and rounded shoulder finish line configurations generally provide improved marginal and internal adaptation when CAD/CAM technologies are utilized for coping fabrication. Chan et al. [34] reported scanner accuracy values ranging from approximately 20 to 40 μm, with calculated linear height percentage errors varying between 0.5% and 1.33%. Additionally, several investigations have documented marginal discrepancies in CAD/CAM restorations within a range of approximately 24 to 110 μm [39–41].

These values are consistent with the results reported by Euan et al. [25], in which the group that scanned definitive casts obtained from conventional impressions presented mean marginal discrepancies of 52.67 μm for rounded shoulder finish lines and 65.07 μm for chamfer configurations. In contrast, the group in which scanning was performed directly on the prepared teeth demonstrated improved outcomes, with marginal discrepancies remaining below 19 μm, specifically 14.99 μm for rounded shoulder and 18.46 μm for chamfer preparations.

Marginal discrepancy lower than 120 μm is often considered clinically acceptable [42]. Thus, studies show that regardless of the type of finish line used in dental preparation (shoulder, chamfer, bevel) the marginal discrepancies are within the clinically acceptable values and allow clinical acceptable marginal integrity.

Unlike the conventional method, in the digital flow a point that can interfere with the accuracy of the scanning is the proximity of the structures adjacent to the dental preparation (teeth and gingival tissue). During interproximal preparation, it is important to avoid positioning the finish line excessively close to adjacent teeth or structures [29, 43]. Properly designed interproximal reduction also contributes to establishing an adequate emergence profile and sufficient space for soft tissue accommodation, thereby enhancing the functional and esthetic outcomes of indirect restorations [29].

With intra- and extracoronal dental preparations, the walls of the interproximal region must be worn to allow the convergence, and the finish line must stay positioned closer to the cervical region, below the region of contact point. According to the dental anatomy and angle of convergence, in this region the interdental space is naturally larger, and the adjacent dental structures are consequently more distant. Some studies have indicated, based on precision analyses, that preparations with deeper finish line locations tend to demonstrate significantly superior performance compared with finish lines positioned more coronally [29, 43, 44].

Although intraoral scanners generally demonstrate adequate capability in capturing deeper regions of tooth preparations, certain limitations remain regarding resolution—namely, the ability to accurately differentiate structures located in close proximity [29]. These limitations may be related to phenomena such as light scattering or optical interferences during data acquisition [44]. From a precision standpoint, positive deviations are expected to exert minimal influence on restoration fit, as such discrepancies can often be compensated by the cement space or by the internal geometry of the restoration. Nevertheless, these inaccuracies may contribute to increased material shrinkage, potentially leading to microleakage and reduced restorative thickness [45]. In contrast, negative deviations present a greater clinical concern, as they may result in improper seating or misalignment of the restoration [29].

According to the region that will be rehabilitated, the finish line is often located at the gingival level or subgingival. When compared to the region of the finish line: supra-, sub-, or epigingivally, the worst results obtained in the digital flow are the preparations with subgegival margins [6, 46].

Salivary contamination may lead to clinically unacceptable increases in marginal discrepancies, and its negative impact on scanning trueness becomes even more pronounced when finish lines are located subgingivally [32, 46]. Additional sources of moisture contamination near preparation margins commonly include blood, gingival crevicular fluid, hemostatic solutions, and residues such as handpiece lubricating oil [47].

Effective management of gingival tissues is therefore essential to achieve accurate impressions, particularly when preparation margins are positioned close to gingival tissues [48]. Under such conditions, optimal gingival displacement combined with strict control of bleeding and salivary flow is required for predictable outcomes, with the double-cord technique frequently recommended to obtain adequate retraction [32]. In the case of the double cord technique, however, the primary cord is often left in the sulcus, allowing persistent expansion of the sulcus during scanning [49]. Earlier studies showed that after the use of the double cord technique, the sulcus still exhibited an expansion of approximately 0.2 mm in the proximal sulcus area after 20 s [50, 51]. This period of gingival retraction (20 s) after the second cord is removed can be interesting for single crowns, but in the multiple crowns it is insufficient. Some techniques may contribute to favor the interproximal regions that are located subgingivally, for example DME, as was previously discussed.

Besides finishing line/preparation margin, tooth surface may also affect the accuracy of IOS for single-tooth preparation impressions. Techniques performed at the preparation surface, aiming to improve adhesion at final cementation, may affect the accuracy of digital imaging.

11.7 IMMEDIATE DENTIN SEALING IN THE DIGITAL WORKFLOW

The complex composition of dentin leads to a challenging adhesion process. An optimal bonding may be achieved by dentin hybridization and the formation of a complete hybrid layer. In this context, the timing for adhesive application is an important issue. IDS consists of applying an adhesive layer on tooth dentin immediately after tooth preparation, providing adhesion to a freshly cut and uncontaminated dentin, which is ideal for bonding [52]. It is an alternative to the conventional delayed dentin sealing (DDS), when the dentin hybridization is performed following the impression

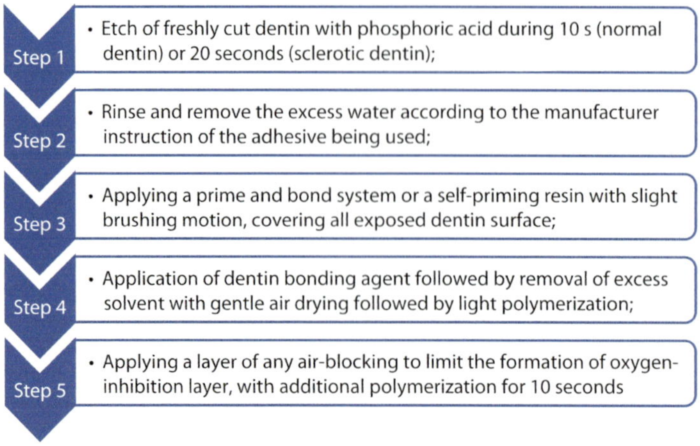

Figure 11.32 Flowchart of the sequence for the IDS technique.

and provisional phase (with the application of interim cement/restoration) and just before the indirect restoration luting procedure. IDS is recommended to be performed when a substantial area of dentin is exposed and should be performed prior to impression making and contamination of the dentin by temporary cement/restorative material [53].

Right after preparation, the dentin fibrils are not collapsed and dentin is also not affected by dehydration or contaminated. Thus, the penetration of dental adhesives after demineralization is facilitated, and the formation of the hybrid layer is optimized [54]. Besides that, the application of adhesive may form a layer which may impair restoration seating and adaptation, but when adhesive is applied before impression making, this layer is already included as part of the preparation and does not interfere with the complete seating of the restoration.

Both total-etch and self-etch dentin bonding agents are indicated for the performance of IDS techniques, where the self-etching systems may present some advantage in blocking the permeability of initially infused dentin [55]. The original technique, proposed by Magne et al. [52], comprises the steps shown in **Figure 11.32**.

The three-step total-etch adhesive is the first option for the cementation of inlays, onlays, and veneers, when some enamel may be involved; the two-step self-etch adhesives are the first option for full crown restorations, decreasing the risk of postoperatory sensibility. Regarding resin cement, both conventional and self-adhesive resin cements beneficiate from IDS [53].

The advantages of IDS are the improved bond strength, reduction of gap formation, decrease in bacterial leakage, and reduction of dentin sensitivity [56]. IDS provides an efficient sealing of dentin, which may provide protection of the pulp from microleakage. The exposition of dentin tubules after enamel removal allow microleakage, and interim or definitive restorations may not be efficient alone in sealing dentin. Thus, sealing dentin with IDS may be considered a preventive procedure for preservation of pulp health.

In addition to all the advantages mentioned, the IDS technique increases the fracture resistance of lithium disilicate veneers when bonded to dentin, attributed to the enhanced bond strength provided. Glass ceramics are dependent on adhesive cementation for final restoration strength. When dentin is exposed during tooth preparation, the use of IDS increases the survival rate of ceramic laminate veneers after 11 years of evaluation [57].

Such advantage would be of great benefit, since the most common cause of failure reported for indirect partial restorations is fracture of the restoration [57]. Clinical survival rates of resin matrix ceramic overlays and endocrowns, combined with IDS, may reach 91.4% after almost four years of clinical function [58]. Ceramic crowns cemented after IDS are associated with the application of an adhesive system and a flowable resin composite, presenting the maximum in vitro bond strength and the highest bond durability in the qualitative bonding performance after the cyclic loading condition simulation of clinical mastication [59]. IDS improves bond strength and bond reliability of glass-ceramic CAD/CAM onlay restorations [60].

However, the literature is not consistent regarding the benefits of IDS in the strength of restorations, showing no effect on fatigue resistance of lithium disilicate occlusal veneers [61]. Clinical studies are necessary for understanding the effectiveness of IDS in enhancing strength of indirect restorations. In addition, IDS may present disadvantages when a digital workflow is intended to be used.

Trueness and precision of IOS may be affected by tooth preparation surface finishing procedures. In addition, IDS may decrease trueness and precision values. The application of adhesive to tooth surface results in a smooth, glazed-like surface, which might modify the reflectance properties of the tooth surface. In this context, the air particle abrasion of the tooth surface provides a more accurate virtual definitive cast. However, few studies are available regarding bond strength values to the air abraded surface before impression making and interim steps [62].

The physical characteristic of tooth surface after IDS might be compared to a wet tooth surface, providing less accurate trueness and precision of the imaging of IOS. The deviations caused in imaging by a wet surface are not related to composition or physical or chemical characteristics of the liquid, and are mainly located at surface irregularities, interproximal area, and margin of the abutments [63]. The same locations present volumetric discrepancy in scanned abutments after IDS [62].

The decrease in trueness of scanning IDS surfaces may be worked around with the application of a composite resin layer after adhesive application. The trueness of scanning of polished resin composite surface is similar to the trueness of scanning the tooth surface [62]. Besides that, the combination of an adhesive system and a layer of composite resin enhance the bond strength values in the long term [64]. Another alternative for enhancing trueness of IDS surfaces of the application of powder previously to scanning. It is recommended to create a uniformly reflective surface and was reported to promote high accuracy [65].

The IDS technique, cavity design optimization, and cervical margin relocation are classified as modern treatment concepts, combining simpler techniques with more predictable and durable results [66]. Clinical studies must be performed to assess the effects of benefits and impairments offered by IDS in a digital workflow. The choice of IDS due to its advantages in restorations' strength, bond strength, dentin sealing, and postoperatory sensitiveness must not affect the precision of IOS significantly, or they will be lost due to incorrect seating and marginal sealing of the indirect restoration.

11.8 CLINICAL CASE 4 (FIGURES 11.33–11.37)

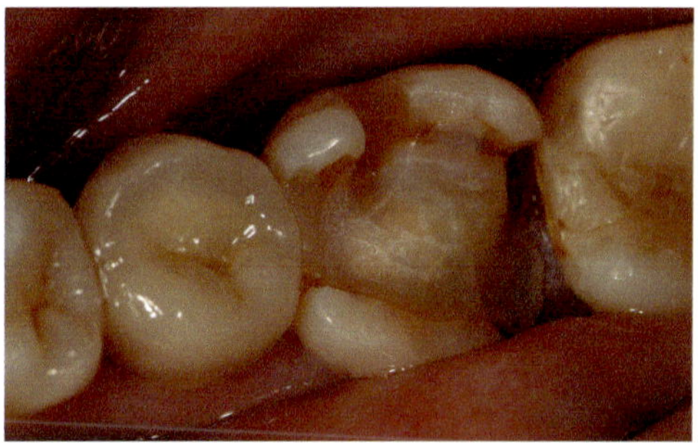

Figure 11.33 Old composite remotion.

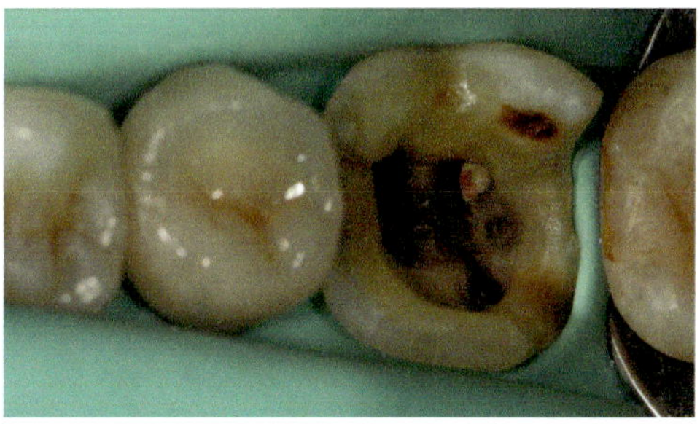

Figure 11.34 Rubber dam isolation. It is very interesting to remove all old composites and adequately clean the dental reminiscent before IDS technique.

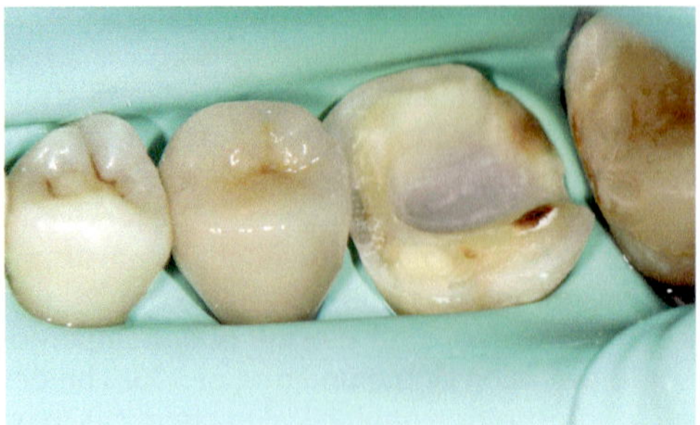

Figure 11.35 IDS (Optibond FL – Kerr followed by Beautifull Flow Plus 00 – Shofu) and dental preparation for intraoral scanning.

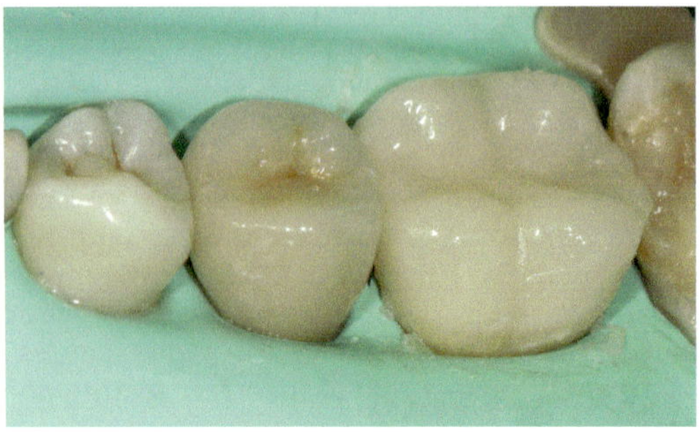

Figure 11.36 Cerec blocks overlay (Dentisply Sirona) adhesively cemented with rubber dam isolation.

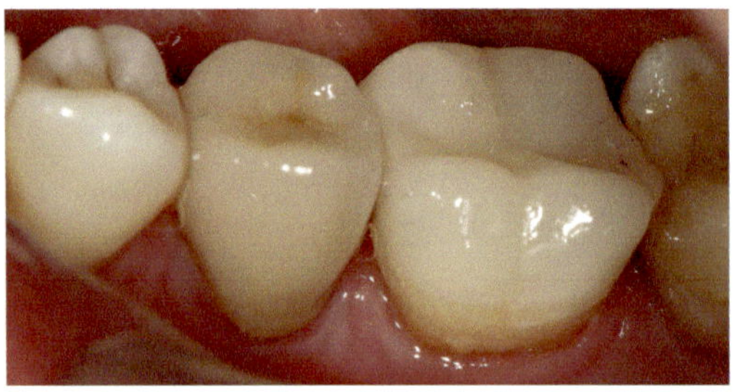

Figure 11.37 Case finalized.

11.9 CLINICAL CASE 5 (FIGURES 11.38–11.43)

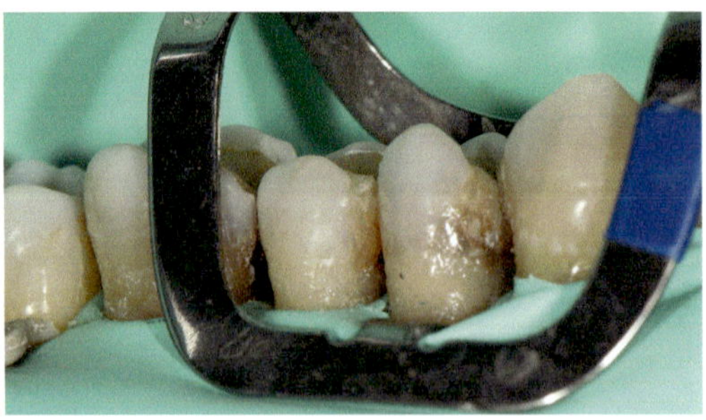

Figure 11.38 Direct inlays composites with marginal infiltration. Teeth: 16, mesial infiltration; 15, distal and mesial infiltration; 14, distal and mesial infiltration.

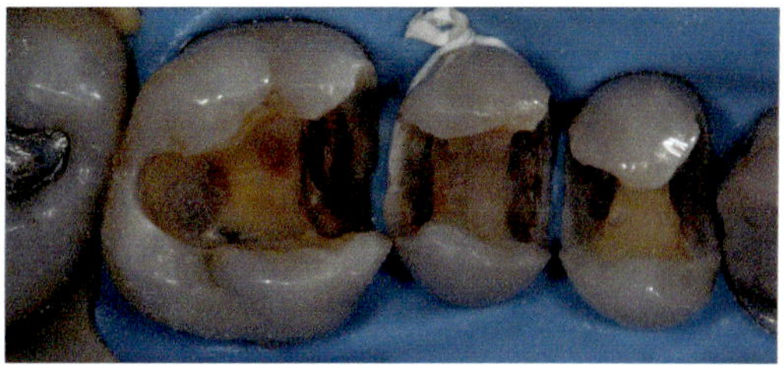

Figure 11.39 Old direct inlay composites with remotion and cleaning of the cavities to receive the IDS technique.

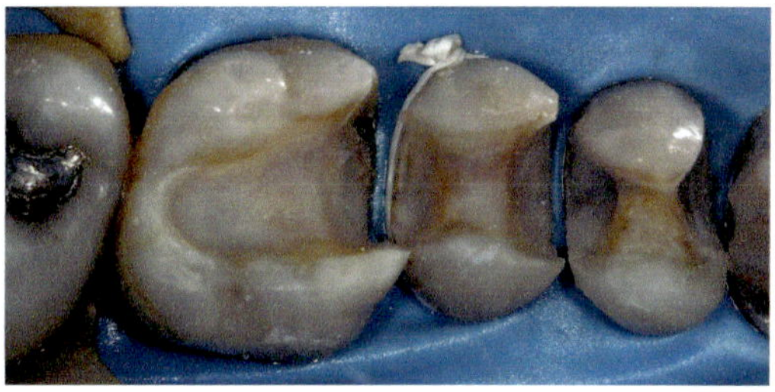

Figure 11.40 IDS (Optibond FL – Kerr and Beautifull Flow Plus 00) and preparations.

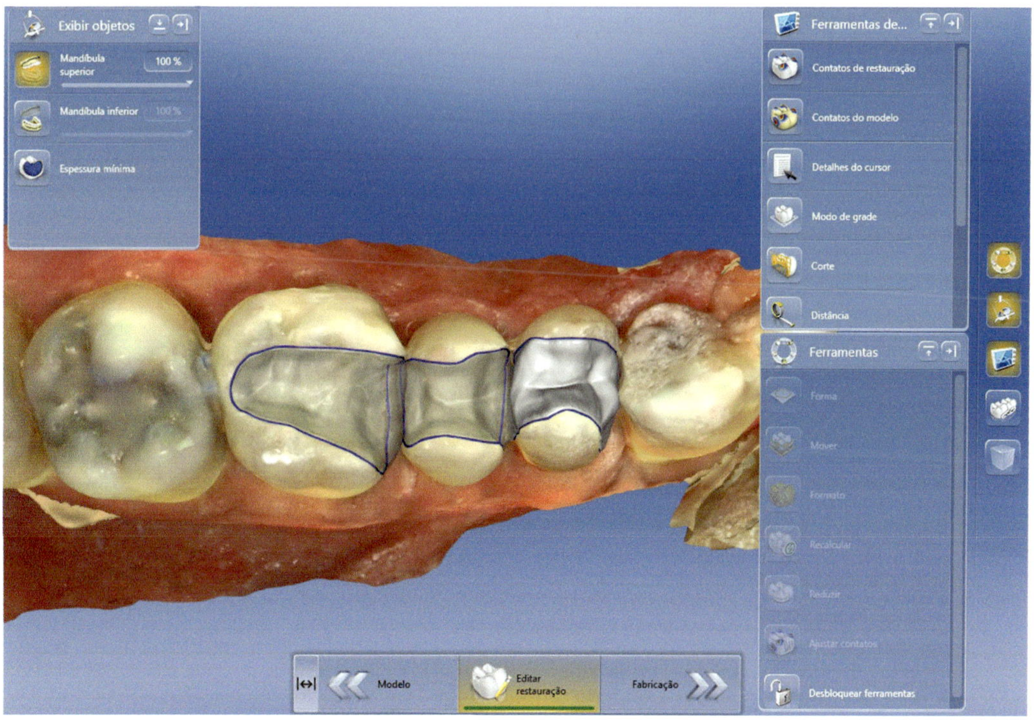

Figure 11.41 Intraoral scanning and virtual restorations (Cerec, Dentsply Sirona).

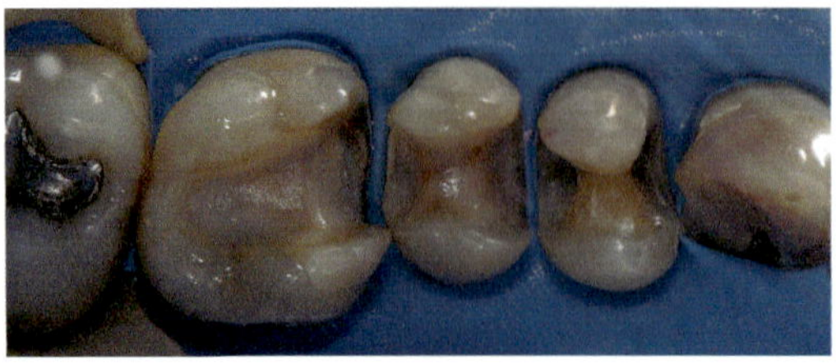

Figure 11.42 Adhesive system application (enamel selective acid etching and universal adhesive application – Gluma Bond Universal – Kulzer).

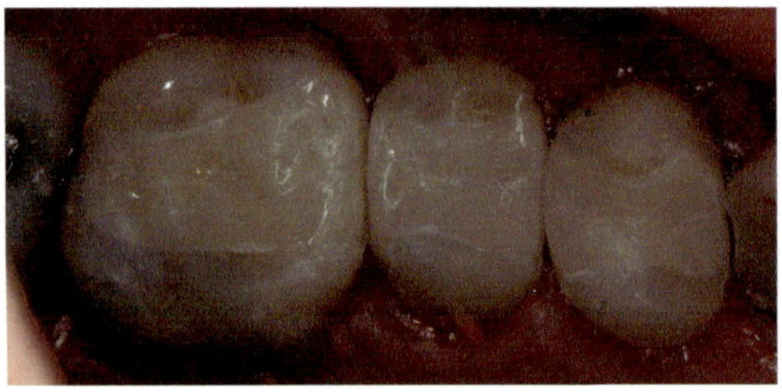

Figure 11.43 Lithium disilicate inlays adhesively cemented. Immediately postoperative at rubber dam remotion (without finishing).

11.10 FINAL CONSIDERATIONS

Different technical and biological characteristics of tooth preparation may affect the digital workflow, especially intraoral scanning accuracy. Elevated margins, walls angles, the finish line, gingival level of preparation margin, and prepared tooth surface may be considered when planning to use the digital workflow, since these aspects may affect the global process from planning to the delivery of the restoration and also the clinical performance.

REFERENCES

1. Aldakheel, M et al. Deep margin elevation: current concepts and clinical considerations: a review. Medicina (Kaunas). 2022;58(10):1482.
2. Eggmann, F et al. Deep margin elevation-present status and future directions. J Esthet Restor Dent. 2023;35(1):26–47.
3. Kielbassa, AM, Philipp, F. Restoring proximal cavities of molars using the proximal box elevation technique: systematic review and report of a case. Quintessence Int. 2015;46(9):751–764.
4. Vichitgomen, J, Srisawasdi, S. Deep margin elevation with resin composite and resin-modified glass-ionomer on marginal sealing of CAD-CAM ceramic inlays: an in vitro study. Am J Dent. 2021;34(6):327–332.
5. Samartzi, TK et al. Deep margin elevation: a literature review. Dent J (Basel). 2022;10(3):48.
6. Ferrari, M et al. The ability of marginal detection using different intraoral scanning systems: a pilot randomized controlled trial. Am J Dent. 2018;31:272–276.
7. Dablanca-Blanco, AB et al. Management of large class II lesions in molars: how to restore and when to perform surgical crown lengthening? Restor Dent Endod. 2017;42(3):240–252.
8. Magne, P, Spreafico, RC. Deep margin elevation: a paradigm shift. Am J Esthet Dent. 2012;2:86–96.
9. Bertoldi, C et al. Clinical and histological reaction of periodontal tissues to subgingival resin composite restorations. Clin Oral Investig. 2020;24(2):1001–1011.
10. Frese, C et al. Proximal box elevation with resin composite and the dogma of biological width: clinical R2-technique and critical review. Oper Dent. 2014;39(1):22–31.
11. Sarfati, A, Tirlet, G. Deep margin elevation versus crown lengthening: biologic width revisited. Int J Esthet Dent. 2018;13(3):334–356.
12. Elsayed, A. Defect-orientated onlay with cavity design optimization and cervical margin relocation: a case report. Int J Comput Dent. 2021;24(1):77–88.
13. Ilgenstein, I et al. Influence of proximal box elevation on the marginal quality and fracture behavior of root-filled molars restored with CAD/CAM ceramic or composite onlays. Clin Oral Investig. 2015;19(5):1021–1028.
14. Bresser, RA et al. Influence of deep margin elevation and preparation design on the fracture strength of indirectly restored molars. J Mech Behav Biomed Mater. 2020;110:103950.
15. Grubbs, TD et al. Efficacy of direct restorative materials in proximal box elevation on the margin quality and fracture resistance of molars restored with CAD/CAM onlays. Oper Dent. 2020;45(1):52–61.
16. Robaian, A et al. Different designs of deep marginal elevation and its influence on fracture resistance of teeth with monolith zirconia full-contour crowns. Medicina (Kaunas). 2023;59(4):661.

17. Zhang, H et al. Effect of proximal box elevation on fracture resistance and microleakage of premolars restored with ceramic endocrowns. PLoS One. 2021;16(5):e0252269. Erratum in: PLoS One. 2021;16(9):e0258038.
18. Grassi, EDA et al. Fatigue behavior and stress distribution of molars restored with MOD inlays with and without deep margin elevation. Clin Oral Investig. 2022;26(3):2513–2526.
19. Juloski, J et al. Cervical margin relocation in indirect adhesive restorations: A literature review. J Prosthodont Res. 2018;62(3):273–280.
20. Mueller, B et al. Effect of immediate dentin sealing on load-bearing capacity under accelerated fatigue of thin occlusal veneers made of CAD-CAM glass-ceramic and resin composite material. Dent Mater. 2023;39(4):372–382.
21. Theisen, CER et al. Quality of CAD-CAM inlays placed on aged resin-based composite restorations used as deep margin elevation: a laboratory study. Clin Oral Investig. 2023;27(6):2691–2703.
22. Roggendorf, MJ et al. Effect of proximal box elevation with resin composite on marginal quality of resin composite inlays in vitro. J Dent. 2012;40(12):1068–1073.
23. Frankenberger, R et al. Effect of proximal box elevation with resin composite on marginal quality of ceramic inlays in vitro. Clin Oral Investig. 2013;17(1):177–183.
24. Alahmari, NM et al. Effects of the cervical marginal relocation technique on the marginal adaptation of lithium disilicate CAD/CAM ceramic crowns on premolars. J Contemp Dent Pract. 2021;22:900–906.
25. Euán, R et al. Marginal adaptation of zirconium dioxide copings: influence of the CAD/CAM system and the finish line design. J Prosthet Dent. 2014;112(2):155–162.
26. Jacobs, MS, Windeler, AS. An investigation of dental luting cement solubility as a function of the marginal gap. J Prosthet Dent. 1991;65(3):436–442.
27. Ahmed, WM et al. Fit of tooth supported zircônia single crowns – a systematic review of the literature. Clin Exp Dent Res. 2020;6(6):700–716.
28. Koulivand, S et al. A clinical comparison of digital and conventional impression techniques regarding finish line locations and impression time. J Esthet Restor Dent. 2020;32:236–243.
29. Baldi, A et al. Does partial adhesive preparation design and finish line depth influence trueness and precision of intraoral scanners? J Prosthet Dent. 2023;129(4):637.e1–637.e9.
30. Falih, MY, Majeed, MA. Trueness and precision of eight intraoral scanners with different finishing line designs: a comparative in vitro study. Eur J Dent. 2023;17(4):1056–1064.
31. Kim, MK et al. The effect of scanning distance on the accuracy of intra-oral scanners used in dentistry. Clin Anat. 2019;32:430–438.
32. Bernauer, SA et al. Influence of preparation design, marginal gingiva location, and tooth morphology on the accuracy of digital impressions for full-crown restorations: an in vitro investigation. J Clin Med. 2020;9:3984.
33. Beuer, F et al. Influence of preparation angle on marginal and internal fit of CAD/CAM-fabricated zirconia crown copings. Quintessence Int. 2009;40:243–250 32.
34. Chan, DC et al. The accuracy of optical scanning: influence of convergence and die preparation. Oper Dent. 2011;36:486–491.
35. Ashraf, Y et al. Influence of preparation type and tooth geometry on the accuracy of different intraoral scanners. J Prosthodont. 2020;29(9):800–804.
36. Suárez, MJ et al. Comparison of the marginal fit of Procera AllCeram crowns with two finish lines. Int J Prosthodont. 2003;16:32.
37. Komine, F et al. Marginal and internal adaptation of zirconium dioxide ceramic copings and crowns with different finish line designs. Dent Mater J. 2007;26:659–664.
38. Shah, N et al. Effect of different finish line preparations on the marginal and internal adaptation of cobalt-chromium metal alloy copings fabricated by using CAD-CAM technology: A systematic review and meta-analysis. J Prosthet Dent. 2022;127(5):716–728.e6.
39. Coli, P, Karlsson, S. Precision of a CAD/CAM technique for the production of zirconium dioxide copings. Int J Prosthodont. 2004;17:80.
40. Nakamura, T et al. Marginal and internal fit of CEREC 3 CAD/CAM all-ceramic crowns. Int J Prosthodont. 2003;16:244–248.
41. Karataşli, Ö et al. Comparison of the marginal fit of different coping materials and designs produced by computer aided manufacturing systems. Dent Mater J. 2011;30:97–102.
42. Sorensen, JA. A standardized method for determination of crown margin fidelity. J Prosthet Dent. 1990;64(1):18–24.
43. Zimmermann, M et al. Local accuracy of actual intraoral scanning systems for single-tooth preparations in vitro. J Am Dent Assoc. 2020;151:127e135.
44. Kim, JH et al. In vitro analysis of intraoral digital impression of inlay preparation according to tooth location and cavity type. J Prosthodont Res. 2021;65:400e406.
45. May, LG et al. Effects of cement thickness and bonding on the failure loads of CAD/CAM ceramic crowns: multi-physics FEA modeling and monotonic testing. Dent Mater. 2012;28:e99ee109.
46. An, H et al. Effect of finish line location and saliva contamination on the accuracy of crown finish line scanning. J Prosthodont. 2024;33(1):86–94.
47. Taneja, S et al. Effect of saliva and blood contamination on the shear bond strength of fifth-, seventh-, and eighth-generation bonding agents: an in vitro study. J Conserv Dent. 2017;20(3):157–160.
48. Tabassum, S et al. Gingival retraction methods: a systematic review. J Prosthodont. 2017;26(8):637–643.
49. Kuhn, K et al. Influence of the gingival condition on the performance of different gingival displacement methods – a randomized clinical study. J Clin Med. 2021;10:2747.
50. Baharav, H et al. The effect of displacement time on gingival crevice width. Int J Prosthodont. 1997;10:248–253.
51. Wellappuli, NC et al. Oral and blood neutrophil activation states during experimental gingivitis. JDR Clin Trans Res. 2018;3:65–75.
52. Magne, P et al. Immediate dentin sealing improves bond strength of indirect restorations. J Prosthet Dent. 2005; 94:511–519.
53. Brigagão, VC et al. Effect of interim cement application on bond strength between resin cements and dentin: Immediate and delayed dentin sealing. J Prosthet Dent. 2017;117(6):792–798.

54. Pashley, EL et al. Dentin permeability: sealing the dentin in crown preparations. Oper Dent. 1992;17:13–20.
55. Sahin, C et al. In-vitro permeability of etch-and-rinse and self-etch adhesives used for immediate dentin sealing. Dent Mater J. 2012;31:401–408.
56. van den Breemer, C et al. Prospective randomized clinical trial on the survival of lithium disilicate posterior partial crowns bonded using immediate or delayed dentin sealing: short-term results on tooth sensitivity and patient satisfaction. Oper Dent. 2019;44:E212.
57. Gresnigt, MMM et al. Performance of ceramic laminate veneers with immediate dentine sealing: An 11 year prospective clinical trial. Dent Mater. 2019;35(7):1042–1052.
58. Vervack, V et al. Clinical evaluation of resin composite CAD/CAM restorations placed by undergraduate students. J Clin Med. 2021;10(15):3269.
59. Nakazawa, M et al. Appropriate immediate dentin sealing to improve the bonding of CAD/CAM ceramic crown restorations. Polymers (Basel). 2022;14(21):4541.
60. Ishii, N et al. Bonding state of metal-free CAD/CAM onlay restoration after cyclic loading with and without immediate dentin sealing. Dent Mater J. 2017;36(3):357–367.
61. Müller, V et al. Influence of proximal box elevation technique on marginal integrity of adhesively luted Cerec inlays. Clin Oral Investig. 2017;21(2):607–612.
62. Revilla-León, M et al. The effect of different tooth preparation finishing procedures and immediate dentin sealing on the scanning accuracy of different intraoral scanners. J Dent. 2023;130:104431.
63. Chen, Y et al. Influence of liquid on the tooth surface on the accuracy of intraoral scanners: an in vitro study. J Prosthodont. 2022;31(1):59–64.
64. Hardan, L et al. Immediate dentin sealing for adhesive cementation of indirect restorations: a systematic review and meta-analysis. Gels. 2022;8(3):175.
65. Nedelcu, RG, Persson, AS. Scanning accuracy and precision in 4 intraoral scanners: an in vitro comparison based on 3-dimensional analysis. J Prosthet Dent. 2014;112:1461–1471.
66. Rocca, GT et al. Evidence-based concepts and procedures for bonded inlays and onlays. Part II. Guidelines for cavity preparation and restoration fabrication. Int J Esthet Dent. 2015;10:392–413.

12 Limitations, Challenges, and Opportunities of Digital Technologies

Taha Fayad

12.1 INTRODUCTION

Digital technologies have significantly transformed the landscape of prosthodontics and restorative dentistry, introducing a paradigm shift characterized by unprecedented precision, customization, and workflow efficiency. From computer-aided design and computer-aided manufacturing (CAD/CAM) systems to three-dimensional (3D) printing and intraoral scanners, digital technologies have become integral components of contemporary dental practices [1–3].

12.1.1 Evolution of Digital Technologies

The evolution from traditional methodologies to the current era of digital dentistry marks a revolutionary progression in the conceptualization and execution of prosthodontic treatments. These technological advancements, exemplified by CAD/CAM systems and 3D printing, have redefined the practice of prosthodontics [1].

12.1.2 Significance of Understanding Limitations and Challenges

While the advantages of digital technologies in prosthodontics are evident, a comprehensive understanding of the associated limitations and challenges is equally imperative. This chapter aims to explore these facets, providing insights into the multifaceted world of digital dentistry. Informed decision-making and improved patient outcomes can be achieved by navigating the evolving landscape with a nuanced comprehension of both promises and complexities [2, 4].

12.1.3 Structure of This Chapter

This chapter explores the opportunities presented by digital technologies, delving into areas such as precision, customization, and workflow efficiency [5]. Subsequently, it addresses challenges encountered during implementation, encompassing initial investments, training requirements, and standardization issues [6, 7]. The chapter further scrutinizes the limitations imposed by materials and biological considerations in digital dentistry [8, 9]. Lastly, a glimpse into future trends and innovations serves as a forward-looking conclusion, emphasizing the dynamic nature of this ever-evolving field [10].

As we embark on this journey through the realms of digital dentistry in prosthodontics and restorative dentistry, the overarching goal is to provide a holistic understanding of the subject matter, fostering a nuanced perspective that acknowledges both the promises and complexities of the digital era in dental practice.

12.2 DIGITAL TECHNOLOGIES IN PROSTHODONTICS: A SNAPSHOT

Digital technologies have become integral to the field of prosthodontics, offering a comprehensive toolbox for clinicians to enhance treatment planning, design, and fabrication processes [1]. This section provides an overview of key digital technologies employed in prosthodontics, underscoring their advantages over traditional methods.

12.2.1 Overview of Key Digital Technologies

The advent of CAD/CAM systems has been transformative in prosthodontics [1]. These systems enable precise digital modeling and the fabrication of restorations, such as crowns and bridges, with exceptional accuracy [2]. Additionally, 3D printing technologies have gained prominence, allowing for the fabrication of intricate dental structures layer by layer [2].

12.2.2 Advantages of Digital Technologies

Digital technologies offer several advantages over traditional methods in prosthodontics. They provide clinicians with the ability to achieve high precision and accuracy in restoration design, leading to improved clinical outcomes [1]. Furthermore, the digital workflow enhances efficiency by reducing manual errors and streamlining the fabrication process [3]. These advancements empower dental professionals to deliver customized and patient-specific prosthetic solutions, aligning with the evolving demands of modern dental practice [4].

As we delve into the subsequent sections, it is crucial to recognize the pivotal role played by these digital technologies in shaping the contemporary landscape of prosthodontics.

DOI: 10.1201/9781003428541-12

12.3 OPPORTUNITIES IN DIGITAL DENTISTRY

Digital dentistry presents myriad opportunities that significantly impact the field of prosthodontics. This section explores key areas where digital technologies provide distinct advantages, including precision and accuracy, customization and personalization, and workflow efficiency.

12.3.1 Precision and Accuracy

One of the notable opportunities afforded by digital dentistry is the unprecedented level of precision and accuracy achievable in prosthodontic treatments. The integration of CAD and CAM systems allows for meticulous digital modeling of restorations, reducing the margin of error inherent in traditional methods [1]. The ability to design and fabricate prosthetic components with sub-millimeter precision enhances the overall quality of care and contributes to favorable clinical outcomes [1, 2].

12.3.2 Customization and Personalization

Digital technologies enable a new era of customization and personalization in prosthodontics. Clinicians can leverage digital workflows to create highly individualized treatment plans tailored to the specific needs and anatomy of each patient [3]. This level of customization extends to the design and fabrication of prosthetic restorations, ensuring an optimal fit and esthetic outcome [3, 4]. Patient-specific solutions enhance patient satisfaction and contribute to the longevity and success of prosthodontic interventions.

12.3.3 Workflow Efficiency

The incorporation of digital technologies into prosthodontic workflows has revolutionized efficiency in treatment processes. Digital impressions, for example, eliminate the need for traditional, time-consuming impression materials and procedures [5]. Moreover, the seamless integration of digital data throughout the treatment pathway, from diagnosis to fabrication, minimizes manual errors and enhances overall workflow efficiency [6]. This not only streamlines clinical processes but also contributes to a more predictable and reproducible treatment outcome.

As we continue to explore the landscape of digital dentistry, it becomes evident that these opportunities pave the way for a more precise, personalized, and efficient approach to prosthodontic care.

12.4 CHALLENGES IN IMPLEMENTING DIGITAL DENTISTRY

While digital dentistry presents numerous opportunities, its implementation is not without challenges. This section delves into key obstacles faced in adopting digital technologies in prosthodontics, including initial investment and training, standardization and compatibility issues, and the learning curve associated with adaptation.

12.4.1 Initial Investment and Training

The transition to digital dentistry necessitates a substantial initial investment in technology and infrastructure. The acquisition of sophisticated equipment, such as CAD/CAM systems and digital scanners, demands a financial commitment that can be challenging for dental practices, particularly smaller ones [1]. Moreover, the integration of digital technologies requires comprehensive training for dental professionals to navigate the complexities of new workflows and software applications [2, 3]. Overcoming the financial and educational barriers is crucial for a successful transition to digital prosthodontics.

12.4.2 Standardization and Compatibility

Another challenge lies in the standardization and compatibility of various digital systems used in prosthodontics. The absence of universal standards can hinder interoperability between different devices and software platforms [1]. This lack of standardization may lead to inefficiencies, requiring additional efforts to ensure seamless communication and data transfer between different components of the digital workflow [3]. Addressing these issues is paramount to establishing a cohesive and integrated digital environment in prosthodontic practice.

12.4.3 Learning Curve and Adaptation

The introduction of digital technologies introduces a learning curve for dental professionals accustomed to traditional methodologies. The adaptation to new software interfaces, digital impression techniques, and CAD/CAM workflows may initially pose challenges in terms of time and proficiency [1, 2]. Overcoming this learning curve requires dedicated training programs and continuous education to ensure a smooth transition and the optimal utilization of digital tools in daily practice [3].

As we navigate through the challenges, it becomes evident that overcoming these obstacles is essential for unlocking the full potential of digital dentistry in prosthodontics.

12.5 LIMITATIONS OF DIGITAL TECHNOLOGIES

While digital technologies in prosthodontics offer numerous advantages, it is essential to critically examine their limitations. This section explores challenges related to material constraints and biological considerations, providing insights into areas where further research and development are needed.

12.5.1 Material Limitations

The materials used in digital dentistry, such as those in CAD/CAM restorations, may have inherent limitations [1]. These limitations can include issues related to the mechanical properties, aesthetics, and long-term stability of the materials [1]. While significant advancements have been made, understanding the constraints of current materials is crucial for clinicians when selecting appropriate options for prosthodontic treatments [1, 2].

12.5.2 Biological Considerations

In addition to material limitations, digital dentistry must address biological considerations to ensure successful outcomes. The response of oral tissues to digitally fabricated restorations, including soft tissue adaptation and biocompatibility, requires thorough investigation [2]. The interaction between the prosthesis and the surrounding biological environment plays a pivotal role in the long-term success of prosthodontic treatments [2]. Continuous research is essential to enhance our understanding of these biological dynamics and improve the performance of digital restorations.

As we explore the limitations, it is important to acknowledge that these challenges represent opportunities for future advancements. Ongoing research and innovation in materials and biological aspects will contribute to overcoming these limitations and further optimizing the efficacy of digital technologies in prosthodontics.

12.6 FUTURE TRENDS AND INNOVATIONS

As digital dentistry continues to evolve, it is essential to anticipate future trends and innovations that will shape the landscape of prosthodontics. This section explores emerging developments and provides a glimpse into the potential trajectory of digital technologies in the field.

12.6.1 Advancements in Materials

One of the exciting prospects for the future involves continuous advancements in materials used in digital dentistry. Ongoing research aims to overcome the limitations of current materials, enhancing their mechanical properties, aesthetics, and long-term stability [1]. The introduction of novel materials, such as bioactive ceramics and polymers, holds promise for further improving the performance and biocompatibility of digitally fabricated restorations [1, 2].

12.6.2 Integration of Artificial Intelligence

The integration of artificial intelligence (AI) is expected to play a significant role in the future of digital dentistry. AI algorithms have the potential to streamline diagnosis, treatment planning, and even aid in the design of prosthetic restorations [3]. Machine learning applications may enhance the predictive capabilities of digital technologies, contributing to more accurate and efficient prosthodontic workflows.

12.6.3 3D Printing Innovations

While 3D printing has already made significant strides, ongoing innovations are expected to further expand its capabilities. Advancements in printing technologies, including the development of faster and more precise printers, will contribute to the broader adoption of 3D printing in prosthodontics. Additionally, the exploration of new materials compatible with 3D printing holds promise for creating increasingly sophisticated dental structures.

12.6.4 Teledentistry and Remote Workflows

The future of prosthodontics may witness an increased integration of teledentistry, allowing for remote consultations, treatment planning, and follow-up care. This shift towards remote workflows has the potential to enhance accessibility to prosthodontic care, particularly in underserved areas. The development of secure and efficient digital communication platforms will be pivotal in facilitating these remote interactions.

As we look towards the future, these trends and innovations underscore the dynamic nature of digital dentistry, continually pushing boundaries and redefining the possibilities within prosthodontics.

12.7 CONCLUSION

As we conclude this exploration of the opportunities, challenges, and future prospects of digital technologies in prosthodontics, it is evident that the integration of digital dentistry has revolutionized the field. The dynamic interplay between precision, customization, workflow efficiency, and emerging innovations underscores the transformative impact of digital technologies on prosthodontic practice.

12.7.1 Summary of Key Points

1. *Precision and Accuracy*: Digital technologies, particularly CAD/CAM systems, have elevated the precision and accuracy of prosthodontic treatments [1]. The ability to achieve sub-millimeter accuracy in restoration design contributes to favorable clinical outcomes [1, 2].
2. *Customization and Personalization*: The era of digital dentistry enables a high degree of customization, with treatment plans and restorations tailored to the unique needs of each patient [3]. This level of personalization enhances patient satisfaction and contributes to the success of interventions [3].
3. *Workflow Efficiency*: The integration of digital workflows streamlines prosthodontic processes, from diagnosis to fabrication [4]. Digital impressions and data transfer minimize manual errors, contributing to a more efficient and predictable treatment pathway.

12.7.2 Addressing Challenges

1. *Initial Investment and Training*: Overcoming the financial barriers associated with the initial investment in digital technologies requires strategic planning. Comprehensive training programs are crucial to equip dental professionals with the skills needed to navigate the complexities of digital workflows [3].
2. *Standardization and Compatibility*: The challenge of standardization and compatibility emphasizes the need for industry-wide standards to ensure seamless interoperability between different digital systems. Efforts to establish protocols for data exchange will contribute to a more integrated digital environment.
3. *Learning Curve and Adaptation*: The learning curve associated with digital technologies necessitates ongoing education and training programs [3]. Addressing this challenge ensures that dental professionals can harness the full potential of digital tools in their daily practice.

12.7.3 Acknowledging Limitations and Future Directions

1. *Material Limitations*: Current materials used in digital dentistry come with inherent limitations. Future advancements in materials, such as bioactive ceramics and polymers, hold promise for overcoming these constraints.
2. *Biological Considerations*: Ongoing research is essential to understand the biological implications of digitally fabricated restorations. This knowledge will guide improvements in biocompatibility and tissue response for enhanced long-term success.

12.7.4 Embracing Future Trends and Innovations

1. *Advancements in Materials*: The continuous evolution of materials in digital dentistry promises to enhance mechanical properties, aesthetics, and long-term stability.
2. *Integration of Artificial Intelligence*: The incorporation of AI into digital workflows presents opportunities for more efficient diagnosis, treatment planning, and design processes.
3. *3D Printing Innovations*: Ongoing advancements in 3D printing technologies, including faster and more precise printers, open new possibilities for prosthodontic applications [2].
4. *Teledentistry and Remote Workflows*: The integration of teledentistry is poised to enhance accessibility to prosthodontic care, particularly in remote or underserved areas.

12.7.5 Looking Ahead

As we peer into the future of digital dentistry in prosthodontics, it is clear that the journey is characterized by continuous innovation and adaptation. The challenges faced today pave the way for solutions, and the opportunities presented by digital technologies hold the potential to redefine the standard of care in prosthodontics.

In the ever-evolving landscape of digital dentistry, this exploration serves as a testament to the transformative power of technology, inspiring dental professionals to embrace change, overcome challenges, and contribute to the ongoing evolution of prosthodontic practice.

REFERENCES

1. Abdelnabi, MH, Swelem, AA. Digital technology in complete denture prosthodontics: a review of literature. Egyptian Dental J. 2017;63/3:2871–2885.
2. Jain, S et al. Physical and mechanical properties of 3D-printed provisional crowns and fixed dental prosthesis resins compared to CAD/CAM milled and conventional provisional resins: a systematic review and meta-analysis. Polymers. 2022;14(13):2691.
3. Binhuraib, H et al. Evaluating the efficiency of complete digital workflow in prosthodontics. J Health Sci. 2023; 3(12):695–700.
4. Rosenstiel, SF et al., eds. *Contemporary Fixed Prosthodontics*. Elsevier, 2022.
5. Joda, T, Brägger, U. Digital vs. conventional implant prosthetic workflows: a cost/time analysis. Clin Oral Implants Res. 2015;26(12):1430–1435.
6. Jahangiri, L et al. Understanding the complexities of digital dentistry integration in high-volume dental institutions. Br Dent J. 2020;229(3):166–168.
7. Fasbinder, DJ. Materials for chairside CAD/CAM restorations. Compendium Continuing Educ Dent. 2010;31(9):15488578.
8. Chuchulska, B et al. Comparative analysis of the mechanical properties and biocompatibility between CAD/CAM and conventional polymers applied in prosthetic dentistry. Polymers. 2024;16(7):877.
9. Chen, YW et al. Artificial intelligence in dentistry: current applications and future perspectives. Quintessence Int. 2020;51(3):248–257.
10. Fortich-Mesa, N, Hoyos-Hoyos, V. Applications of teledentistry in dental practice: a systematic review. Rev Facultad Odontol Universidad Antioquia. 2020;32:77–88.

Index

Note: Page numbers in **bold** and *italics* refer to tables and figures, respectively.

E

F

G

H

I

T

U

V

W

X

For Product Safety Concerns and Information please contact our
EU representative GPSR@taylorandfrancis.com Taylor & Francis
Verlag GmbH, Kaufingerstraße 24, 80331 München, Germany